Electrotherapy in Rehabilitation

Contemporary Perspectives in Rehabilitation

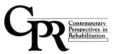

Steven L. Wolf, Ph.D., F.A.P.T.A.
Editor-in-Chief

PUBLISHED VOLUMES

Thermal Agents in Rehabilitation - Volume 1
Susan L. Michlovitz, M.S., P.T.

Cardiac Rehabilitation: Basic Theory and Application - Volume 2
Frances Brannon, Ph.D., Mary Geyer, M.S., Margaret Foley, R.N.

The Biomechanics of the Foot and Ankle - Volume 3
Robert Donatelli, M.A., P.T.

Pharmacology in Rehabilitation - Volume 4
Charles D. Ciccone, Ph.D., P.T.

Wound Healing: Alternatives in Management - Volume 5
Luther C. Kloth, M.S., P.T., Joseph M. McCulloch, Ph.D., P.T. and
Jeffrey A. Feedar, B.S., P.T.

Thermal Agents in Rehabilitation, 2nd Edition - Volume 6
Susan L. Michlovitz, M.S., P.T.

Electrotherapy in Rehabilitation

Meryl Roth Gersh, M.M.Sc., P.T.
Associate Professor
Department of Physical Therapy
Eastern Washington University
Cheney, Washington

F. A. DAVIS COMPANY • **Philadelphia**

F. A. Davis Company
1915 Arch Street
Philadelphia, PA 19103

Printed in the United States of America

Last digit indicates print number: 10 9 8 7 6 5 4 3

Note: As new scientific information becomes available through basic and clinical research, recommended treatments and drug therapies undergo changes. The author(s) and publisher have done everything possible to make this book accurate, up-to-date, and in accord with accepted standards at the time of publication. However, the reader is advised always to check product information (package inserts) for changes and new information regarding dose and contraindications before administering any drug. Caution is especially urged when using new or infrequently ordered drugs.

Library of Congress Cataloging-in-Publication Data

Gersh, Meryl R.
    Electrotherapy in rehabilitation/Meryl Roth Gersh
        p.   cm.   (Contemporary perspectives in rehabilitation ; v. 7)
    Includes bibliographical references and index.
    ISBN 0-8036-4025-0 (hardbound:alk. paper)
    1. Electrotherapeutics.   I. Title.   II. Series.
    [DNLM: 1. Electric Stimulation Therapy — methods.   2. Physical
Therapy.   3. Rehabilitation.   W1 CO769NS v. 7 / WB 495 G381e]
    RM871.G47   1992
    615.8′45 — dc20

                                                                              91-28188
ISBN-8036-4025-0

Foreword

In the last twenty years physical therapists have witnessed an exponential growth in the research literature on the use of electrical stimulation for physical rehabilitation. This proliferation corresponds with an upsurge in the number of companies creating the products from which this body of knowledge has emerged. From the clinical perspective, physical therapists need only look at the multifold increase in the use of electrical stimulation as an adjunct to treatment to realize that the myriad of applications in electrotherapeutics is now commonplace in the physical therapy clinic.

This widespread acceptance is even more remarkable when we consider the state of electrotherapeutic education only 2 decades ago. Ideally, electrical stimulation techniques were taught by an instructor with clinical experience in the use of electricity for both thermal therapy and muscle excitation and a thorough understanding of biophysics and neurophysiology. All too often the instructor was that person most comfortable with the machinery and best able to convey information without eliciting fear of electric "shock" in the heart of the learner. The major desideratum seemed to be a thorough grounding (so to speak) in the safe use of the devices.

Such concern was, of course, valid. For many students and clinicians of my generation, uncertainty about the operation of a device and the fearful anticipation of stimulus escape and a painful shock often reduced our ability to learn about and from the modality. Only a handful of teachers managed to overcome the "fear factor" well enough to inculcate psychomotor skills, let alone to teach the decision-making process or to address the need for efficacy studies.

Today's electrotherapy teachers and their students are more sophisticated. Most instructors are well versed in biophysics and have gained hands-on experience with the equipment through clinical experience or postgraduate education. Given this evolutionary stage the time is right for an electrotherapeutic text that rises to the intellectual challenge of today's student, clinician, and teacher.

One cannot refute the contribution of some excellent texts on the subject of clinical electrotherapy. Until this book, however, none has placed the learning experience so squarely within the context of contemporary society and economy. Today, both clinician and student must be prepared to 1) provide a rationale for the use of any piece of equipment, including electrostimulation instruments; 2) use documentation and the relevant references to convince physician colleagues and third-party payers of the need for and efficacy of a treatment approach; and 3) rely upon a well-defined, logical, decision-making approach to formulating treatment choices and alternatives. The strength of *Electrotherapy in Rehabilitation* is that it addresses all three of these concerns in a more dedicated and comprehensive manner than its predecessors.

In editing this volume, Meryl Gersh has aimed for and achieved consistency among the various presentations that conforms with the philosophical basis of the entire *Contemporary Perspectives in Rehabilitation* series. The reader is not merely spoon-fed a mass of facts, but presented with information in a format that tests and reinforces reasoning skills. The clinical chapters contain real cases, presented to challenge the thinking of student and clinician, and each chapter is replete with up-to-date references. In the Preface, Meryl clearly lays out the *specific* elements of the work that set it apart from its competitors.

Readers who have enjoyed the content and appreciated the format of preceding volumes in this series will not be disappointed. Every student or clinician looking for a comprehensive treatise and standard reference on electrotherapeutics in physical therapy will be delighted. This book will serve as a constant companion

Steven L. Wolf, Ph.D., F.A.P.T.A.
Series Editor

Preface

In June, 1986, at the American Physical Therapy Association Annual Conference in Chicago, I casually suggested to Steve Wolf that he update a previously published electrotherapy text. The next day I found myself appointed editor of *Electrotherapy in Rehabilitation*, a volume in the *Contemporary Perspectives in Rehabilitation (CPR)* series, of which Steve is editor-in-chief. Lesson number one: keep all fertile ideas away from Steve Wolf! Thus, an editor is born.

The use of electrotherapeutic interventions in physical therapy has increased significantly in the past twenty years. Innovative evaluative and therapeutic technologies that use electrical interfaces have found their way to the professional marketplace in ever-increasing numbers. Recent advances in microprocessors and computers have contributed to this development. The pace of development, however, means that many clinicians did not receive training in the underlying principles or critical application of contemporary electrotherapy during entry-level physical therapy education. Practitioners often rely on manufacturers' representatives and sales personnel as their primary resources for education in this area. Objective evaluation is often conspicuously absent during many of these educational exchanges.

The purposes of this text are: (1) to introduce the reader to applications of therapeutic electricity; (2) to provide the underlying rationale for the selection, application, and evaluation of these applications; (3) to review critically the contemporary literature in order to evaluate the clinical efficacy of these applications; and (4) to provide guidelines for the selection, evaluation, and application of these treatment techniques as part of a comprehensive patient management plan. Each of the applications chapters is developed using a problem-solving approach, in a style consistent with other texts in the *Contemporary Perspectives in Rehabilitation* series.

The primary audience for this text is the physical therapist — student, clinician, and educator. The student will gain an understanding of the physiologic bases of electrotherapeutic interventions, an appreciation for the critical evaluation of literature, and an understanding of the operation and application of various electrotherapeutic procedures. Clinicians will enhance their understanding of the principles underlying the application and evaluation of electrotherapeutic procedures and devices. The physical therapist educator will find this text a well-organized and well-referenced resource upon which to develop an electrotherapeutic procedures course for both entry-level and advanced curricula. Other health care professionals who incorporate electrotherapy into their practices will also find this text to be a valuable resource.

The text is organized in three parts. Section I, Neurophysiologic Bases for Application of Therapeutic Electricity, includes a review of the physiologic mechanisms underlying neuromuscular excitation and an update on the neurophysiologic theories of pain perception and modulation. Applications of these principles to clinical problems are suggested and referenced to the appropriate chapters.

Section II, Application of Electrical Currents, presents information on device characteristics, selection, evaluation, and safety, as well as a critical analysis of the application of electrotherapeutic interventions. Chapter 3 presents a comprehensive review of electrical principles and an analysis of the components of electrical stimulation and recording devices, along with essential guidelines for evaluation and maintenance of electrical safety.

Chapter 4 reviews principles and techniques of electrophysiologic evaluation. The inclusion of traditional electrophysiologic tests such as Reaction of Degeneration, measurement of rheobase and chronaxie, and determination of a strength-duration curve provides an historical perspective as well as the basis for a detailed presentation of contemporary evaluation techniques. Motor point charts appear on p. 400 for the reader's convenient reference.

Chapters 5 through 9 discuss the rationale, operation, and application of electrotherapeutic techniques for pain control, circulatory enhancement, and neuromuscular reeducation and strengthening. Each chapter presents the biophysical principles underlying the application, a critical review of the literature regarding the scope and efficacy of the application, guidelines for patient selection, evaluation and treatment, a summary of contraindications and precautions associated with the application, and a case history to illustrate the key points of the chapter. Chapter 10 offers a model for the critical evaluation of innovative devices and techniques as well as a vision of the future of electrotherapy in rehabilitation.

Section III, Clinical Decision Making, offers the reader the opportunity to synthesize the principles and practices presented in the text and to apply this information to the comprehensive management of patients with orthopedic or neurologic impairment. Chapter 11 integrates electrotherapeutic applications into the comprehensive patient care plans for two patients with acute orthopedic injuries. Principles of evaluation, treatment selection, application, assessment, and modification are reviewed. In Chapter 12 a similar model is presented for patients with chronic central nervous system dysfunction.

One of the great challenges in the study of electrotherapy is the lack of clear, consistent terminology. Throughout this text, we have made a concerted effort to use terminology consistent with the document, Electrotherapeutic Terminology, developed by the Section on Clinical Electrophysiology of the American Physical Therapy Association (1990).

In summary, *Electrotherapy in Rehabilitation* provides a clear, comprehensive, analytical review of the underlying principles and clinical applications of contemporary electrophysiologic evaluation and treatment techniques. I hope that the information in this text will augment students' comprehension of electrotherapy, facilitate clinicians' critical utilization of these techniques, foster the continued evaluation of treatment efficacy, and ultimately improve the quality of care offered to the patients we serve.

Meryl Roth Gersh, M.M.S., P.T.
Editor

Acknowledgments

The completion of a multiauthored text is a labor of dedication, professionalism, and commitment to the ideal that the whole is truly greater than the sum of its parts. I am privileged to thank the following people who have shared their talents, expertise, and precious time to complete this project:

All the contributing authors for their knowledge, patience, and fortitude

Steven L. Wolf, Editor-in-Chief, mentor, and friend, for his enthusiasm over the peaks, his unfailing support through the valleys, and his constant confidence in my abilities

Susan L. Michlovitz, for sharing her wisdom, experience, and perspective throughout the process

The manuscript reviewers, in particular George Hampton, Martha Trotter, Dale R. Fish, Billie Nelson, and Jane Gierhart for their rigorous reviews and always constructive criticism

The staff at F.A. Davis Company, in particular Senior Editor Jean-François Vilain, for their guidance, encouragement, and support

Linda Bracey for her typing and retyping of portions of the manuscript

My students at Eastern Washington University, whose thoughtful questions and quest for excellence in education inspired and sustained my commitment to this project

My colleagues at Eastern Washington University and in the Section on Clinical Electrophysiology, whose encouragement helped me meet the challenges of editorship

My husband, Bob Gersh, and my children, Andy and Jill, for their patience, confidence, and humor—especially in the face of dreaded deadlines.

To my family — Bob, Andy, and Jill;
my mother, Norma Roth, and in
memory of my father, Keith J. Roth

Contributors

JOHN P. CUMMINGS, Ph.D., P.T.

Associate Professor
Program in Physical Therapy
State University of New York
Health Science Center
Syracuse, New York

JULIE DeVAHL, M.S., P.T.

Clinical Resources Manager
Chattanooga Group, Inc.
Hixson, Tennessee

MERYL ROTH GERSH, M.M.Sc., P.T.

Associate Professor
Department of Physical Therapy
Eastern Washington University
Cheney, Washington

JAMES L. HANEGAN, Ph.D.

Professor of Biology
Eastern Washington University
Cheney, Washington

LUTHER C. KLOTH, M.S., P.T.

Associate Professor
Program in Physical Therapy
Marquette University
Milwaukee, Wisconsin

CARL G. KUKULKA, Ph.D., P.T.

Associate Professor
Physical Therapy Graduate Program
The University of Iowa
Iowa City, Iowa

DEBORAH E. LeCRAW, M.M.Sc., P.T.

Medical College of Georgia
Augusta, Georgia

BARBARA M. MYKLEBUST, Ph.D., P.T.

Assistant Professor of Neurology and Physical Medicine and
    Rehabilitation
Medical College of Wisconsin
    Chief, Prosthetic and Sensory Aids Service
    Director, Laboratory of Sensory-Motor Performance
Veterans Administration Medical Center
Milwaukee, Wisconsin

CHARLENE NELSON, M.A., P.T., E.C.S.

Associate Professor
Division of Physical Therapy
The School of Medicine
University of North Carolina at Chapel Hill
Chapel Hill, North Carolina

ROBERTA PACKMAN-BRAUN, M.Ed., P.T.

Clinical Specialist in Electrotherapy
Department of Physical Therapy
Moss Rehabilitation Hospital
Philadelphia, Pennsylvania

SUSAN W. STRALKA, M.S., P.T.

Director of Physical Therapy
The Campbell Clinic
Memphis, Tennessee

STEVEN L. WOLF, Ph.D., P.T., F.A.P.T.A.

Editor-in-Chief
Associate Professor
Department of Rehabilitation Medicine
Emory University School of Medicine
Atlanta, Georgia

Contents

Neurophysiologic Bases for Application of Therapeutic Electricity

CHAPTER 1

Principles of Neuromuscular Excitation

Carl G. Kukulka, Ph.D., P.T.

The purpose of this chapter is to provide an overview of the physical concepts underlying neuromuscular excitation by describing the physiologic and electrical events associated with the percutaneous application of electrical stimulation. This approach requires a rudimentary understanding of electricity and cellular neurophysiologic processes. No attempt is made to provide an exhaustive review of these topics, which is best left to textbooks, two of which are highly recommended. That by Jewett and Raymer[1] is appropriate for all levels of readers and has been drawn upon heavily for the description of membrane phenomena. A more quantitative, advanced treatment of this subject may be found in the text by Jack, Noble, and Tsien.[2]

Most textbooks on electrotherapy contain an obligatory chapter on the principles of nerve and muscle excitation. This inclusion implies a need to distribute what is presumably important information, but is it important, and is it necessary? It may be neither important nor necessary for a technician trained in the prescribed placement of electrodes and setting of stimulus parameters. It is a different situation for the physical therapist who plans the treatment, evaluates its effectiveness, and makes adjustments throughout its course. The physical therapist must decide upon the appropriate placement of electrodes and the adjustments of stimulus parameters. The physical therapist must ask, What am I trying to accomplish in my treatment? Rational answers to this question can only come from a knowledge and appreciation of the electrical and physiologic events associated with the treatment.

A problem arises, though, in defining the limits within which this basic information may be applied. The information presented in this chapter is exclusively derived from carefully controlled experiments, many of which are not readily applicable to the complex clinical situations encountered by the practitioner. Therefore, an attempt is made not only to provide the essential information for understanding nerve and muscle excitation, but also to provide some indication of the clinical relevance of this information. Ongoing basic and clinical research will further advance our understanding of neuromuscular excitation and ultimately our clinical skills in neuromuscular rehabilitation.

The main theme of this chapter is stated as follows: Excitation of nerve and muscle requires that currents flow. An understanding of neuromuscular excitation requires keeping track of currents that flow in the aqueous fluids of biological tissues. The physiologic and biophysical principles presented here should provide the reader with the information necessary to keep track of the currents and to interpret the physiologic consequences of these currents. In so doing, an appreciation should be gained for what happens when electric stimuli are applied to a person.

PROPERTIES OF ELECTRICALLY EXCITABLE CELLS

Electrical Concepts Specific to Bioelectrical Phenomena

The most useful models to describe excitable membrane phenomena are electric circuits. A general appreciation of these models requires an understanding of three elements: resistors, capacitors, and batteries; and three concepts: voltage, current, and charge.

Figuratively speaking, charge may be thought of as the substance that is either stored or moved. When charge is stored, it represents a potential to do work (i.e., it provides the driving force for producing a charge flow). This storage of charge is termed *voltage*, while the flow of charge is termed *current*. For devices such as electrical stimulators, charge is described in terms of the presence or absence of electrons and current flow is with respect to electron flow. In aqueous systems, such as nerve and muscle, it is customary to speak of charge in terms of the storage or flow of ions, such as Na^+, K^+, and Cl^-. The conversion from the electron flow of the stimulator to the ionic flow of the biological tissue occurs at the electrode-tissue interface.

Current flow through a resistor is typically described in terms of the hydraulic analogy of water flowing through a pipe. For example, decreasing the diameter of the pipe, increases the resistance, thereby reducing water flow; increasing the pipe diameter decreases the resistance, resulting in an increased water flow. Current flow through a capacitor, a concept of critical importance in understanding how a neuron or muscle fiber is excited, is not as intuitively obvious and requires more detailed consideration.

Most of us are familiar with a battery, which is an element that stores charge in the form of a potential chemical energy. If a circuit is completed between the two poles of a battery, the stored energy is released to drive a current. A capacitor is similar to a battery in that it also is capable of storing charge. The main difference between the two is that in the battery, charge is stored in the form of potential chemical energy, while in the capacitor, charge is stored in the form of a charge asymmetry. The physical makeup of a capacitor consists of two conducting plates separated by a nonconducting medium, the dielectric. Currents are actually physically restricted from flowing through the capacitor. If charges were to pass through the capacitor, the capacitor would be considered damaged. What do we mean when we speak of current flow *through* a capacitor?

When we speak of a capacitive current, we do not mean that charge on one side is actually displaced to the other side. Rather, when a capacitor is connected to a circuit, which allows current to flow, charge builds up on one plate of the capacitor and leaves the other plate. During any specific time period, as much charge builds up as leaves. The alternating charge buildup and release behave like a current passing through all parts of

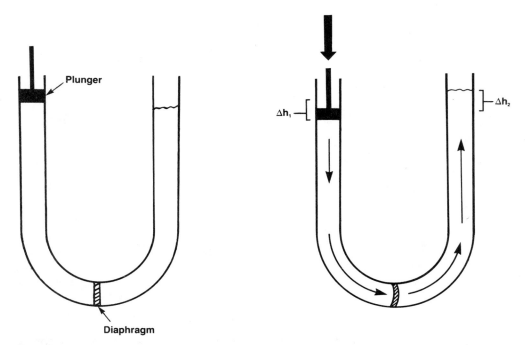

FIGURE 1-1. (*A*) Hydraulic analogy of a capacitor consisting of U-shaped, water-filled tube, partitioned into two chambers by a rubber diaphragm. (*B*) Downward pressure on a plunger (analogous to a voltage) produces movement of water against the diaphragm. The shock wave is transferred into the adjoining chamber, with the resultant flow of water in that chamber. The changes in water levels in each chamber ($h_1 = h_2$) are representative of the consequence of the current flows. The result is as if a current "flowed" across the membrane.

the circuit. Even though no charge has physically passed through the capacitor, the effective current flow throughout the circuit is *as if a current flowed through the capacitor.*

If this concept is still mysterious, consider again a hydraulic analogy.[3] Consider a U-shaped tube filled with water (Fig. 1-1). The tube is divided into two chambers (the two conducting plates of the capacitor) by a rubber diaphragm (the dielectric of the capacitor) which does not allow water to pass from one side to the other (see Fig. 1-1*A*). A plunger is inserted into one end of the tube and is pushed inward (see Fig. 1-1*B*). The driving force of the plunger (voltage) creates water flow (current) which causes the diaphragm to protrude into the adjoining chamber. This protrusion creates water flow (current) in the adjoining chamber, yet no water was transferred across the diaphragm. Currents were generated on both sides of the diaphragm (capacitor) as if water flowed through it (capacitor current).

Two final considerations requiring brief comment are that of the *direction* of current flow and the necessity of having a *completed circuit* so that current can flow. Throughout this chapter, *current flow* is described in the direction of *movement of positive charge.* First, all concepts could equally be described for current flow in the direction of movement of negative charge. The use of the former is conventional and allows for a greater consistency in the presentation of the subject. Second, current flow can only occur if a completed circuit exists. Therefore, in keeping track of current flows one must always be cognizant of the fact that *current flows in a loop.* Interruption of the loop interrupts current flow.

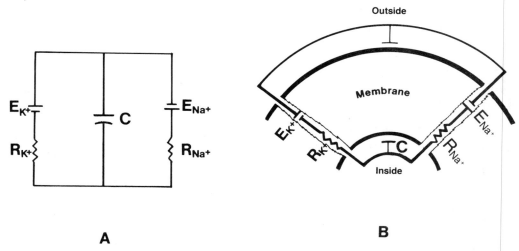

A   **B**

FIGURE 1–2. (*A*) Electrical model of an excitable membrane. Composed of two batteries (E_{Na+} and E_{K+}), two resistors (R_{Na+} and R_{K+}), and a capacitor (*C*). (*B*) Incorporation of the electrical model into a segment of the membrane. (Adapted from Jewett and Raymer.[1])

In summary, when we consider tissue excitability we think in terms of electrical circuits and electrical elements. The function of these circuits requires a manipulation of charge. For electrical devices, charge is electrons, while in aqueous tissue, charge is represented by ions. We will speak of charge flow (current) through resistors, capacitors, and batteries, and charge storage (voltage) across capacitors and batteries. The direction of current flow is described as the direction of movement of positive charge. Finally, we must never lose sight of the important fact that charge can only flow if there is a completed circuit.

Membrane Properties of Excitable Tissues

To understand how nerve or muscle can be excited by an externally applied stimulus, an appreciation of excitable membranes surrounding these tissues is necessary. A model of the membrane is presented in Figure 1–2. This model consists of five elements: The Na^+ and K^+ batteries (E_{Na+} and E_{K+});* the Na^+ and K^+ resistors (R_{Na+} and R_{K+}); and a capacitor (C), charged positive on the outside and negative inside. Although ions other than Na^+ and K^+ exist in the intracellular and extracellular medium of aqueous systems, a good general appreciation of membrane excitability can be obtained solely in terms of Na^+ and K^+ influences. A problem often encountered upon initial presentation of this model is in relating the electrical elements of the model to their physical counterparts in the biological medium. The question therefore is, where in the membrane are the resistors, batteries and capacitors?

The membrane is a lipid bilayer imbedded with proteins. There is speculation as to the actual configuration of the proteins and lipids,[4] but for our purposes, the structure

---

*In that a battery signifies a voltage, the convention has been to represent the Na^+ and K^+ batteries by the letter E, the symbol for a voltage in biological systems.

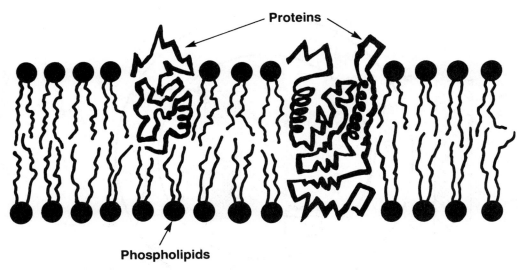

Proteins

Phospholipids

FIGURE 1–3. Schematic representation of the cross-sectional view of the lipid protein model of the membrane. The phospholipids are arranged in a bilayer with their polar, spherical heads facing outward, and their wavy, fatty acid chains facing inward. The proteins are depicted as folded polypeptide chains, imbedded within or throughout the bilayer. (Adapted from Singer and Nicholson.[4])

might be visualized as presented in Figure 1–3. We earlier defined a capacitor as an element consisting of two conducting plates separated by an insulator, the dielectric. The high concentration of electrically insulating lipids within the membrane acts as an excellent dielectric. The intracellular and extracellular fluids readily allow the flow of charge and may therefore be thought of as conducting plates. This unique combination of a conducting media separated by an insulated area results in a membrane acting as a capacitor.

The dielectric properties of the membrane are similar to that of glass of the same dimensions and therefore should not allow ionic flow. Yet, we know that ions do move through the membrane. This movement is believed to occur through select portions of the membrane, which are conceptualized as holes or pores within the membrane. Since these pores offer a finite resistance to ionic flow, they act as resistors and are modeled as such in our membrane circuit. The two ions of major interest to us are Na^+ and K^+, and therefore, two resistors (R_{Na^+} and R_{K^+}) are depicted in the model.

The batteries are somewhat more difficult to conceptualize, although we may begin by stating that they are a consequence of the differences in ionic concentrations between the inside and outside of the cell membrane. Whenever the concentrations of a given substance are unequal between two regions, if the substance is allowed to flow, it will move from the region of higher concentration to the region of lower concentration. In nerve and muscle cells, the K^+ concentration is much greater inside the cell than outside. If K^+ were allowed to flow, it would flow down this concentration gradient (i.e., from higher to lower concentration), and move out of the cell (Fig. 1–4). This outward movement of K^+ would create a positive charge buildup outside the cell membrane, which would eventually counter any further outward flow of K^+. This separation of charge is a storage of potential chemical energy which, if released, would drive a current; this is the definition of a battery given earlier. Because ion flow across the

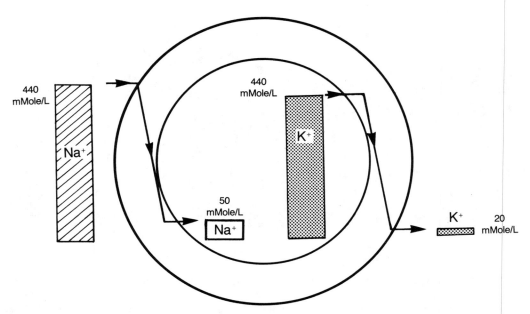

FIGURE 1–4. Depiction of the concentration gradients for K^+ and Na^+ for a typical excitable cell. K^+ is more highly concentrated inside than out, and if allowed to flow, would move from inside out. Na^+ is more highly concentrated outside than in, and if it were allowed to flow, it would move from outside in.

membrane can occur only at the pores, the "battery" must reside at the pores. A combination of two factors, therefore, which make up the battery are the pores, which allow ionic flow, and the ionic concentration difference, which provides the driving force for ionic flow.

The Na^+ battery is also characterized by a concentration difference and the ability of Na^+ ions to diffuse across the membrane at the pores. The polarity of this battery is opposite to that of the K^+ battery because the concentration gradient is in the opposite direction, that is, Na^+ flows from outside in (Fig. 1–4). The battery is developed to resist further movement of an ion down its concentration gradient. Na^+ is more highly concentrated outside the cell than inside and therefore would diffuse into the cell. A positive charge buildup inside the cell would develop to resist further Na^+ influx. The Na^+ battery in this model is therefore of opposite polarity compared to the K^+ battery.

THE RESTING POTENTIAL

A microelectrode can be inserted into a nerve or muscle cell, and when connected to appropriate recording devices, a voltage can be measured. This voltage is termed the resting potential. By convention it is determined as the potential of the inside of the cell relative to the outside and therefore is expressed as a negative value. The resting potential is nearly equal to the potential of the K^+ battery (E_{K^+}). The reason that K^+ has a strong influence in determining the resting potential is that the membrane is more than 10 times more permeable to K^+ than to Na^+. Therefore, K^+ is freer to move; it does so down its concentration gradient and thereby establishes an electrical potential which will resist further K^+ outflow.

If the K^+ battery is related to the resting potential, what is the Na^+ battery related to? Remember, the Na^+ battery is of opposite polarity to that of the K^+ battery. The only time in which the membrane potential reverses polarity is during the rise of the action potential. It is during this time that the membrane potential approximates (but falls slightly short of) the Na^+ battery.

The development of the membrane potential, as a good first approximation, can therefore be attributed to two major factors: a selective permeability of the membrane to K^+ and a concentration gradient favoring outward K^+ movement. A more complete description of the membrane potential, which includes the role of Na^+ in this phenomenon, may be found in textbooks of cellular physiology; the one by Kuffler and Nicholls[5] is highly recommended. The magnitude of the potential is the voltage required to counteract further movement of K^+ down its concentration gradient. It is important to realize that this description explains the development of the resting potential. To understand what happens when an electrical stimulus is applied to a person, we need to understand how the membrane potential is maintained and how it can be excited to generate action potentials.

It was previously stated that the potential that builds due to K^+ leaving the cell reaches a point at which further K^+ movement is counteracted. This does not mean that no K^+ leaves the cell. There actually is movement of K^+ out of the cell, but that movement is balanced by an active metabolic pump which returns K^+ in to the cell. Therefore, once the membrane potential is established, there is no *net* K^+ movement. This condition, in which there is no net transfer of ions, is referred to as a *steady state*.

A similar situation exists for Na^+. Na^+ tends to move in accordance with its concentration gradient, thus entering the cell. At this time an active pump extrudes Na^+ from the cell. Therefore, under resting conditions, there are both K^+ and Na^+ currents, but because of the pumps, no net transfer of ions occurs. The result is that the resting potential is maintained. It should be emphasized that all currents so far described have been through the membrane pores and none through the membrane capacitance. *The only way to alter the membrane resting potential is to discharge the capacitor (i.e., produce a capacitive current).* This process is described below.

THE ACTION POTENTIAL

Key points from our study of the resting potential are also applicable to the understanding of the action potential. First, the action potential will develop when the membrane allows passage of specific ions. Second, these ions will diffuse down their concentration gradients. Third, currents will flow in completed circuits, and finally, one path of the current flow must be through the capacitor which signifies a change in the membrane potential.

At this point it is necessary to return to the circuit model of the membrane and the tracking of currents. Figure 1–5 provides a qualitative description of these current flows for different phases of the action potential. Four phases of the action potential are depicted: (1) the resting state (resting potential), (2) initial depolarization of the membrane, (3) peak of the action potential, and (4) decline of the action potential (repolarization).

1. The membrane is at rest and is characterized by events previously described. A steady-state inward flow of Na^+ and outward flow of K^+ result in no net transfer of charge. No capacitive current is induced, and therefore the membrane potential remains stable.

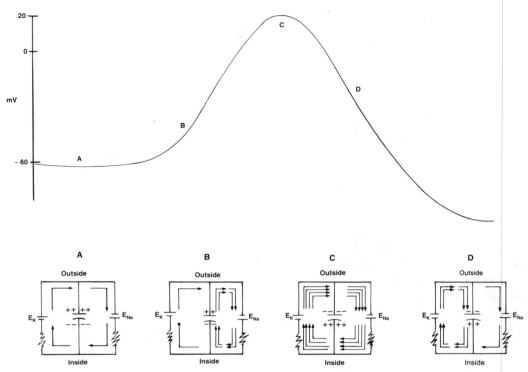

FIGURE 1–5. Spatial representation of the action potential. The directions of current flow for different phases of the action potential are given $(A-D)$ using the electrical model of the membrane. Predominance of a specific current path is depicted by the number of arrows around a loop. Note that the membrane potential is only changing when current passes *through the capacitor* (B). (Adapted from Jewett and Raymer.[1])

2. The membrane suddenly becomes more permeable to Na$^+$, resulting in an inward Na$^+$ current (double arrows in figure). The inside plate of the capacitor therefore becomes more positively charged due to Na$^+$ influx, while the outside plate becomes less positively charged. This charge movement on the inside and outside of the cell produces a current (capacitive current) which behaves *as if* charge actually moved through the capacitor. The net result is depicted as a completed circuit consisting of an inward Na$^+$ current and an outward capacitive current.

3. At the peak of the action potential, the membrane has reversed polarity, with the inside now positive with respect to the outside. The membrane permeability is very high for both Na$^+$ and K$^+$, and therefore large currents are generated (quadruple arrows). The completed circuit is strictly with the Na$^+$ and K$^+$ currents. Without a capacitive current, no change in the membrane potential is seen. This condition exists for only an instantaneous fraction of a millisecond and signifies the peak of the action potential.

4. The membrane has switched from an enhanced Na$^+$ permeability to an enhanced K$^+$ permeability. Large K$^+$ currents are generated, and in a process similar to that described in 2, an inward capacitive current is induced. The net result is the return of the membrane potential to more negative values, inside with respect to outside.

Three important concepts are derived from this description. First, an ionic current always flows down the ion's concentration gradient (i.e., from an area of greater concentration to an area of lesser concentration); these currents are inward for Na^+ and outward for K^+. Second, the membrane potential only changes when there is a capacitive current. When the capacitive current is outward, the membrane depolarizes (becomes more positive inside). When the capacitive current is inward, the membrane hyperpolarizes (becomes more negative inside). Third, all currents flow in complete circuits with the total current flow across the membrane at any given time being zero (i.e., the total outward current always equals the total inward current).

NERVE AND MUSCLE EXCITATION INDUCED BY EXTERNALLY APPLIED STIMULATION

Stimulation of Peripheral Nerves

A major emphasis of action-potential generation is based on the fact that the membrane can only be depolarized (excited) when an outward capacitive current is induced. This fact is the basis by which an externally applied electrical stimulus excites the underlying tissue. That is, the *purpose of an electrical stimulus is to induce an outward capacitive current across the membrane.*

Figure 1–6 depicts a circuit diagram representing electrical stimulation of a peripheral nerve using electrodes placed on the overlying skin. One possible path for current flow (direction of movement of positive charges) is from the anode (positive pole) of the stimulator into the axon through the membrane, through the axoplasm (R_i), and back out of the axon through the membrane at the cathode (negative pole) of the stimulator. An alternative current pathway, through the subcutaneous tissue (R_o), is also possible (dashed line). If this resistance (R_o) is too low, which occurs if the electrodes are spaced too closely to each other, then the majority of the stimulating current would be shunted through the subcutaneous tissue, the path of least resistance. Even under the most ideal conditions some current does pass through this path, which is one of the reasons that relatively large voltages are required for stimulation via surface electrodes. The current pathway through R_o is neglected in the remaining discussion, but its effect should not be forgotten when attempting to optimize stimulation effectiveness.

What happens when this circuit is initially energized? Again, it is important to remember that all current flow in aqueous solutions is due to ionic movement. At the anode (Fig. 1–6B), the positive charge placed on the surface repels the positive ions of the extracellular region toward the surface of the membrane and positive ions of the intracellular region away from the inside of the membrane. At the cathode (Fig. 1–6C), positive ions in the extracellular region are attracted to the surface, while those of the intracellular region are attracted to the inside of the membrane. The subsequent effect of these intracellular and extracellular currents is a net inward capacitive current at the anode and an outward capacitive current at the cathode. Again, remember that a major point in the description of action-potential generation is that the membrane can only be excited (depolarized) when an outward capacitive current is induced. This condition occurs at the cathode and signifies the onset of membrane depolarization.

The discussion thus far has focused strictly on capacitive currents as the initial membrane event that occurs upon energizing this circuit. Following this initial event, ionic currents arise. At the cathode, the ionic currents are the same as those described

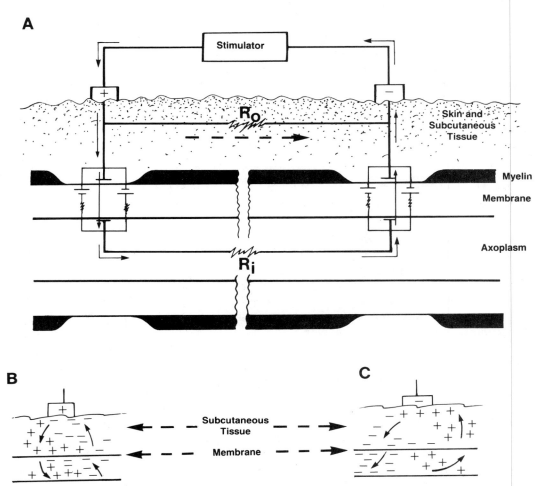

FIGURE 1–6. (*A*) Electrical schematic diagram for an externally applied electrical stimulus. Two current paths are depicted; one through the extracellular medium (R_o) and a second through the axon core (R_i). See text for details. Note that the direction of capacitive currents is inward at the anode (+ pole) and outward at the cathode (− pole). Comparison of the electrical networks at these poles with Figure 1–5B and 1–5D reveals that the membrane will depolarize at the cathode and hyperpolarize at the anode. (Adapted from Jewett and Raymer.[1]) (*B*) Ionic flow at the anode consists of extracellular positive charges being driven toward the membrane and intracellular positive charges away from the membrane. Negative charges flow in the opposite direction. The result is a net inward capacitive current at the anode. (*C*) Ionic flow at the cathode consists of extracellular positive charges being driven away from the membrane and intracellular positive charges toward the membrane. The result is a net outward capacitive current at the cathode.

previously for action-potential generation (Fig. 1–5). That is, an initial inward Na^+ current associated with the accompanying outward capacitive current leads to further depolarization of the membrane (Fig. 1–5B). As the membrane potential approaches the value of the Na^+ battery (Fig. 1–5C), a reversal occurs in ionic flow. In this instance, an outward K^+ current is generated, accompanied by an inward capacitive current. This inward capacitive current acts to restore the membrane potential to its resting level.

The reader is reminded that the purpose of this chapter is to gain an understanding of neuromuscular excitation by keeping track of the currents; if you need clarification, retrace the current paths presented. Remember that first, the membrane can only become excited if an outward capacitive current is induced, and second, current can only flow if there is a completed circuit.

When an electrical stimulus is applied to a peripheral nerve the initial excitation occurs under the cathode since it is at this site that an outward capacitive current is generated. If the excitation is of sufficient magnitude, a subsequent inward Na^+ current together with the outward capacitive current gives rise to the action potential. When an action potential is generated in the periphery, it will propagate both away from and toward the spinal cord. In subsequent sections events that occur with transmission of the action potential toward the spinal cord will be discussed.

Reflex Activation and Synaptic Transmission

This discussion is restricted to a single emphasis that is important for later comprehension of reflex recruitment of motoneurons: Ionic currents that are generated at a synapse produce a voltage change in the postsynaptic cell. If this voltage change is of sufficient magnitude to make the resting potential less negative, an action potential will be generated in the postsynaptic cell. Details of the mechanisms underlying synaptic transmission may be found in standard neurophysiology texts.[1,5] A two-neuron chain is used here to illustrate this point simply (Fig. 1–7). Neuron X represents a presynaptic cell whose axon forms a synapse on the postsynaptic cell, neuron Y. An electrode inserted into neuron Y records a resting membrane potential. If the sensitivity of the recording amplifier is increased sufficiently, spontaneous fluctuations in the membrane potential would also be recorded (Fig. 1–7B). These fluctuations, termed miniature end-plate potentials (MEPPs) are of similar amplitude and duration. They are the consequence of the spontaneous release of single packets of neurotransmitters from neuron X and neuron Y.

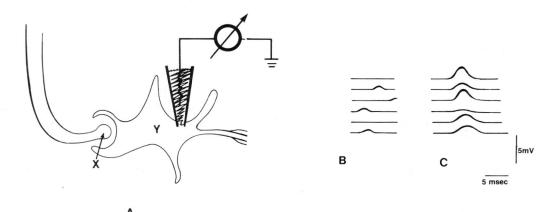

FIGURE 1–7. (A) Schematic representation of an intracellular recording setup for recording postsynaptic events in postsynaptic cell, Y. (B) Spontaneous fluctuations (miniature epsps) in the membrane potential of neuron Y. (C) Summation of miniature epsps, induced by synaptic activation between X and Y, results in a large excitatory postsynaptic potential (EPSP) in Y.

An action potential conducted down neuron X would produce a much larger change in the membrane potential of Y (Fig. 1–7C) than that of the MEPPs. This potential in neuron Y is the result of the release of several packets of transmitters from neuron Y, each of which would produce a single MEPP, but together summate to produce the larger potential, termed an excitatory postsynaptic potential (EPSP). The important consideration here is that a release of neurotransmitter produces a current across neuron Y which was recorded as a voltage change, the EPSP.

It should be emphasized that a single EPSP is never sufficient to produce a large enough change in the membrane potential to generate an action potential. Rather, several EPSPs, generated either by the activation of the same synapse or at different synapses, must summate to produce a sufficient voltage change to reach the threshold for generation of an action potential.

Whenever an electrical stimulus is applied to the skin surface, it has the potential to activate neurons within the spinal cord by the processes just described. Centrally located neurons which may be activated include the alpha motoneurons which supply skeletal muscle and interneurons of somatic and visceral pathways. Which centrally located neurons are activated depends upon the types of peripheral neurons activated by the stimulus. To understand which peripheral neurons are activated preferentially by a particular stimulus requires an appreciation of the types of afferent fibers that may be found in a peripheral nerve.

Afferent Fiber Types

In the two-neuron chain of Figure 1–7, the large postsynaptic neuron (Y) could be an alpha motoneuron or an interneuron of the spinal cord. The presynaptic neuron (X) could be a peripheral afferent fiber or, again, an interneuron. For the purposes of this discussion, assume that neuron Y is an alpha motoneuron and neuron X, a peripheral afferent. The synaptic input at a motoneuron, depicted here as the sole input, is actually much more elaborate. It has been estimated that a typical motoneuron has about 5500 synapses on its cell body and dendrites.[6] These synapses represent both direct and indirect connections from peripheral afferents as well as from central nervous system (CNS) regions. The peripheral afferent input is of interest to the physical therapist employing electrical stimulation.

Table 1–1 provides a summary of the afferent fiber types that may be found in a peripheral nerve. The focus of classification is often with regard to fiber diameter and is presented here for both the I through IV classification of David Lloyd[7] and the A and C classification of Gasser and Erlanger.[8] The striking feature of fiber size is that the fibers span a 20-fold range of diameters. The table further depicts the peripheral receptor associated with the afferent, the site of origin of the afferent, the most effective stimulus for activation, and the associated reflex action. At the extremes of this spectrum of fiber sizes are the large-diameter muscle afferents and small-diameter pain fibers. This convenient categorization of afferents according to size and experimentally based categorization according to function has provided the basis for much speculation on the physiologic rationale underlying the effectiveness of therapeutically applied electrical stimulation such as transcutaneous electrical nerve stimulation (TENS) for pain control and neuromuscular electrical stimulation (NMES) for muscle re-education. The biophysical principles underlying these interventions are discussed in Chapters 5 and 7, respectively. At the core of this rationale is the known physiologic fact that neuron excitability is largely determined by neuron size, as presented below.

TABLE 1–1 Classification of Afferent Fiber Types*

Afferent Fiber Size		Fiber Size and Conduction Velocity	Peripheral Origin	Receptors	Effective Stimulus	Reflex Action
Aα	Ia	12–20 μm 70–120 m/sec	Muscle	Muscle spindle primary ending	Muscle stretch	Monosynaptic excitation of agonists and synergists Disynaptic inhibition of antagonists
	Ib	12–20 μm 70–120 m/sec	Muscle	Golgi tendon organ	Muscle contraction	Disynaptic inhibition of agonists and synergists Disynaptic excitation of antagonists
Aβ	II	5–12 μm 30–70 m/sec	Extensor muscle	Muscle spindle secondary ending	Muscle stretch	Monosynaptic and polysynaptic excitation of agonists and synergists
Aγ			Flexor muscle	Muscle spindle secondary ending	Muscle stretch	Monosynaptic and polysynaptic excitation of flexors and inhibition of extensors (flexion withdrawal)
			Skin	Touch/pressure	Mechanical deformation of skin	Polysynaptic excitation of flexors and inhibition of extensors (flexion withdrawal)
Aδ	III	2–5 μm 12–30 m/sec	Muscle	Unknown (pain?) Pain (cold and hot)	Noxious Noxious temperature changes	Polysynaptic excitation of flexors and inhibition of extensors (flexion withdrawal)
C	IV	0.5–1 μm 0.5–2 m/sec	Muscle and skin	Pain	Noxious	

*Adapted from Henneman,[6] p 764.

Excitation of Neurons Based on Size

Under ideal conditions, neuron excitation depends upon the size of the neuron and the type of electrical stimulus that is applied.[2] For our purposes, assume that the stimulus is a rectangular pulse and therefore excitability is dependent solely on fiber diameter and not different types of stimulus pulse forms. It is necessary at this point to distinguish between excitation produced by intracellular versus extracellular stimulation. This distinction is necessary because the order of excitation, whether from small to large neurons or large to small, is determined by the type of stimulation used. Intracellular stimulation may be performed in the laboratory by impaling a neuron with a micropipette and injecting current into it, or (more physiologically) by inducing synaptic transmission. Extracellular stimulation on the other hand is performed by placing electrodes on the surface of neurons, or, as in the clinic, on the skin overlying the nerve. In the clinic, electrical stimuli are applied to the axons extracellularly. Nonetheless, intracellular excitation of cell bodies occurs as a result of synaptic activation from afferent volleys entering the spinal cord. Why then is the order of activation of neurons of different sizes different for intracellular and extracellular stimulation?

An appreciation of the rules by which neurons are excited under these two stimulating conditions requires consideration of three factors:

1. The resistance of a neuron-to-current flow is largely dependent upon the neuron's size. For cell bodies, size is expressed as the diameter of the cell body. For axons, size is expressed as the total diameter of the axon plus its myelin sheath. Neurons with small cell bodies have small-diameter axons while neurons with large cell bodies have large-diameter axons. Small neurons have a larger resistance than large neurons.
2. Both large and small neurons require the same absolute voltage change to bring them to threshold.
3. For intracellular stimulation, the currents generated are assumed to be equal for large and small neurons. For extracellular stimulation, the currents generated are not equal but are influenced largely by the resistance of the neuron. Because a small neuron has a larger resistance than a large neuron, for any specific voltage, less current flows through the small neuron than through the large neuron.

Looking more closely at how two different-sized neurons are activated for intracellular versus extracellular stimulation can be informative. For intracellular stimulation (Fig. 1–8A), equal currents are generated at both the large and small neuron (Factor 3 above). The important point is that we are trying to create a voltage change (depolarization) by passing current through a resistance. The relationship among these three variables is expressed by Ohm's law:

$$E = IR$$

where E is the voltage, I is the current, and R is the resistance. The resistance of the small neuron is greater than that of the large neuron (Factor 1), yet the currents are equal (Factor 3). Therefore, according to Ohm's law, the voltage change associated with intracellular excitation of the small neuron will be greater than that for the large neuron (Fig. 1–8A). Since both neurons need a similar voltage change to reach threshold (Factor 2), the larger voltage change that occurs in the small neuron will bring it closer to

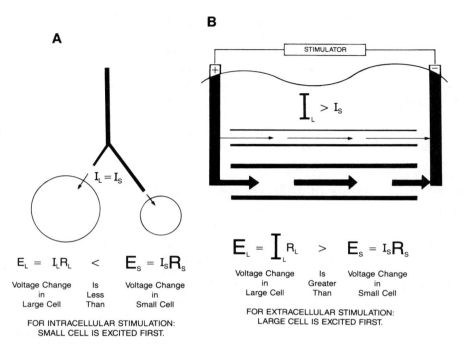

FIGURE 1–8. Relative relationships among voltage (E), current (I), and intracellular resistance (R) for two hypothetical neurons of different sizes (L = large, S = small). The relationship among these three variables is expressed by Ohm's law, $E = IR$. The relative influence of each of these variables is schematically depicted by their size in the equations. For intracellular stimulation (A), current flow is equal for both large and small cells. For extracellular stimulation (B), current flow is directly proportional to axon size. This relationship can be used to predict which neuron will discharge first for either intracellular (A) or extracellular (B) stimulation. (A) The two neurons receive the same synaptic input and their currents are therefore equal. Since the resistance of the large cell is smaller than that of the small cell, the voltage change in the large cell is less than the voltage change in the small cell, and the small cell therefore fires first. (B) Two neurons are excited by the same extracellular stimulation but a disproportionate current flows through each. This disproportionate current flow is the determining factor in the voltage change occurring in each cell, offsetting the effect of different resistances. The result is a voltage change in the large neuron greater than that in the small neuron, and the large neuron will therefore fire before the small.

threshold than the large neuron. Therefore, for intracellular stimulation the small neuron is activated (reaches threshold) before the large neuron.

With extracellular stimulation, current flow through two different-sized neurons is not equal, but rather is determined by the diameter of the neuron (Fig. 1–8B). Less current will flow through the small neuron than the large neuron. In this situation, the differences in current flows predominate over the differences in resistance in determining the voltage changes in the two neurons. The result is that a greater voltage change occurs for the larger neuron than for the smaller neuron because of the larger current flow through the larger neuron. The larger neuron is more readily excited by a large voltage change than is the smaller neuron. Therefore, for extracellular stimulation, the larger neuron is activated at lower stimulus intensities than the smaller neuron.

In summary, the excitability of neurons, under ideal conditions, is dependent upon the diameter of the axon or cell body. For synaptic activation (intracellular stimulation), excitation is from smaller to larger neurons, whereas for extracellular, or direct activation of a peripheral nerve, excitation is from larger to smaller neurons. One should understand that these orders of excitation are determined under ideal conditions. When a therapist applies an electrical stimulus to a patient, the conditions depart from the ideal. One reason for this departure is the inability to apply the electrical stimulus directly to the nerve. In addition, the order of excitation for synaptic activation is critically dependent upon the assumption that equal synaptic currents are generated at all cells. This assumption also cannot be guaranteed in a clinical situation.

Clinical Implications of Size Dependence in Afferent Excitation and Order of Neuron Recruitment

The major clinical concern arising from a size-dependent factor affecting neuron excitation is the ability to selectively activate a given group of neurons. Most textbooks indicate that by careful selection of waveform parameters, the clinician may selectively activate large-diameter afferents to control pain[9] or to selectively activate motoneurons to produce muscle contractions with the least amount of discomfort.[10]

The physiologic rationale for this selectivity is based upon the well-established relationship between strength of stimulation and duration of the stimulus. Figure 1–9 depicts the excitability characteristics of three of the afferent fiber types listed in Table 1–1. Note that the X axes for each of the fiber populations are vastly different. The shortest pulse durations are sufficient for exciting the large-diameter A fibers, whereas much larger pulse durations are needed for exciting the small-diameter C fibers. The

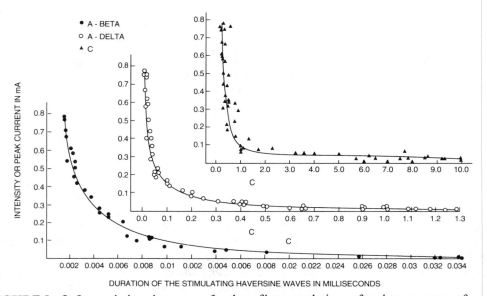

FIGURE 1–9. Strength duration curves for three fiber populations of saphenous nerve of a cat. The two parameters of stimulation, stimulus intensity and stimulus pulse duration, are plotted against each other to depict the combination of these two parameters needed to produce just measurable evoked neural responses in nerve. (From Li and Bak,[15] with permission.)

clinical implication here is that by choosing electrical pulses of very short duration, one should be able to preferentially activate large-diameter fibers.

This selective activation is certainly true for the ideal conditions of an isolated nerve preparation for results such as those presented in Figure 1–9. For the extremes in fiber diameter (the Aβ and Aδ versus C fibers) a gross selective activation may possibly be obtained when using clinical stimulators. By selecting a short enough pulse duration, such as 0.01 to 0.05 ms, one should be able to preferentially activate larger motoneurons before the small pain-conducting fibers, thereby minimizing pain perception during treatments in which induced muscle contraction is sought. The clinical applications of electrically induced muscle contractions for pain control or neuromuscular re-education are reviewed in Chapters 5 and 7, respectively.

The frequent interpretations of TENS-induced pain relief by selective activation of large-diameter afferents is somewhat more tenuous. Although theoretically plausible from the standpoint of an isolated nerve preparation (Fig. 1–9), the ability of clinically applied stimulation to selectively activate neurons is complicated by several factors. The first is the inability to apply a uniform current to all axons of a peripheral nerve. Axons closest to the electrodes tend to be exposed to a greater current density than those lying more deeply. Smaller diameter, superficially located axons can therefore be excited before larger, deeply located axons. Secondly, rarely in a clinical setting does one apply the stimulus exclusively to the trunk's peripheral nerves. Rather, large-pad electrodes are placed over the skin surface resulting in the stimulation of terminal branches of axons as well as peripheral nerve trunks. A size-dependent recruitment of neurons in this case is unpredictable and requires experimental verification. This problem is discussed in more detail in the following section. A final problem arises from the lack of experimental evidence testing the effectiveness of clinically used waveforms to excite neurons. To appreciate this problem requires a closer examination of how strength-duration curves are derived.

The strength-duration curves in Figure 1–9 succinctly and quantitatively depict the two most important factors, pulse strength (amplitude) and duration, which determine tissue excitability. A third factor, implicit to all depictions of strength-duration curves, is the manner in which the stimulus is applied. The two most easily quantifiable waveforms used are rectangular pulses and sine waves.[12,13] Both waveforms, when used under the controlled conditions of an isolated nerve preparation, are capable of demonstrating a separation of fiber-type responses based upon differences in axon diameters.[14,15] There appears to be little or no experimental verification of selective neuron activation for the complicated waveforms and electrode placements used in TENS therapy. These complicating factors in the clinical applications of TENS therapy warrant caution in the interpretation of TENS studies solely in terms of selective activation of afferent fiber types.

EXCITATION OF ALPHA MOTONEURONS

Neuromuscular electrical stimulation (NMES) is a class of stimulation which has recently regained popularity in attempts to restore normal muscle function. Although both sensory and motor fibers are excited with this stimulation, the focus of this discussion will be exclusively on the consequences of direct and reflexive activation of the motor fibers. The comments made previously in the section on afferent excitability would be equally applicable to this discussion of NMES.

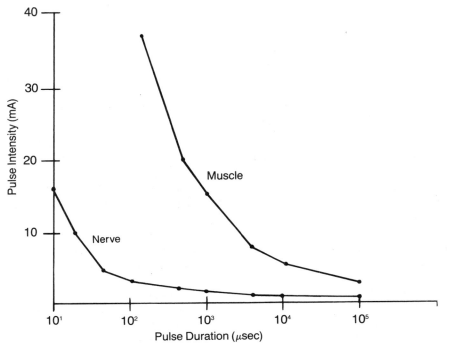

FIGURE 1-10. Difference in excitability between nerve and muscle as exemplified by their strength duration curves. The excitability of nerve tissue is possible even for the shortest pulse durations (.01 – .1 msec). Excitation of muscle is not possible at these short pulse durations, and for longer durations, much larger currents are needed compared with nerve. (Adapted from Mortimer.[11])

Direct and Reflex Activation of Motoneurons

When an electrical stimulus is applied to the muscle belly of an innervated muscle, activation of the muscle is most likely due to the excitation of the terminal motor axons within the muscle. This preferential activation is the result of the much lower threshold of excitation for nerve versus muscle and is exemplified by the divergence in the strength-duration curves for these two tissues (Fig. 1 – 10). The question arises as to how the muscle fibers are activated by electrical stimulation. Although this question probably has never been directly addressed for the clinical types of stimulation generally used, an attempt is made here to provide some theoretical speculation on what may occur. Further consideration of excitation of nerve and muscle is presented in Chapter 4, "Electrical Evaluation of Nerve and Muscle Excitability."

To simplify this discussion, assume that rectangular electrical pulses are applied directly to a peripheral nerve rather than application of a diffuse stimulation over the muscle belly. The stimulation, if of sufficient intensity, will generate action potentials in the axons of the peripheral nerve. Action potentials will be conducted both toward the spinal cord and toward the muscle. For the sensory axons stimulated, conduction toward the muscle (antidromic) will terminate in action-potential annihilation and, therefore, is of no consequence to this discussion. Likewise, motor-axon conduction back to the spinal cord (antidromic) will result in action-potential annihilation at the motoneuron cell body. Therefore, the action-potential conduction of particular interest to this discussion (with the exception of F waves, see Chapter 4) is that of sensory conduction toward the spinal cord and motor conduction to the muscle (orthodromic).

For direct stimulation of a peripheral nerve, a size-dependent order of axon recruitment can often be demonstrated. The first fibers recruited are of the group A classification: these include both muscle afferents and alpha motoneurons. Certain peripheral nerves are reported to have a larger disparity between the size of the large diameter motor and sensory fibers, with the sensory fibers being the larger. In these nerves, such as the tibial nerve to the soleus muscle, the lowest threshold electrical response recorded in the muscle is a reflex-generated response. Figure 1–11A depicts a hypothetical example of this reflex in response to increasing intensities of stimulation. The major point of interest here is the decrease in the latency of the response (line a–a') with increasing intensities of stimulation. Such a finding indicates that for increasing intensities of stimulation, the motoneurons recruited reflexly are progressively faster in their conduction velocity. These faster conducting neurons are also of larger axon diameter (Table 1–1), and therefore the order of reflex recruitment as depicted in Figure 1–11A, top to bottom, must be from small to large. This size-dependent reflex recruitment would be predicted based upon the earlier discussion of the effect of neuron size on excitation with intracellular stimulation.

Figure 1–11C shows a hypothetical example of the order of direct excitation of motoneurons. In this case, the muscle chosen is one in which no reflex response can be demonstrated, such as the thenar muscle, *adductor pollicis*. As the intensity of ulnar nerve stimulation is increased, the direct motor response (M wave) is recorded in the muscle. This response is seen to increase in amplitude for increasing stimulus intensity, but without change in its latency of response (line c–c'). The interpretation is that the fastest conducting fibers are those initially activated, followed by excitation of the slower conducting fibers which become incorporated into the response at a slightly longer latency. Again, based upon the direct relationship between conduction velocity and axon size, the order of excitation for direct activation of motoneurons would be from largest to smallest. This size-dependent *direct* recruitment would also be predicted from the earlier discussion of axon size and order of excitation to extracellular stimulation.

Mechanical Consequences of Motoneuron Recruitment

The mechanical consequences of the difference in excitation for direct motor-axon stimulation versus reflex excitation is demonstrated in Figure 1–11B and 1–11D. As the stimulus intensity in increased for *reflex* activation of the motoneurons (Fig. 1–11B), the twitch responses become progressively larger. The point of major interest here, is that the time from stimulus onset to peak twitch tension (see line b–b') becomes progressively shorter for increasing stimulus intensity. This pattern of progressive shortening in the time-to-peak tension is reversed when the motoneurons are *directly* stimulated (Fig. 1–11D). In this case, the time-to-peak tension progressively increases for increases in stimulus intensity. Interpretation of these findings requires examination of the properties of the muscle fibers supplied by the motoneurons.

A single motor axon, prior to termination in a muscle, diverges into numerous endings, each of which forms a junction with a single muscle fiber. A single motor axon and all the muscle fibers supplied by it have been termed the motor unit.[16] Motor units

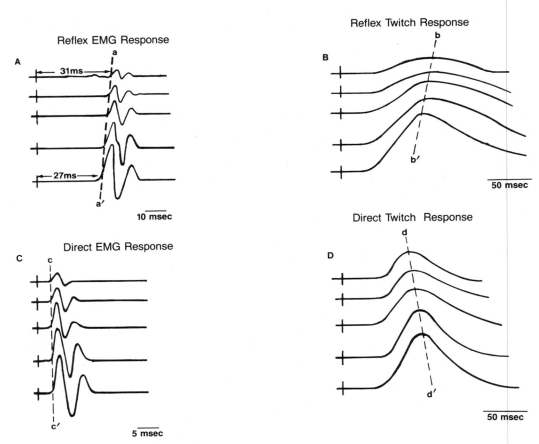

FIGURE 1–11. (*A*) Reflex EMG responses for progressive increase in intensity of stimulation of a peripheral nerve. Stimulus intensity increases in all traces from top to bottom. As stimulus intensity is increased, the reflex response increases in amplitude and decreases in the latency (a–a'). The decrease in latency (from 31 msec in top trace to 27 msec in bottom trace) is indicative of the progressive recruitment of larger diameter, faster conducting motoneurons. (*B*) Corresponding twitch responses for the EMG of A. Progressive recruitment of larger motoneurons results in an increase in the twitch amplitude together with a shortening in the time to peak tension (b–b'). (*C*) Direct EMG response for progressive increases in stimulation of a peripheral nerve. As stimulus intensity is increased, the direct response increases in amplitude with no change in the latency (c–c'). The lack of a latency change is indicative of the larger, faster conducting fibers being recruited first followed by the progressive recruitment of the smaller, slower conducting motoneurons. (*D*) Corresponding twitch responses for the EMG of C. Progressive recruitment of the smaller motoneurons results in an increase in the twitch amplitude together with a prolonging of the time to peak twitch tension (d–d').

have been classified according to numerous histochemical staining characteristics as well as their mechanical twitch properties.[17] Of particular interest to the interpretation of the findings of Figure 1–11*B* and 1–11*D* are the twitch properties of the different motor units and the size of the axons supplying each of them.

Although various classification schemes have been used to classify motor units into three, four, or more types, it is most informative for this discussion to look at the two extremes. The key points here are that the largest diameter motoneurons consist of the largest axons which supply muscle fibers that produce the largest twitch tensions, have the shortest time to maximum tension, but are most readily fatigued. At the opposite end of the spectrum are the small motoneurons, consisting of small-diameter axons which supply muscle fibers that produce the smallest twitch tensions, have the longest time to maximum tension, but are highly fatigue resistant. The peak twitch tension and time-to-peak tension help to explain the findings of Figure 1–11B and 1–11D.

In Figure 1–11B, the motoneurons are excited reflexly in the order of small to large, as depicted in Figure 1–11A. These small motoneurons supply muscle fibers that produce small twitch tensions that take the longest time to reach maximum twitch tension. As the intensity of stimulation is increased, larger motoneurons are recruited, each of which progressively produces greater twitch tensions but of shorter contractile times. The result as depicted in Figure 1–11B is a progressive increase in twitch tension with a shortening in the time-to-peak tension (see line b–b'). Figure 1–11D can be interpreted in a similar manner, but with the understanding that the order of excitation for direct stimulation is reversed; recruitment in this instance is from large to small.

Clinical Implications of Direct versus Reflex Excitation of Motoneurons

If electrical stimuli of progressively larger amplitudes are applied to a peripheral nerve, the sequence of motor-unit recruitment should, at the lower stimulus intensities, be a reflex recruitment of small-to-large units. At higher stimulus intensities, the motoneurons would be directly excited, in which case additional recruitment would progress from large to small motoneurons. This phenomenon actually occurs only in select muscles (i.e., soleus) where submaximal electrical stimuli applied to the peripheral nerve will evoke a reflex response (H reflex) and maximal electrical stimuli will recruit the smaller motor axons, producing a direct motor response in the muscle (M-response of motor nerve conduction velocity (NCV) testing). The more typical response seen is that of direct recruitment of larger, faster conducting motoneurons (Fig. 1–11D). Therefore, at low intensities of stimulation, motor-unit activation would be biased to the large, fast-twitch, fatigable units. Only at higher intensities would the small, slow-twitch, fatigue-resistant motor units be activated. Direct stimulation would be highly unlikely to selectively activate the small, slow-twitch units. These are the units which are believed to be active most often in typical activities of daily living,[18] whereas the large-twitch units would be activated during less frequent, high-force or high-velocity activities.

The problem with this prediction is that it is based upon the ability to stimulate a nerve directly and upon the ability to apply a uniform current to all axons within the nerve. Clinically, the typical means of neuromuscular stimulation is via pad electrodes placed over wide regions of the skin. Terminal nerve fibers are most likely being stimulated, but whether a size-dependent recruitment occurs is speculative. This uncertainty results from never really knowing whether stimulation is being delivered to the main axon of the motor unit or to its terminal endings. Activation is dependent upon the anatomic arrangement of the axon and terminals relative to the stimulating electrodes. This arrangement varies from muscle to muscle and person to person.

From a clinical perspective, the recruitment of motoneurons by cutaneously applied electrical stimulation is unpredictable in terms of the size of motoneurons and types of motor units activated. The goals of treatment can only be stated in general, qualitative terms based on observation of the quality and quantity of the induced muscle contraction and not the selective activation of one fiber type over another. (Further research of this topic appears to be needed.) Clinical considerations related to these issues are presented in detail in Chapters 7 and 8 on electrical stimulation of muscle.

SUMMARY

This chapter primarily reviews selected topics in electricity and cellular neurophysiology and discusses the application of this information to an understanding of clinical electrostimulation. An attempt has been made to present the basic information needed to obtain a better understanding of clinical electrostimulation as it is presently practiced. Electricity is discussed in qualitative terms and reduced to a review of three elements, resistors, capacitors, and batteries, and three concepts, charge, voltage, and current. The elements are incorporated into a model of the cell membrane, and the concepts are used to describe the excitability of the membrane. The major point of this discussion is that the only way to alter the membrane resting potential, and thereby excite the tissue, is to induce a current across the membrane's capacitance. The function of an electrical stimulus is to induce such a current.

The second half of this chapter provides an overview of selected topics in physiology that facilitate an understanding of the physiologic consequences of electrical stimulation. Considerable attention is given to the effects of neuron size on excitability of the tissue because this topic is frequently of clinical importance. The excitability of neurons, under ideal conditions, is demonstrated to be dependent upon the diameter of the axon or cell body. For synaptic (intracellular) excitation, the order of excitation is from small to large neurons, whereas for extracellular stimulation, the excitation order is from large to small neurons. These size-dependent factors, however, are demonstrated under ideal, experimentally controlled conditions. In the clinic these exacting conditions are not met. An attempt is made to describe some of the limitations in applying the size-dependent excitation effects to clinical practice. The major point of this discussion is that, in a clinical setting, one can obtain a gross selective activation of large-diameter fibers versus small-diameter fibers but probably only for the extremes in fiber size. Uncertainties in determining the structures being stimulated (axon terminals versus peripheral nerve trunks), the nonuniform current density about the tissue, and a lack of experimental evidence of the effectiveness of clinically used waveforms of stimulation represent problems in predicting the effectiveness of clinical electrical stimulation. These uncertainties indicate the need for enhanced research effort in this important area of therapeutic intervention.

REFERENCES

1. Jewett, DL and Raymer, MD: Basic Concepts of Neuronal Function. Little, Brown & Co, Boston/Toronto, 1984.
2. Jack, JJB, Noble, D, and Tsien, RW: Electric Current Flow in Excitable Cells. Clarendon Press, Oxford, 1983.
3. Clamann, HP: Original idea for the hydrolic analogy of the capacitor. Personal communication.
4. Singer, SJ and Nicolson, GL: The fluid mosaic model of the structure of cell membranes. Science 175:720, 1972.
5. Kuffler, SW and Nicholls JG: From Neuron to Brain. Sinauer Assoc, Inc, Sunderland, MA, 1976.
6. Henneman, E: Organization of the spinal cord and its reflexes. In Mountcastle, VB (ed): Medical Physiology, ed 14. CV Mosby, St Louis, 1980, p 762.
7. Lloyd, DPC: Neuron patterns controlling transmission of ipsilateral hind limb reflexes in cat. J Neurophysiol 6:293, 1943.

8. Gasser, HS and Erlanger, J: The role played by the sizes of the constituent fibers of a nerve trunk in determining the form of its action potential wave. Am J Physiol 80:522, 1927.
9. Mannheimer, JS and Lampe, GN: Clinical Transcutaneous Electrical Nerve Stimulation. FA Davis, Philadelphia, 1984, p 210.
10. Benton, LA, Baker, LL, Bouman, BR, and Waters, RL: Functional Electrical Stimulation: A Practical Clinical Guide. Rancho Los Amigos Hospital, Downey, CA, 1981, p 73.
11. Mortimer, JT: Motor prostheses. In Brooks, VB (ed): Handbook of Physiology, Section 1, The Nervous System, Vol II, Motor Control, Part 1. Williams & Wilkins, Baltimore, 1981, p 155.
12. Alon, G: Principles of electrical stimulation. In Nelson, RM and Currier, DP (eds): Clinical Electrotherapy. Appleton & Lange, Norwalk, CT, 1987, p 29.
13. Geddes, LA: A short history of the electrical stimulation of excitable tissue including electrotherapeutic applications. Physiologist 27 (Suppl):1, 1984.
14. Erlanger, J and Gasser, HS: Electrical Signs of Nervous Activity. University of Pennsylvania Press, Philadelphia, 1968, p 40.
15. Li, CL and Bak, A: Excitability characteristics of the A and C fibers in a peripheral nerve. Exp Neurol 50:67, 1976.
16. Liddell, EGT and Sherrington, CS: Recruitment and some other factors of reflex inhibition. Proc R Soc London [Biol] 97:488, 1925.
17. Burke, RE: Motor units: anatomy, physiology, and functional organization. Handbook of Physiology, Section 1, The Nervous System, Vol II, Motor Control, Part 1. In: Brookes, VB (ed) Williams & Wilkins, Baltimore, 1981, p 345.
18. Monster, AW, Chan, HC, and O'Connor, D: Activity patterns of human skeletal muscles: Relation to muscle fiber type composition. Science 200:314, 1978.

SUGGESTED READINGS

Geddes, LA: A short history of the electrical stimulation of excitable tissue including electrotherapeutic applications. Physiologist 27(Suppl):1, 1984.

An excellent monograph reviewing the history of electrical stimulation for all levels of readers. A superb job of relating cellular concepts of neuron properties, such as membrane time constants to electrodiagnostic measures, e.g., strength-duration curves.

Jack, JJB, Noble, D, and Tsien, RW: Electric Current Flow in Excitable Cells. Clarendon Press, Oxford, 1983.

Advanced, quantitative treatment of the cellular processes of excitable cells.

Jewett, DL and Raymer, MD: Basic Concepts of Neuronal Function. Little, Brown & Co., Boston/Toronto, 1984.

An excellent self-study text of neurophysiological and biophysical concepts. It is designed to be used by students with a variety of scientific backgrounds. Entry-level as well as graduate students will enhance their levels of understanding of the subject.

Katz, B: Nerve, Muscle, and Synapse. McGraw-Hill, New York, 1966.

This brief textbook (169 pages) has withstood the test of time and continues to be a superb introduction to the subject of electrical excitability in nerve and muscle; it contains the basic essentials.

CHAPTER 2

Principles of Nociception

James L. Hanegan, Ph.D.

Pain has been viewed by physiologists as a distinct sensation from temperature and other cutaneous senses.[1,2] Pain can also be defined as a response related to actual or impending tissue damage from the initial stimulus. Physical pain is often accompanied by emotional overtones, somatic and autonomic effects, and avoidance or escape behaviors. Reaction to pain differs widely among individuals and is influenced by the age, sex, and personality of the individual, and the etiology and duration of the pain.

Stimuli that can cause pain are mechanical (pressure), electrical (shock), thermal (radiant heat), and chemical (e.g., bradykinin). Responses to the painful stimuli are commonly measured by physiologic, verbal, or behavioral responses. We can define pain in terms of stimulus parameters and sensory or motor responses, but pain goes beyond mere sensibility because of its psychologic and cultural components.

Sternbach[3] emphasized that pain is an abstract term referring to many different phenomena. He categorized these phenomena into neurologic, physiologic, behavioral, subjective, and psychiatric experiences. Each category represents a different level of experience and uses different methods of observation, description, and measurement.

Modern theories of pain tend to be multidisciplinary in their approach and fall into three general categories: (1) the anatomic and physiologic bases of pain, which focus on the location and interpretation of intensity of noxious stimuli as well as the neuroanatomic circuitry involved; (2) the motivational and behavioral bases, which include the emotional responses as well as the goals and expectations of the individual; and (3) the psychiatric component, which looks at the past experience of the individual, the present sensation of pain, and its future implications. The early concept of pain perception was based on the stimulus-response model and provides historical perspective to our understanding of pain today. However, with the merging of physiology and psychology we understand that pain is not simply another of the several senses. Rather, it constitutes a response to an extraordinary variety of stimulus conditions. The pain response is susceptible to modification by neural mechanisms which modify the emotional reaction to pain sensation. We are just beginning to understand these modulatory capabilities of the central nervous system.[4]

The purpose of this chapter is to facilitate an understanding of the anatomy and

26

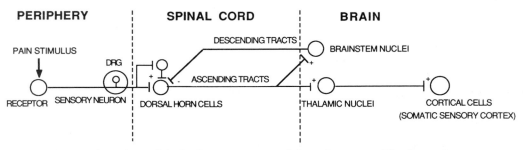

FIGURE 2–1. Overview of the basic components of the pain system. The first order or sensory neurons are found in the peripheral nervous system and their cell bodies are located in the dorsal root ganglia (DRG). The second order neurons that form the ascending pain paths are found in the spinal cord and project to the thalamus and other brain-stem nuclei. The third order neurons project from the thalamus to the sensory and association areas of the cerebral cortex.

physiology of the pain system as it relates to electrotherapy. Figure 2–1 provides an overview of the anatomy of the pain system and shows the basic components of this system. Noxious stimuli excite receptors in the skin and deep tissues. The receptors may be specialized or simply free nerve endings of afferent (sensory) neurons. The afferent neurons carry the pain message to the spinal cord and terminate on interneurons within the dorsal horn. These dorsal horn neurons make local connections within the spinal cord, receive input from higher centers through descending tracts, and form the ascending sensory tracts that project to the brain. The ascending tracts project to many different nuclei within the brain stem where further processing of the sensory information takes place. A major nucleus is the thalamus, which relays the pain message to the cerebral cortex where conscious localization of pain occurs. The following sections will discuss in detail the anatomic and physiologic properties of each of these components of the pain system.

We will begin by reviewing the clinical aspects of pain and the different forms of pain expression that may be treated by electrotherapy. Most individuals are familiar with the different sensations of pain but this brief review will provide a common framework for understanding the underlying physiologic and neuroanatomic principles of the pain system.

CLINICAL DEFINITIONS OF PAIN

Pain is not fully understood at the neurophysiologic level, and our understanding of pain at the clinical level is incomplete. It is recognized, however, that several distinct clinical pain states exist. These are classified as acute, chronic, referred, and psychogenic pain. These are not totally separate classes because one type may merge with another or evolve into another over a period of time.

Acute Pain

It seems obvious that pain enables an organism to sense tissue damage and avoid further harm, thus facilitating survival. The damage to tissue by mechanical, chemical, or thermal agents directly activates neurons signaling the presence of noxious stimuli.

This initial phasic stage of pain takes on a tonic persistence until healing can occur. The tonic phase of pain may occur following abrupt injury and may serve to enforce rest or quiet behavior, promoting healing and recovery.[5] Damage to tissue results in muscle guarding in which the patient protects the damaged area from excessive movement, promoting healing. The development of muscle spasm associated with tonic pain imposes involuntary rest of an area and can lead to dysfunction, rather than healing. Acute pain can be thought of as both a sensation of actual or impending tissue damage and as an indication for rest.[6]

Mechanical injury is not simply an initial stimulus to be recorded by nociceptive units and transmitted to the central nervous system. The injury directly alters the activity of the neurons in the pain pathways from the peripheral receptors to their central connections and can induce changes in their predicted function. Some neurons become more excitable and others become less sensitive.[7,8] In damaged tissue, reflexes are activated which alter blood flow, cause changes in the permeability of capillaries, and effect changes in tissue chemistry. These effects, which lead to healing, may be initiated by neurons called C fibers, which are thought to release substance P or other local tissue hormones at the site of tissue damage.[9]

When axons are cut or smashed in an injury, small sprouts begin to grow out of the neuron at the site of damage. The properties of these sprouts differ from normal neurons by, (1) becoming spontaneously active, producing paresthesia; (2) becoming mechanically sensitive, which adds to the tenderness of the damaged region; and (3) becoming sensitive to norepinephrine by the development of alpha receptors on the neural membranes.[10] This last effect may explain the development of sympathetic nervous system hypersensitivity or reflex sympathetic dystrophy following nerve injury.

Changes initiated by injury also occur in the dorsal root ganglia, the site where the cell bodies of the sensory nerves are located, and in the dorsal horn cells of the spinal cord. The dorsal horn cells receive input from the sensory neurons and project in sensory tracts to other regions of the central nervous system. The sensory neurons in the dorsal root ganglia may become more sensitive to mechanical stimuli, increasing their activity by propagating more action potentials to the dorsal horn cells, or become more sensitive to local tissue chemicals at the injury site.[11,12] Output from dorsal horn cells is modified by afferent input from nociceptors and larger neurons projecting from mechanoreceptors. In addition, the activity of these dorsal horn cells can be modified by descending pathways from higher centers in the brain. Direct electrical stimulation of the periaqueductal gray matter (PAG) and the reticular formation in animals produces analgesia characterized by behavioral changes, and inhibition of the dorsal horn cells. The inhibition may result from the activity of endogenous opiates or through inhibiting neurotransmitters such as 5-hydroxytryptamine (5-HT, also called serotonin) or gamma-aminobutyric acid (GABA).[13] The pain message seems to be transmitted to the dorsal horn cells in the spinal cord, but the message is blocked at this level and is not transmitted in the spinal cord to the higher conscious centers in the brain.

Therefore, the system that responds and signals to the central nervous system the onset of acute pain, undergoes changes in function because of the presence of noxious stimuli or damage to tissue. Normally, activation of the pain receptors and their sensory neurons triggers appropriate local reflexes to the pain stimulus and signals the higher conscious centers of the location and intensity of the stimulus. However, depending upon conditions within the nervous system, the pain message may be blocked from reaching consciousness, or the individual may become more sensitive to the injury and the pain sensation may remain long after noxious stimuli have been removed.

Chronic Pain

This pain sensation persists beyond the period of time required for healing and can become very destructive because of the negative psychological, physiologic, and social consequences to the individual. In this condition, the pain does not serve a positive role in triggering escape or withdrawal behaviors to prevent further harm, nor does it serve to promote recovery. Chronic pain can develop out of acute pain or appear insidiously.

Cannon[14] demonstrated that pain was one of the sensations capable of provoking the "fight or flight" response, under which the sympathetic division of the autonomic nervous system is activated. The vagal nerve, which is the major pathway for the parasympathetic division of the autonomic nervous system, is also inhibited in this response. The sympathetic response prepares the organism metabolically and physiologically for immediate action. In acute pain the sympathetic nervous system activity and adrenal gland secretions are roughly proportional to the intensity of the noxious stimuli. In chronic pain, which may last for months or more, there is a change in the pattern of the sympathetic and adrenal mechanisms.[6] There appears to be habituation of the sympathetic responses to moderate chronic pain with the appearance of vegetative signs. Individuals show delayed sleep onset and frequent awakening. Individuals may isolate themselves to avoid interpersonal conflict. Pain tolerance is lowered, thus with additional noxious stimuli the individual may appear to overreact in a given situation. Eating patterns change with either a diminished or heightened appetite, and a general decrease in motor activity is observed. The individual adopts the role of the sick and behaviors of a chronic invalid, which are extremely difficult to extinguish or modify.[6]

There may be a central mechanism that enhances the vegetative behavior associated with chronic pain. Depletion of serotonin (5-HT) in the central nervous system is associated with changes in sleep patterns, depression, and lowered pain tolerance. Since serotonin is involved as a neurotransmitter in the inhibitory pathways of pain modulating systems, a reduction of this transmitter at the central level would enhance the responses to painful stimuli.[15] The use of serotonergic antidepressants, those substances that mimic or enhance the effects of serotonin, can reverse the vegetative signs and may possess analgesic properties which elevate the pain threshold.[16]

Somatic and Visceral Pain

A distinction must be made between pain arising from the body surface and that from the viscera. Pain arising from the body wall may be either superficial or deep. Superficial pain arises from the skin and is localized. The pain may be mediated through the faster conducting A-delta afferent neurons or the slower C fibers. Both afferents respond to stimuli which are potentially damaging to tissue. If tissue damage or inflammation already exists, then the pain threshold is generally lowered in the afferent fibers.

Deep pain arises from the muscles, joints, fascia, tendons, and periosteum. It tends to be more diffuse but can be localized. It may last for longer periods of time and is often accompanied by muscle spasms, which are themselves a source of pain. Deep pain is thought to be mediated through C fibers, although there is probably overlap between deep and superficial receptor systems.

Visceral pain arises from organs in the abdominal and thoracic cavities either from the visceral or the parietal membranes. Pain originating in the viscera is often poorly localized and is characterized as an aching or gripping sensation associated with sympathetic effects, such as the pain associated with angina pectoris. Visceral pain is not generally associated with skeletal muscle spasms or superficial tenderness. A-delta fibers innervate the peritoneum, pleura, and pericardium. In these organs parietal pain is sharp and fairly well localized. It is also accompanied by superficial tenderness and reflex rigidity, as seen in the abdominal rigidity of acute appendicitis.

Referred Pain

The pain initiated in deep body structures may be localized at sites some distance from the actual location of pathologic origin. The pain is said to be referred to a distant anatomic site. The mechanisms which account for this referral of pain are based on the anatomic arrangement of dermatomes, scleratomes, and myotomes, and the convergence of cutaneous and visceral afferents with the spinal cord (Table 2–1). An area of skin whose sensory receptors feed predominantly into a given dorsal root is called a dermatome. Visceral pain such as that which occurs during appendicitis, inflammation of the gall bladder, or obstructive stones in the urinary tract is referred to specific cutaneous areas because certain viscera and dermatomes share a common spinal cord segment. The brain may interpret pain that is visceral in origin as cutaneous pain. For example, kidney pain may be referred to dermatomes T_{10} and T_{11}. Pain in the pleura over the diaphragm (innervated by phrenic nerve C_3–C_5) may be referred to the neck and shoulder, where C_3–C_5 dermatomes are found. The afferent input to the spinal cord from visceral receptors synapses on the spinothalamic neurons in the dorsal horn that also receive afferent input from the skin. This convergence produces sensations that are interpreted as arising from the skin and not the viscera. Knowledge of these patterns

TABLE 2–1 Segmental Input of General Visceral Afferents to the Spinal Cord

Visceral Organ	Spinal Segment
Head and neck	T1–5
Upper limb	T10–L2
Heart	T1–5
Bronchi, lung	T2–4
Esophagus	T5–6
Stomach	T6–10
Small intestine	T9–10
Large intestine to splenic flexure	T11–L1
Splenic flexure to rectum	L1–2
Liver and gall bladder	T7–9
Pancreas	T6–10
Ureter	T11–L2
Suprarenal	T8–L1
Testis and ovary	T10–11
Epidymis, vas deferens, seminal vesicles	T11–12
Urinary bladder	T11–L2
Prostate and urethra	T11–L1
Uterus	T12–L1
Fallopian tube	T10–L1
Spleen	T6–10

Adapted from Williams, et al.: Gray's Anatomy. Churchill Livingstone, New York, 1989.

of convergence of visceral and cutaneous pathways is obviously important in making a correct diagnosis of the anatomic source of pain and may influence treatment approaches. In addition it may also serve to explain how electrostimulation placed at seemingly remote sites may inhibit visceral pain.

Emotional or Psychogenic Pain

Evidence for emotionally induced pain does not extend beyond clinicians' reports.[17] Merskey[18] described two forms of psychogenic pain derived from psychological factors; pain which occurs during hallucinations and pain associated with conversion hysteria. Chronically anxious and depressed people appear to be vulnerable to pain. Fear, anxiety, and depression are capable of amplifying pain and environmental stress can give rise to or amplify pain.[19,20] Emotional stress may be associated with increased pain by activating biological systems that are also responsive to noxious stimuli. Anxiety, depression, anger, and aggressive behavior may provoke substantial autonomic, visceral, and skeletal activity, which can enhance pain sensations. The neuroendocrine and autonomic nervous system changes induced by psychological stress have been associated with diseases of the cardiovascular, digestive, and respiratory systems.[21] These somatic changes induced by stress may lead to acute and chronic pain conditions. Patients often focus on the somatic evidence of pain and are reluctant to discuss underlying psychological stress, making accurate diagnosis of the cause of pain and successful treatment extremely difficult.

We may now turn to the anatomic and physiologic aspects of the pain system. We will begin with a discussion of the development of the major pain theories which provide the foundation for our present knowledge of the pain system.

PAIN THEORIES

Many different mechanisms of pain perception and transmission have been proposed and subjected to experimental analysis. Experimentation has validated some of these mechanisms and refuted others. Since pain has both physical and psychological components, it is extremely difficult to study under strictly controlled conditions. Three major theories of pain have emerged; each has elements that withstand scientific testing. These theories have provided insight into the pain process and have stimulated critical analysis of the mechanisms involved.

Specificity Theory

The specificity theory proposes the existence of a specific system of pain receptors and pathways within the peripheral nervous system. This theory evolved in part from the doctrine of specific nerve energies proposed by Muller,[22] which states that different sets of nerve fibers, when stimulated, elicit different sensations by virtue of their central connections. In this scheme, a given set of nerve fibers always elicits an identical sensation no matter how it is excited. Muller proposed that specific receptors have a low threshold for a particular stimulus (adequate stimulus) but could respond to other forms of stimuli if these were of higher intensity. Von Frey[23] expanded Muller's concept to

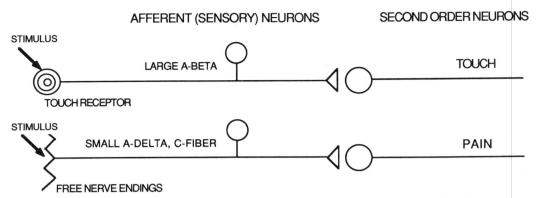

FIGURE 2–2. The specificity theory. Receptors have different adequate stimuli and the sensations perceived are determined by the central connections.

include four distinct types of sensation at the skin: warmth, cold, touch, and pain. Von Frey used histological evidence to identify the specialized peripheral receptors for the different sensations. He identified free nerve endings as pain receptors based on their widespread distribution in the skin. Pain is perceived when noxious or harmful stimuli activate the free nerve endings in the skin (Fig. 2–2). The nerve impulses are conducted through specific pathways to pain centers in the brain. The difficulty with this theory is that it does not account for the finding that many different forms of stimuli can be perceived as painful. Extreme heat, cold, pressure, and a variety of chemicals can all be painful stimuli. Therefore, Von Frey's evidence of four basic receptors is inadequate to account for the variety of painful stimuli. This difficulty led to a different interpretation of pain perception — that of pattern theory.

Pattern Theory

This early theory, first formalized by Goldscheider in 1894[24] (also referred to as the intensity theory), is based on empirical observation. The absence of specific pain receptors, pathways, or groups of neurons dedicated to the transmission of painful stimuli is its basic assumption. Rather, the theory attributes the sensation of pain to the pattern or frequency and intensity of stimulation applied that excite touch, pressure, or temperature receptors in the skin. If the stimulus is of sufficient intensity and frequency, regardless of the energy form, the sensation is perceived as painful (Fig. 2–3). Summation of neural impulses that result from excessive stimulation is relayed to cerebral structures concerned with localization and interpretation of intensity. The temporal and spatial summation of impulses is thought to be the basic mechanism underlying this theory and may occur at different points along the pathways from the skin to the cerebral levels.

Gate Control Theory

The gate control theory of pain perception, first proposed by Melzack and Wall[25] in 1965, has undergone refinement to account for recent experimental findings. This theory incorporates the concepts of specificity and patterning of impulses and empha-

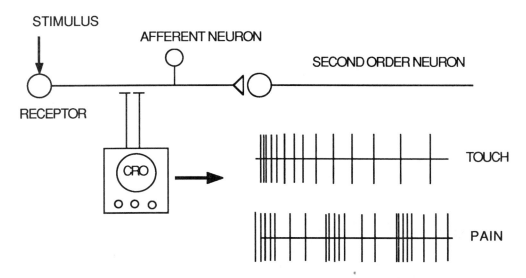

STIMULUS

AFFERENT NEURON

SECOND ORDER NEURON

RECEPTOR

CRO

o o o

TOUCH

PAIN

RECORDED PATTERN OF ACTION POTENTIALS

FIGURE 2–3. The pattern theory: the response of the neuron is shown by recording action potentials with a cathode ray oscilloscope (CRO). With light touch the response is a uniform train of action potentials. With noxious stimulation the neuron responds with bursts of impulses that are perceived as painful. (Adapted from Newton, RA: Contemporary views on pain and the role played by thermal agents in managing pain symptoms. In Michlovitz, SL (ed): Thermal Agents in Rehabilitation. FA Davis, Philadelphia, 1986.)

sizes the importance of centrally located cells concerned with transmission and modification of pain messages. Information concerned with pain impulses transmitted from the first centrally located cells in the spinal cord depends upon three factors: (1) the arrival of nociceptive messages or impulses at the level of the spinal cord, (2) the convergent effect of other peripheral afferent impulses, which may enhance or diminish the pain message, and (3) the presence of control mechanisms within the central nervous system which can influence the activity of the first central cells (dorsal horn cells) of the spinal cord. The gate control system is a rapidly activated mechanism which influences afferent input to the central cells. These cells in turn activate effector systems and eventually evoke sensations through ascending pathways to higher brain centers. The gate control system consists of four distinct components: (1) afferent neurons, (2) neural interactions within the dorsal horn of the spinal cord, (3) transmission cells or T cells, and (4) descending controls from higher brain centers.

The gate itself consists of small inhibitory internuncial cells in the *substantia gelatinosa* (SG) of the dorsal horn and the T cells which relay information to higher centers. The level of activity of the T cells is determined by the balance of input from large-diameter A-beta and A-alpha and small-diameter A-delta and C-afferent neurons (Fig. 2–4). The activity of the T cells can also be influenced by descending neurons from higher control centers. Input from small-diameter afferents will activate the T cell and be perceived as pain arising from the receptive fields of these small afferents. The activity of the small afferents inhibits the internuncial cells by reducing presynaptic inhibition at the T-cell junction. When the larger afferents are concurrently activated, they will also directly activate the T cell. However, these afferents also stimulate the small SG cells, which decrease the input to the T cell from both large and small afferent fibers by

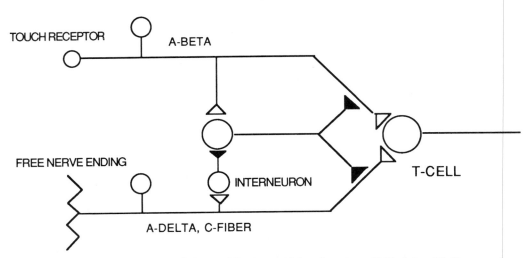

FIGURE 2–4. The gate control theory. The large (A-beta) and small (A-delta, C) fibers project to the substantia gelatinosa (SG) and to the first central transmission cells (T-cell). The small fiber input to the SG is inhibitory through a small interneuron. The solid black triangles represent inhibitory synapses and the open triangles represent excitatory synapses. An ascending pathway to higher centers is shown. (Adapted from Melzack, R and Wall, PD.[25])

presynaptic inhibition. Therefore, input from the large-diameter afferents, in effect, closes the *gate* and blocks transmission of impulses from the small afferent pain fibers.

The gate control mechanisms occurring in the dorsal horn are not quite as simple as those described by Melzack and Wall[25] because descending pathways from higher centers can influence the activity of the gate mechanism, resulting in either increased or decreased transmission of pain messages. These effects of central pain-modulating systems will be discussed in a later section.

PAIN RECEPTORS

Skin

Perl[10] discussed the basic problem of establishing the existence of pain receptors (nociceptors) first hypothesized by Sherrington.[26] Several small-diameter sensory neurons have been described that require strong stimulation for activation, but others can also be activated by gentle tactile stimuli. Because the threshold of many different cutaneous receptors may be exceeded by noxious stimuli, true nociceptive units must be uniquely activated by noxious stimuli. Different tissues and individuals may have different thresholds to noxious stimuli, and therefore, comparisons of the results of pain-receptor studies are difficult.

It is now widely recognized that specialized receptors in the skin signal actual or potential tissue damage. These receptors are the free nerve endings which are morphologically the least differentiated of the cutaneous receptors. Free nerve endings are able to respond to mechanical, thermal, and chemical stimuli. Pain is signaled by two types of peripheral afferent neurons, small, myelinated A-delta neurons and smaller, unmyelinated C neurons.[27] Lynn[28] described three well-defined types of nociceptors in terms of their response to different stimulus modalities: (1) high-threshold mechanoreceptors (HTM) which respond to strong mechanical stimulation but do not respond in normal skin to heat, irritant chemicals, or extreme cold; (2) polymodal nociceptors (PMN) which respond to strong mechanical stimuli and also to noxious heat and irritant chemicals; and (3) cold nociceptors which respond consistently to severe cold but usually not to other noxious stimuli.

The HTM receptors are different from other specialized mechanoreceptors of the skin. True mechanoreceptors do not signal information about noxious or painful stimuli.[29] Torebjork and Ochoa[30] used small electrodes to selectively stimulate afferent neurons or receptors in human subjects. They demonstrated that stimulation of nociceptive afferent neurons is perceived as pain, whereas high-frequency stimulation of specialized mechanoreceptors is not painful.

The HTM units are distributed as discrete points spread over the skin and respond to strong pressure. The receptive fields of the HTM units are small and circular in shape, usually less than 2 mm in diameter. The fields are separated from each other by skin which cannot be excited by equivalent noxious stimuli, and there are up to 50 distinct fields per afferent neuron.[10] The conduction velocity of the propagated action potential in the HTM unit varies from 2.5 to 52.5 m/sec.[31] These units are served by small, myelinated A-delta fibers. The responses to pressure adapt slowly, with little or no dynamic response during the onset of the stimulus. The sensitivity of the HTM units increases following mild injury. The increase in sensitivity results in an abnormal background activity of variable frequency in the receptor.

PMNs are characterized by slow adaptation to firm pressure. They show a short latency response to noxious heating (44° to 50°C) and are also excited by potassium chloride, histamine, and substance P. The conduction velocities for these PMN units range from 0.4 to 1.0 m/sec, characteristic of C fibers. In PMN units the threshold for activation decreases with repeated heat stimulation.[32] The increase in sensitivity of these slower conducting C-fiber units may be responsible for hyperalgesia in injured skin. A summary of fiber types, conduction velocities, and adequate stimuli for the different receptors is provided in Table 2–2.

TABLE 2–2 Afferent Fiber Types in Peripheral Nerves

Type	Group	Diameter (μm)	Conduction Velocity (m/sec)	Tissue	Receptor Type
A	I	12–20	72–120	Muscle	Muscle spindle, primary endings
				Muscle	Golgi tendon organ
A	II	6–12	36–72	Muscle	Muscle spindle, secondary endings
A	III	1–6	6–36	Skin	Touch receptors
				Muscle	Pressure, pain
				Skin	Touch, pressure, pain
C	IV	0.4–1.2	0.5–2.0	Muscle	Pain
				Skin	Touch, temperature, pain

Adapted from Willis, WD, Jr and Grossman, RC: Medical Neurobiology. CV Mosby, St Louis, 1973.

Muscle

Skeletal muscle is also innervated by nociceptive units. Group IV muscle receptors respond to irritant chemicals, strong local pressure, and heating.[33] The C-fiber units belonging to these receptors appear to end as simple free endings associated with connective tissue or blood vessels.[34] In addition to group IV afferents, there are group III afferents (A-delta) with both polymodal and mechanical nociceptive properties. Therefore, in addition to nociceptors found in the skin, deep muscle tissue is also innervated by pain-sensitive units, possibly accounting for the pain of muscle spasm or the soreness associated with excessive use.

Joints

There are numerous encapsulated receptive units in and around joints for detection of the mechanical properties of joint movement. There are also A-delta fibers which respond to noxious stimuli.[35] These subcutaneous receptors in muscles and joints have receptive fields which appear to be similar to those of cutaneous receptors; that is, they are spotlike and distributed in the subcutaneous tissue. Although these receptors have been shown to be distinct from cutaneous nociceptors, there is some overlap of the receptive fields from the skin and deeper tissue.[36] There does not appear to be a distinct anatomic division between superficial and deep receptors.

In summary, the peripheral mechanisms of pain perception are complicated. A-delta and C fibers both conduct impulses arising from noxious and non-noxious stimuli. High-threshold receptors respond to well-defined noxious stimuli. Low-threshold receptors appear to respond to both noxious and non-noxious stimuli. Irritant substances can also cause pain but it is not clear at this time if chemicals, such as histamine, substance P, adenosine triphosphate (ATP), serotonin, bradykinin, and the prostaglandins, play a primary role in activating nociceptors or an intermediary role as sensitization agents following initial noxious stimulation.[37,38]

Cutaneous nociceptors with receptive fields in undamaged skin have essentially no background activity. This changes dramatically after application of skin-damaging stimuli. The increase in frequency and duration of the background activity is partially related to the amount of skin damage. The C-fiber polymodal nociceptors appear to play a more prominent role in the increased background activity due to damage than do the myelinated A-delta fibers. The A-delta fibers are probably responsible for the initial acute sense of pain. They respond to specific modalities, with optimal responses to intense mechanical stimuli. The second or persistent pain in the absence of continued noxious stimulation is thought to be signaled by the increased background activity of the C fibers. These units tend to be polymodal and summate slowly over time.

The mechanisms for differentiating painful from nonpainful stimuli reside in more central locations of the nervous system than the afferent input to the dorsal horn of the spinal cord.

AFFERENT INPUT AND DORSAL HORN CELLS OF THE SPINAL CORD

The cell bodies of the primary sensory neurons lie in the dorsal root ganglia. At the spinal cord level, afferent neurons have axons which reach the spinal cord through segmentally organized dorsal roots. The small A-delta and unmyelinated C fibers group together in the lateral portion of the dorsal root. These axons bifurcate and travel several segments, ascending and descending, within Lissauer's tract before entering the spinal gray matter.[39,40] In addition, up to 20 percent of the unmyelinated afferent neurons carrying pain messages enter the spinal cord through the ventral root.[41,42] This may account for the fact that some patients who have had dorsal rhizotomies to relieve pain do not experience relief.[43]

A-delta and C fibers terminate in the outermost lamina, or marginal zone, which correspond to Rexed lamina 1 (Fig. 2–5). They also terminate in the *substantia gelatinosa* (Rexed lamina 2). Some A-delta neurons terminate on interneurons in the deeper layers of Rexed lamina 5. The termination of the A-delta neurons and C fibers within these laminae do not limit their activities to these zones. Interneurons within lamina 5 have

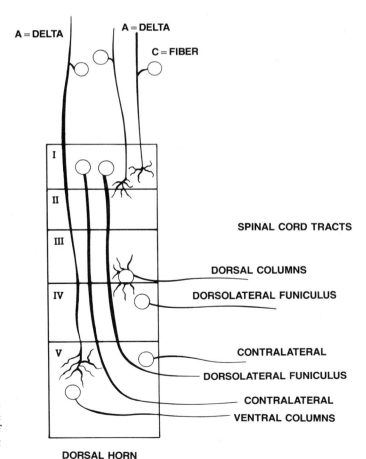

FIGURE 2–5. Termination of the afferent input to the dorsal horn and the sites of origin of the ascending tract neurons.

dendrites which extend to the outermost layer of the dorsal horn (lamina 1) and could therefore be excited by afferent neurons which terminate in lamina 1.[10]

The cells in the dorsal horn do not passively transmit the pain messages received from the primary sensory neurons to higher centers. Dorsal horn cells process the information received and integrate the local autonomic and somatomotor reflexes initiated by painful stimuli. In addition these cells are instrumental in the inhibitory and facilitating mechanisms of pain modulation from higher control centers.

Within the dorsal horn are interneurons which respond to three general types of peripheral stimulation: (1) low-threshold mechanosensitive (LTM) which respond only to low-threshold innocuous stimuli such as touching or brushing the skin; (2) nociceptive specific (NS) which are only excited by high-threshold noxious stimuli; and (3) wide dynamic range (WDR), whose firing rate is increased by innocuous stimuli but further augmented in response to noxious stimuli (Table 2–3).

The receptive field of WDR cells in the skin typically consists of a central area in which both low threshold and noxious stimuli excite the cell, whereas low threshold stimuli in the surrounding area are inhibitory and noxious stimuli are excitatory. The ability of low threshold stimuli in the periphery of the receptive field to inhibit the firing of cells excited by noxious stimuli, is the keystone of the gate control theory of Melzack and Wall[25] discussed previously. In man, low intensity electrical stimulation of low threshold afferents in peripheral nerves or in the dorsal columns can increase the pain threshold and may be effective in the treatment of pain. This inhibition may be mediated through lamina 1 interneurons or through changes in the excitability of C fibers.

Large interneurons found in lamina 4 are generally of the LTM type and receive input from A-delta fibers.[44] Lamina 5 interneurons receive input from many different

TABLE 2–3 Characteristics of Dorsal Horn Interneurons

Type of Interneuron	Required Stimulus	Location in Dorsal Horn	Receptive Field of Interneuron
Nonclassified interneurons		Forms connections between laminae 1 and 5 and between other laminae	No specific field
Low-threshold mechanical cells	Low-threshold stimuli	Laminae 3 and 5	Large fields, input from noxious and low-threshold stimuli converge on these cells
Nociceptive cells	High-threshold noxious stimuli	Laminae 1 and 5	Small distinct field for noxious stimuli
Wide dynamic range (WDR) cells	Variety of stimuli, frequency of action potentials varies with stimulus intensity	Laminae 1, 2, and 5	Central area of receptive field responds to low threshold and pain. Surrounding area, pain stimuli and low-threshold stimuli inhibit the interneuron

TABLE 2-4 Afferent Input to Dorsal Horn Cells

Receptor	Sensory Neuron	Lamina	Dorsal Horn Cells
LTM*	A-beta	V	Wide dynamic range
HTM†	A-delta	V	Wide dynamic range
Heat	A-delta	V	Wide dynamic range
Polymodal	C	V	Wide dynamic range
HTM	A-delta	I, V	Nociceptive specific
Heat	A-delta	I, V	Nociceptive specific
Polymodal	C	I, V	Nociceptive specific

*LTM, low-threshold mechanical.
†HTM, high-threshold mechanical.
Adapted from Synder-Mackler, L and Robinson, AJ: Clinical Electrophysiology. Williams & Wilkins, Baltimore, 1989.

receptors but WDR cells are the most numerous with fewer NS cells present. The WDR cells have large peripheral receptive fields and respond to noxious and non-noxious stimuli from visceral and somatic sources.[45-53] The response to noxious stimuli is not a simple rate-dependent response. Low intensity stimulation does not cause low-firing rates, and noxious stimuli, high-firing rates. Different ascending pathways to the brain originating from the WDR cells in the dorsal horn may be utilized to differentiate noxious from innocuous stimuli.[54]

The convergence of visceral and cutaneous noxious stimuli on WDR cells may be the basis of referred pain (Table 2-4). Noxious stimuli arising from the viscera and projecting to WDR cells in the dorsal horn may be interpreted at higher levels as arising from cutaneous sources which also project to these same WDR cells. The sensory processing systems in the cerebral cortex may be habituated to receiving sensory information from cutaneous receptors and cannot discriminate between the normal route of stimulation through the skin and visceral input. Thus, when the viscera are the site of origin of noxious stimuli, the stimuli are perceived as arising from the skin.

The convergence of sensory input on WDR or NS cells in the dorsal horn may also provide a mechanism in which stimulation of one part of the body influences or modulates the effects of stimuli from other remote areas of the body. For example acupuncture-point stimulation at apparently remote sites can be effective in relieving certain types of pain. This may not be the only mechanism operating; endogenous opiates may also play a significant role and are discussed in the section on pain modulation in this chapter.

SPINAL CORD PATHWAYS TO HIGHER CENTERS

The contralateral spinothalamic tract is the major nociceptive ascending pathway from the dorsal horn. The cells of origin of this pathway are highly concentrated in laminae 1 and 5 of the dorsal horn. These cells are presumed to be of the NS and WDR type. A second major projection system is the dorsal column postsynaptic spinomedullary system. This pathway is an ipsilateral system traveling the dorsal columns to the dorsal column nuclei.[55,56] Neurons of this pathway originate in laminae 2 and 4 which generally correspond to LTM and WDR cells.[57,58]

TABLE 2–5 Ascending Pain Pathways of the Spinal Cord

Ascending Tract	Laminae of Origin	Proposed Cells	Termination
Contralateral spinothalamic and trigeminothalamic tracts	1, 5	Nociceptive specific, wide dynamic range	Ventroposterior lateral nucleus of the thalamus
Ipsilateral dorsal column (spinomedullary system)	2, 4	Low-threshold mechanical	Dorsal column nuclei

The spinothalamic tract (STT) is essential for the transmission of both noxious and thermal input to higher centers.[59,60] The neurons in the STT are myelinated, and the pathway is multimodal, without distinct separation for noxious and innocuous sensations. Contemporary evidence suggests that only one pathway exists rather than a lateral pathway for pain and temperature, and a ventral pathway for light touch.[61] The STT terminates in the thalamic nuclei, principally the ventroposterolateral (VPL) nucleus (Table 2–5).[62-65]

The thalamus acts as a general relay station for sensory information and has precise projections to specific cortical areas. The thalamic neurons are arranged in aggregates which receive input from particular areas in the periphery and project to neurons arranged in columns in the cerebral cortex. Electrical recordings from neurons within the somatosensory cortex have shown that these cells can be excited by noxious stimuli.[66] The overall pathway from the periphery is probably through A-delta sensory neurons which activate spinal cord cells in laminae 1 and 5.[67] These cells project the pain message through the spinothalamic tract to the ventroposterolateral nucleus of the thalamus, and from this relay station to the somatosensory cortex. This pathway is essential to discriminate the site of origin of the pain stimulus on the body's surface.

Two types of cells found in the sensory association area of the cortex of the monkey were described by Kenshalo and Isensee.[68] One type had a high threshold with a small contralateral receptive field. The other type had a very large receptive field and was activated by noxious and innocuous stimuli. It was suggested that the high-threshold cells were driven by the ventrobasal complex of the thalamus and function in the sensory discriminative aspect of pain. These cells with a small sensory field would allow for fine localization of the site of origin of the pain stimulus. The low-threshold wide-range cells would provide information on the intensity of the stimulus. These investigators[68] have demonstrated the existence of cells within the cortex which characterize the pain message in terms of location and relative intensity.

The spinothalamic tract also synapses via collateral branches on neurons in the periaqueductal gray nucleus. This area of the brain stem is important in modulating the response to pain. Spinothalamic neurons which arise in the deeper lamina (7 and 8) of the dorsal horn project through the intralaminar thalamus, which relays input to most of the cortex, particularly the prefrontal areas. Synapses in this pathway are morphine sensitive, and this pathway also appears to mediate the affective components of pain.[67]

In primates, stimulation of VPL cells in the thalamus can inhibit responses of the spinothalamic cells in the lumbar region of the spinal cord.[69] The significance of this inhibitory response may be that the thalamic neurons projecting to other brain-stem nuclei modulate the activity of the spinal neurons that receive the primary sensory input in the dorsal horn.[61] This response provides one of the basic mechanisms for neural modulation of pain by the analgesia systems of the brain and spinal cord. This concept is presented in detail in Chapter 5.

Additional ascending pathways involved in the transmission of noxious stimuli have been described. The spinoreticular tracts are of particular interest because electrical stimulation of the mesencephalon in animals result in analgesia, and many neurons in the reticular formation are activated by noxious stimuli.[70-73] WDR and NS neurons of the dorsal horn are responsible for input to the neurons of the reticular formation. Since WDR and NS neurons are known to receive input from A-delta and C-fiber primary afferents, it is logical to assume that the reticular formation is involved in the assessment of noxious stimuli or serves as a relay to more rostral structures.

CENTRAL NERVOUS SYSTEM COMPONENTS OF PAIN MODULATION

There are several mechanisms involved in the central nervous system modulation of pain. The discovery of endogenous opiates stimulated recent basic research on analgesia systems. The early evidence for intrinsic analgesia systems was demonstrated by electrical stimulation of the PAG which produced suppression of pain.[74-77] Studies have shown that the PAG is rich in endogenous opiates and opiate receptors.[78-83]

Numerous endogenous opiates with physiologic properties have been identified in the central nervous system. Methionine and leucine enkephalins are pentapeptides and were the first opiates that fit the criteria for an endogenous substance that, when released, inhibited pain perception.[84-86] These pentapeptides have a half-life of 2 minutes. They are located in many different brain structures associated with neurons containing substance P or 5-HT and probably play a role in pain modulation by altering afferent input to spinal neurons or altering the excitability of dorsal horn neurons.[86]

B-endorphin is a 31-amino-acid chain with a half-life of 4 hours. B-endorphin is a powerful CNS suppressant, resulting in catatonia, analgesia, and behavioral disturbances.[86] It is concentrated in the pituitary gland and may be released in response to severe stress. In addition to their role in pain modification the endogenous opiates may function as neurotransmitters, neurohormones, and systemic hormones since they are also synthesized in several endocrine glands.[87]

Using cat and rat animal models, Mayer and Watkins[88] describe different classes of endogenous analgesia based on neural and opiate-mediated systems. The criteria they used to classify analgesia as opiate-mediated included naloxone reversibility and cross tolerance to morphine. Unlike the endogenous opiates, morphine is an alkaloid, not a peptide. Morphine and the endogenous opiates bind to specific receptor sites on the surface of neurons and exert their effects by influencing subsequent neural activity. This binding can be blocked by naloxone, which competes for the same receptor sites. Naloxone is therefore antagonistic to morphine and the endogenous opiates and has been used extensively in identifying the anatomic locations and physiologic activity of these centrally active opiates.

The endogenous opiates can inhibit activation of individual neurons. However, in animal experimental situations using intact systems, the opiates appear to exert their effect by activation of central pain-modulating systems rather than by direct inhibition of the pain-transmission neurons of the dorsal horn.[89-93] Electrical stimulation of the PAG produces widespread analgesia.[94] The PAG projects to nuclei in the rostroventral medulla, including the nucleus *raphis magnus* (NRM). The NRM has descending projections to the dorsal horn cells of the spinal cord through the dorsal lateral funiculus. It is hypothesized that cells in the rostroventral medulla activated by endogenous opiates, or through input from the PAG, modulate the activity of the pain-transmission neurons in the dorsal horn of the spinal cord. The modulating effect may be via direct inhibition of the pain-transmission neurons or through activation of small inhibitory neurons. These inhibitory neurons act on either the primary afferent pain neurons or the central pain-transmission neurons through enkephalinergic synapses.[95-98]

Electrical stimulation of the brain has been used to illustrate both opiate and nonopiate classes of analgesia. The final common link in all classes of analgesia is the dorsal lateral funiculus since lesions of this descending pathway attenuate all analgesic manipulations.

THE APPLICATION OF ELECTRICAL STIMULATION FOR PAIN RELIEF

Transcutaneous electrical nerve stimulation (TENS) is a means of utilizing electrical energy to stimulate the nervous system across the surface of the skin and is effective in relieving some types of pain. TENS is capable of activating both large and small nerve fibers conveying a variety of sensory information to the CNS. The gate control theory of Melzack and Wall,[25] based on an understanding of the neurophysiology of the dorsal horn, provides one possible explanation for the effectiveness of TENS. Pathological activation of small A-delta and C fibers will inhibit the small interneurons in the *substantia gelatinosa* and activate transmission cells which transmit impulses to higher centers where the conscious sensation of pain is perceived. According to the gate control theory, TENS applied at comfortable intensities will preferentially activate larger A-alpha and A-beta fibers which have lower electrical thresholds than the smaller pain fibers. Activation of these large-diameter neurons will facilitate the small interneurons of the *substantia gelatinosa*, which block the small fiber input to the transmission cells by presynaptic inhibition. Thus pain is blocked through electrical stimulation by closing the *gate* to small-diameter afferent input.

Melzack and Casey[99] proposed a modification of the basic gate control theory in which the sensory input through the anterolateral spinothalamic projection system to the cortex provides the sensory discriminative aspect of pain. Activation of reticular and limbic structures through dorsal column and dorsolateral tracts gives rise to the motivational drive and the unpleasant sensation that triggers appropriate motor responses. Higher centers in the neocortex monitor the input from these two systems in terms of past experience. The interaction of these systems may comprise a *central control trigger* which activates the descending mechanisms capable of modifying sensory input at the level of the dorsal horn. The output of the dorsal horn T cells is transmitted through the two ascending systems and is dependent on the balance of activity in large- and small-diameter afferents operating through the gate mechanism. According to this model, TENS may operate by preferentially stimulating large afferent fibers, which, in turn, activate the central control trigger. Turning on the trigger mechanism would modulate the sensory input through descending controls operating on the gate mechanism or on the T cells directly.

It is important to remember that the gate control system operating within the dorsal horn is not the only CNS mechanism capable of modulating painful sensations and that TENS may function at several levels of control within the CNS or in the periphery. One simple proposal is that TENS operates through antidromic stimulation of the afferent neurons. Antidromic stimulation of small afferent fibers may simply block the transmission of impulses from the nociceptors to the spinal cord. Antidromic conduction is also thought to initiate the release of substance P from sensory neurons in the vicinity of arterioles stimulating vasodilation. This is the basis of the *triple response* (red reaction, wheal, and flare) when the skin is stroked firmly with a pointed instrument. Increased blood flow to damaged tissue could dissipate pain-producing substances such as bradykinin, histamine, or substance P.

Another possible mechanism is that TENS activates the sympathetic nervous system. This activation of peripheral sympathetic neurons would also cause vasomotor responses, leading to changes in tissue chemistry. Painful stimuli cause diffuse noradrenergic discharge, leading to generalized cutaneous vasoconstriction. However in skeletal muscle tissue, in addition to the vasoconstrictor noradrenergic fibers, there are sympathetic vasodilator fibers which act on cholinergic receptors causing vasodilation. When these neurons are activated, the resulting increased blood flow to damaged muscle tissue could dissipate pain-producing substances.

Another intriguing postulate is that TENS may operate via opiate-mediated pain-modulating systems. Basbaum and Fields[89] proposed a feedback loop in which small-fiber afferent input travels through ascending systems to the thalamus and higher centers as well as to the nucleus *reticularis gigantocellularis* (RGC). The RGC projects to the PAG, which provides descending input to the dorsal horn via tracts through the nucleus *raphis magnus* and the nucleus *reticularis magnocellularis*. These descending pathways are inhibitory to neurons in the dorsal horn and are probably opiate-mediated. The presence of endorphins and enkephalins in the brain stem and the dorsal horn has been established. Direct electrical stimulation of the opiate-rich PAG is known to produce analgesia over large regions of the body, which can be reversed by naloxone.[94,100,101] TENS may exert its analgesic effect via this opiate-mediated inhibitory system by activation of brain-stem nuclei. Electrical stimulation applied at a site some distance from the actual damaged or pain-producing tissue can still be effective. Lending support to this idea is the fact that high intensity, low frequency electrical stimulation at acupuncture sites has been shown to result in increased endorphin release in cerebrospinal fluid.[102,103] The source of these endorphins, however, has not been determined.

The application of TENS to obtain relief from pain is effective, and the relief persists beyond the period of treatment. The site of application of TENS may be within the affected dermatome or at a distant site. There is great variability in duration of application, frequency, amplitude, and other stimulus characteristics in effective treatment reported in the literature. TENS probably activates both opiate and nonopiate pain-modulating systems, which has led to the complex literature associated with electroanalgesia.

SUMMARY

The role of small A-delta and C fibers is well established in the peripheral mechanisms of pain perception. The mode of activation of the nociceptors associated with these fibers remains unclear. There are both direct effects of heat and mechanical stimulation, as well as indirect effects mediated through the release of a variety of chemical substances. Most A-delta and C fibers terminate in the outer margins of the dorsal horn, although some project to deeper regions of the spinal gray matter. The neurotransmitters of these neurons is unknown but one candidate is substance P, which may also be involved in the nociceptive activating system.

There are both pain-specific and nonspecific or polymodal neurons in the dorsal horn. There is evidence for convergence of cutaneous and visceral afferents on both types of dorsal horn neurons, providing a reasonable model for referred pain and pain modulation via electrostimulation. Several ascending tracts are responsible for pain transmission. The spinothalamic tract appears to be involved with discriminative aspects of pain sensation and other senses as well. The spinoreticular tract has its origins primarily in the outer lamina of the dorsal horn and may be involved in motivational aspects of pain perception and response. Dorsal columns are also implicated in pain transmission and may be involved in motivational aspects and the unpleasant sensation of pain, or in activating pain-modulating systems.

The modulation of pain appears to occur at several levels within the central nervous system. Large cutaneous fiber inhibition of small pain fibers occurs at the segmental level (gate control theory). Pain inhibition at the spinal cord may operate through endogenous opiates functioning as either presynaptic or postsynaptic neurotransmitters. The brain stem is also involved in pain modulation through descending systems, influencing segmental levels of the spinal cord. Direct electrical stimulation of the PAG triggers generalized anesthesia and is probably mediated through serotonin, norepinephrine, and endogenous opiates acting as neurotransmitters. Enhanced understanding of pain-modulating systems has provided additional treatments for patients with pain, including the application of TENS, electroacupuncture, and direct brain stimulation.

The pain system is not a simple heterogeneous sensory system with a well-defined adequate stimulus. The system responds to complex stimuli mediated through parallel ascending tracts with multiple levels of modulation available within the CNS. The pain system responds through a variety of motor outputs and activates a wide range of physiologic and emotional responses. As our understanding of the interactions of peripheral and central mechanisms of pain expands, we will be more effective in our treatment of the patient with pain.

REFERENCES

1. Mountcastle, VB: Pain and temperature sensibilities. In Mountcastle, VB (ed): Medical Physiology, Vol 1, ed 13, CV Mosby, St Louis, 1974, p 348.
2. Hardy, JD, Wolff, HG, and Goodell, H: Pricking pain threshold in different body areas. Proc Soc Exp Biol Med 80:425, 1952.
3. Sternbach, RA: Pain: A Psychophysiological Analysis. Academic Press, New York, 1968.
4. Kruger, L: Introduction. In Kruger, L and Liebeskind, JC (eds): Advances in Pain Research and Therapy, Vol 6. Raven Press, New York, 1984, p XIX.
5. Wall, PD: On the relation of injury to pain. Pain 6:253, 1979.
6. Sternbach, RA: Acute versus chronic pain. In Wall, PD and Melzack, R (eds): Textbook of Pain. Churchill Livingstone, New York, 1984, p 173.
7. Miller, JC, Boureau F, and Albe-Fessard, D: Human nociceptive reactions: Effects of spatial summation of afferent input from relatively large diameter fibers. Brain Res 201:465, 1980.
8. Perl, ER, et al.: Sensitization of high threshold receptors with unmyelinated C-afferent fibers. In Iggo, A and Ilyensky (eds): Somatosensory and Visceral Receptor Mechanisms, Progress in Brain Research, Vol 43, 1976, p 263.

9. Wall, PD: Mechanisms of acute and chronic Pain. In Kruger, L and Liebeskind, JC (eds): Advances in Pain Research and Therapy, Vol 6. Raven Press, New York, 1984, p 95.

10. Perl, ER: Characterization of nociceptors and their activation of neurons in the superficial dorsal horn: First steps for the sensation of pain. In Kruger, L and Liebesskind, JC (eds): Advances in Pain Research and Therapy, Vol 6. Raven Press, New York, 1984, p 23.

11. Wall, PD and Devor, M: The effect of peripheral nerve injury on dorsal root potentials and on transmission of afferent signs into the spinal cord. Brain Res 209:95, 1981.

12. Barbut, D, Polak, JM, and Wall, PD: Substance P in spinal cord dorsal horn decreases following peripheral nerve injury. Brain Res 205:289, 1981.

13. Gibson, SJ, et al.: The distribution of nine peptides in rat spinal cord, with special emphasis on the substantia gelatinosa and on the area around the central canal (lamina X). J Comp Neurol 201:65, 1981.

14. Cannon, WB: Bodily Changes in Pain, Hunger, Fear and Rage. Appleton, New York, 1929.

15. Messing, RB and Lytle LD: Serotonin-containing neurons: Their possible role in pain and analgesia. Pain 4:1, 1977.

16. Sternbach, RA, et al.: Effects of altering brain serotonin activity on human chronic pain. In Bonica, JJ and Albe-Fessard, D (eds): Advances in Pain Research and Therapy, Vol 1. Raven Press, New York, 1976, p 601.

17. Craig, KD: Emotional aspects of pain. In Wall, PD and Melzack, R (eds): Textbook of Pain. Churchill Livingstone, New York, 1984, p 153.

18. Merskey, H: Psychological aspects of pain. Postgrad Med J 44:297, 1968.

19. Weisenberg, M: Pain and pain control. Psychol Bull 84:1008, 1977.

20. Sternbach, RA: Pain Patients; Traits and Treatment. Academic Press, New York, 1974.

21. Selye, H: The Stress of Life. McGraw-Hill, New York, 1976.

22. Muller, J: Handbuch der Physiologie des Menschen, Vol 2, Berlin 1840, p 249.

23. Von Frey, YM: Beitrage zur Physiologica des Schmerzsinns. Berlin Koenigl Saechs Ges Wiss 46: 185,1894.

24. Goldscheider, A: Veber den Schmerz. In Physiologischer und Klinischer Hinsicht. Hirschwald, Berlin, 1894.

25. Melzack, R and Wall, PD: Pain mechanisms: A new theory. Science 150:971, 1965.

26. Sherrington, CS: The Integrative Action of the Nervous System. Scribner, New York, 1906.

27. Adrian, ED: The messages in sensory fibers and their interpretation. Proc R Soc Lond [Biol] 109:1, 1931.

28. Lynn, B: Cutaneous nociceptors. In Holden, AV and Winlow, W (eds): The Neurobiology of Pain. Manchester University Press, Manchester, 1984, p 97.

29. Perl, ER: Is pain a specific sensation? J Psychiatr Res 8:273, 1971.

30. Torebjork, HE and Ochoa, JL: Specific sensations evoked by activity in single identified sensory units in man. Acta Physiol Scand 110:445, 1980.

31. Lynn, B and Carpenter, SE: Primary afferent units from the hairy skin of the rat hind limb. Brain Res 238:29, 1982.

32. Kumazawa, T and Perl, ER: Primate cutaneous sensory units with unmyelinated (C) afferent fibers. J Neurophysiol 40:1325, 1977.

33. Kumazawa, T and Mizumura, K: The polymodal C-fiber receptor in the muscle of the dog. Brain Res 101:589, 1976.

34. Stacy, MJ: Free nerve endings in skeletal muscle of the cat. J Anat 105:231, 1969.

35. Burgess, PR and Clark, FJ: Characteristics of knee joint receptors in the cat. J Physiol 203:317, 1969.

36. Mense, S, Light, AR, and Perl, ER: Spinal terminations of subcutaneous high threshold mechanoreceptors. In Brown, AG and Rethelyi, M (eds): Spinal Cord Sensation. Scottish Academic Press, Edinburgh, 1981, p 79.

37. Chahl, LA: Mechanism of pain and analgesic compounds. In Beers, RF and Basset, EG (eds): Advances in Pain Research and Therapy, Vol 1. Raven Press, New York, 1979, p 273.

38. Keele, CA and Armstrong, D: Substances Producing Pain and Itch. Edward Arnold & Co, London, 1964.

39. Ranson, SW: The tract of Lissauer and the substantia gelatinosa Rolandi. Am J Anat:1697, 1914.

40. Ranson, SW: The course within the spinal cord of the nonmedullated fibers of the dorsal roots: A study of Lissauer's tract in the cat. J Comp Neurol 23:259, 1913.

41. Bessou, P and Perl, ER: Responses of cutaneous sensory units with unmyelinated fibers to noxious stimuli. J Neurophysiol 32:1025, 1969.

42. Van Hess, J and Gybels, JM: Pain related to single afferent C fibers from human skin. Brain Res 48:397, 1972.

43. Coggeshall, RE, et al.: Unmyelinated axons in human ventral roots, a possible explanation for the failure of dorsal rhizotomy to relieve pain. Brain 98:157, 1975.

44. Wall, PD: The laminar organization of dorsal horn and effects of descending impulses. J Physiol 188:403, 1967.

45. Wagman, IH and Price, DD: Responses of dorsal horn cells of Macaca Mulatta to cutaneous and sural nerve A and C-fiber stimuli. J Neurophysiol 32:803, 1969.

46. Mendell, L: Physiological properties of unmyelinated fiber projections to the spinal cord. Exp Neurol 16:316, 1966.

47. Hillman, P and Wall, PD: Inhibitory and excitatory factors influencing the receptive fields of lamina V spinal cord cells. Exp Brain Res 9:284, 1969.
48. Price, DD and Wagman, IH: The physiological roles of A and C-fiber inputs to the dorsal horn of M. Mulatta. Exp Neurol 29:383, 1970.
49. Pomeranz, B, Wall, PD, and Weber, WV: Cord cells responding to fine myelinated afferents from visceral muscle and skin. J Physiol (Lond) 199:511, 1968.
50. Foreman, RD: Viscerosomatic convergence onto spinal neurons respond to afferent fibers located in the inferior cardiac nerve. Brain Res 137:164, 1977.
51. Hancock, MB, Foreman, RD, and Willis, WD: Convergence of visceral and cutaneous input onto spinothalamic tract cells in the thoracic spinal cord of the cat. Exp Neurol 47:240, 1975.
52. Selzer, M and Spencer, WA: Convergence of visceral and cutaneous afferent pathways in the lumbar spinal cord. Brain Res 14:349, 1969.
53. Selzer, M and Spencer, WA: Interactions between visceral and cutaneous afferents in the spinal cord: Reciprocal primary afferent fiber depolarization. Brain Res 14:349, 1969.
54. McMahon, SB: Spinal mechanisms in somatic pain. In Holden, AV and Winlow, W (eds): The Neurobiology of Pain. Manchester University Press, Manchester 1984, p 159.
55. Rustioni, A: Non-primary afferents to the nucleusgracilis from the lumbar cord of the cat. Brain Res 51:81, 1973.
56. Rustioni, A, Hayes, NL, and O'Neill, S: Dorsal column nuclei and ascending spinal afferents in macaques. Brain 102:95, 1979.
57. Bennett, GJ, et al.: The cells of origin of the dorsal column postsynaptic projection in the lumbrosacral enlargements of cats and monkeys. Somatosensory Res 1983.
58. Dubner, R, et al.: Neural circuitry mediating nociception in the medullary and spinal dorsal horn. In Kruger, L and Liebeskind, JC (eds): Advances in Pain Research and Therapy, Vol 6. Raven Press, New York, 1984, p 151.
59. White, JC and Sweet, WH: Pain and the Neurosurgeon: A Forty Year Experience. Charles, C Thomas, Springfield, IL, 1969, p 1032.
60. Price, DD, et al.: Spatial and temporal transformation of input to spinothalamic tract neurons and their relation to the somatic sensations. J Neurophysiol 41:933, 1978.
61. Ralston, HJ: Synaptic organization of spinothalamic tract projections to the thalamus, with special reference to pain. In Kruger, L and Liebeskind, JC (eds): Advances in Pain Research and Therapy, Vol 6. Raven Press, New York, 1984, p 183.
62. Berkley, K: Spatial relationships between the terminations of somatic sensory and motor pathways in the rostral brain stem of cats and monkeys. Part I. Ascending somatic sensory inputs to lateral diencephalon. J Comp Neurol 193:283, 1980.
63. Boivie, J: Anatomical observations on the dorsal column nuclei, their thalamic projection and the cytoarchitecture of some somatosensory thalamic nuclei in the monkey. J Comp Neurol 178:17, 1980.
64. Boivie, J: Thalamic projections from lateral cervial nucleus in monkey: A degeneration study. Brain Res 198:13, 1980.
65. Friedman, DP and Jones, EG: Thalamic input to areas 3a and 2 in monkeys. J Neurophysiol 45:59, 1981.
66. Kenshalo, DR, et al.: Responses of neurons in primate ventral posterior lateral nucleus to noxious stimuli. J Neurophysiol 43:1594, 1980.
67. Bowsher, D: Central pathways and mechanisms of pain sensations. In Holden, AV and Winlow, W (eds): The Neurobiology of Pain. Manchester University Press, Manchester, 1984, p 209.
68. Kenshalo, DR and Isensee, O: Responses of primate SI cortical neurons to noxious stimuli. J Neurophysiol 50:1479, 1983.
69. Gerhart, KD: Inhibition of primate spinothalamic tract neurons by stimulation in ventral posterior lateral (VPL) thalamic nucleus: Possible mechanisms. J Neurophysiol 49:406, 1983.
70. Reynolds, DV: Surgery in the rat during electrical analgesia induced by focal brain stimulation. Science 64:444, 1969.
71. Casey, KL: Responses of bulboreticular units to somatic stimuli eliciting escape behavior in the cat. Int J Neurosci 2:15, 1971.
72. LeBlanc, HJ and Gatipon, GB: Medial bubloreticular responses to peripherally applied noxious stimuli. Exp Neurol 42:264, 1974.
73. Benjamin, RM: Single neurons in the rat medulla responsive to nociceptive stimulation. Brain Res 24:525, 1970.
74. Hosobuchi, Y, Adams, JE, and Linchitz, R: Pain relief by electrical stimulation of the central grey matter in humans and its reversal by naloxone. Science 197:183, 1977.
75. Richardson, DE and Akil, H: Pain reduction by electrical brain stimulation in man. J Neurosurg 47:178, 1977.
76. Barbo, NM: Studies of PAG/PVG stimulation for pain relief in humans. In Fields, HL and Besson, JM (eds): Pain Modulation: Progress in Brain Research, Vol 77. Elsevier, New York, 1988.
77. Myerson, BA: Problems and controversies in PVG and sensory thalamic stimulation as treatment for pain. In Fields, HL and Besson, JM (eds): Pain Modulation: Progress in Brain Research, Vol 77. Elsevier, New York, 1988.

78. Hokfelt, T, et al.: Immunohistochemical analysis of peptide pathways possibly related to pain and analgesia: Enkephalin and substance P. Proc Natl Acad Sci USA 74:3081, 1977.
79. Sar, M, et al.: Immunohistochemical localization of enkephalin in rat brain and spinal cord. J Comp Neurol 182:17, 1978.
80. Atweh, SF and Kuhar, MJ: Autoradiographic localization of opiate receptors in rat brain. Part II. The brain stem. Brain Res 129:1, 1977.
81. Hiller, JM, Pearson, J, and Simon, EJ: Distribution of stereospecific binding of the potent narcotic analgesic ectorphine in the human brain: Predominance in the limbic system. Res Commun Chem Pathol Pharmacol 6:1052, 1973.
82. Pert, CB, Kuhar, MJ, and Snyder, SH: Opiate receptor: Autoradiographic localization in rat brain. Proc Natl Acad Sci USA 73:3729, 1976.
83. Reichling, DB, Kwiat, GC, and Basbaum, AI: Anatomy, physiology and pharmacology of the periaqueductal gray—contribution to antinociceptive controls. In Fields, HL and Besson, JM (eds): Pain Modulation: Progress in Brain Research, Vol 77. Elsevier, New York, 1988.
84. Hughes, J: Isolation of an endogenous compound from the brain with pharmacological properties similar to morphine. Brain Res 88:295, 1975.
85. Snyder, SH: Opiate receptors in the brain. N Engl J Med 296(5):266, 1977.
86. Simon, EJ and Hiller, JM: The opiate receptors. Annu Rev Pharmacol Toxicol 18:371, 1978.
87. Terenius, L: The endogenous opioids and other central peptides. In Wall, PD and Melzack, R (eds): Textbook of Pain. Churchill and Livingstone, New York, 1984, p 133.
88. Mayer, DJ and Watkins, LR: Multiple endogenous opiate and nonopiate analgesia systems. In Kruger, L and Liebeskind, JC (eds): Advances in Pain Research and Therapy, Vol 6. Raven Press, New York, 1984, p 253.
89. Basbaum, AI and Fields, HL: Endogenous pain control mechanisms: Review and hypothesis. Annu Neurol 4:451, 1978.
90. Levine, JD, et al.: A spinal opioid synapse mediates the interaction of pain and brainstem sites in morphine analgesia. Brain Res 236:85, 1982.
91. Yaksh, TL, Al-Rodhan, NRF, and Jensen, TS: Sites of action of opiates in production of analgesia. In Fields, HL and Besson, JM (eds): Pain Modulation: Progress in Brain Research, Vol 77. Elsevier, New York, 1988.
92. Frederickson, RCA and Chipkin, RE: Endogenous opioids and pain: status of human studies and new treatment concepts. In Fields, HL and Besson, JM (eds): Pain Modulation: Progress in Brain Research, Vol 77, Elsevier, New York, 1988.
93. Le Bars, D and Villanueva, L: Electrophysiological evidence for the activation of descending inhibitory controls by nociceptive afferent pathways. In Fields, HL and Besson, JM (eds): Pain Modulation: Progress in Brain Research, Vol 77. Elsevier, New York, 1988.
94. Adams, JE: Naloxone reversal of analgesia produced by brain stimulation in the human. Pain 2:161, 1976.
95. Fields, HL, et al.: Nucleus raphe magnus inhibition of spinal cord dorsal horn neurons. Brain Res 126:441, 1971.
96. Willis, WD: Anatomy and physiology of descending control of nociceptive responses of dorsal horn neurons: Comprehensive review. In Fields, HL and Besson, JM (eds): Pain Modulation, Progress in Brain Research, Vol 77, Elsevier, New York, 1988.
97. Ruda, MA: Spinal dorsal horn circuitry involved in the brain stem control of nociception. In Fields, HL and Besson, JM (eds): Pain Modulation: Progress in Brain Research, Vol 77. Elsevier, New York, 1988.
98. Duggan, AW and Morton, CR: Tonic descending inhibition and spinal nociceptive transmission. In Fields, HL and Besson, JM (eds): Pain Modulation: Progress in Brain Research, Vol 77. Elsevier, New York, 1988.
99. Melzack, R and Casey, KL: Sensory motivational and central control determinants of pain. In Kenshalo, DR (ed): The Skin Senses. Charles C Thomas, Springfield, IL, 1968.
100. Hosobuchi, Y, Adams, J, and Linchitz, R: Pain relief by electrical stimulation of the central grey matter in humans and its reversal by naloxone. Science 197:183, 1977.
101. Lewis, VA and Gebhart, GF: Evaluation of the periaqueductal central gray (PAG) as a morphine specific locus of action and examination of morphine induced and stimulation produced analgesia coincident at PAG loci. Brain Res 124:283, 1977.
102. Sjolund, B, Terenius, L, and Eriksson, M: Increased cerebrospinal fluid levels of endorphines after electroacpuncture. Acta Physiol Scand 100:382, 1977.
103. Sjolund, BH and Eriksson, MBE: Electro-acupuncture and endogenous morphines. Lancet 2:1085, 1976.

SUGGESTED READINGS

Besson, JM and Chaouch, A: Peripheral and spinal mechanisms of nociception. Physiol Rev 67(1):187, 1987.

Bond, MR: Pain: Its Nature, Analysis, and Treatment. Churchill Livingstone, New York, 1984.

Fields, HL and Besson, JM (eds): Pain Modulation: Progress in Brain Research, Vol 77. Elsevier, New York, 1988.

Fields, HL, et al. (eds): World Congress on Pain 4th Proceedings: Advances in Pain Research and Therapy, Vol 9. Raven Press, New York, 1985.

Holden, AV and Winlow, W (eds): The Neurobiology of Pain. Manchester University Press, Manchester, 1984.

Kruger, L and Liebeskind, JC (eds): Neural Mechanisms of Pain: Advances in Pain Research and Therapy, Vol 6. Raven Press, New York, 1984.

Michel, TH (ed): Pain: International Perspectives in Physical Therapy, Vol 1. Churchill Livingstone, New York, 1985.

Wall, PD and Melzack, R (eds): Textbook of Pain. Churchill Livingstone, New York, 1984.

SECTION II

Application of Electrical Currents

CHAPTER **3**

Electrodiagnostic and Electrotherapeutic Instrumentation: Characteristics of Recording and Stimulation Systems and the Principles of Safety

Barbara M. Myklebust, Ph.D., P.T.
Luther C. Kloth, M.S., P.T.

A wide range of biomedical devices is currently available to physical therapists for electrodiagnostic and electrotherapeutic purposes. For several reasons, it is often difficult to make a decision about which piece of equipment is the preferred device for a particular application. Features, such as the type of electrode or display device, vary among manufacturers. A range of stimulating and/or recording characteristics are available among devices intended for a similar application. Because of a lack of uniformity in terminology among clinicians, biomedical engineers, and the vendors of equipment, some performance characteristics may not be described adequately. Furthermore, the optimal parameters for physiologic effect have not been determined for some techniques and devices.

The purpose of this chapter is to outline instrumentation features which are com-

This work has been supported in part by Veteran's Administration Rehabilitation Research and Development. The authors thank the following persons, without whom this endeavor could not have been completed: Joel B. Myklebust, PhD, PE, Thomas Prieto, PhD, Thomas Swiontek, PhD, and the Standards Committee of the Section on Clinical Electrophysiology of the American Physical Therapy Association.

mon to electrotherapeutic and electrodiagnostic instruments, and to help in the selection process for the optimum piece of equipment for a clinic or a particular patient application. The advantages and disadvantages of device options are also discussed. A brief review of engineering terminology to describe signal characteristics and device functions is presented, and general requirements for safety of the patient and the therapist are summarized.

DIAGNOSTIC SYSTEMS FOR RECORDING ELECTRICAL SIGNALS

Biomedical instruments can record a variety of types of electrical signals from a patient. A physiologic response may be recorded as an electrical signal which is *derived from the patient* (Fig. 3–1A), such as the electroencephalogram (EEG). Alternatively, the electrical response may result from an *applied electrical stimulus,* as in measuring nerve signals in a nerve conduction study or the somatosensory evoked potential (Fig. 3–1B), or from an *applied mechanical stimulus,* as in measuring surface-muscle electrical signals or electromyograms (EMGs) in response to a tendon tap. The electrical signal of interest has inherent characteristics (e.g., amplitude and frequency ranges) which dictate how that signal must be processed (Table 3–1). That signal can be visualized on an oscilloscope.

The following section reviews features that are common to instruments which record and display electrical signals: the applied stimulus (if any), the recording electrodes, the signal processor which "conditions" (amplifies and filters) the recorded signal, and devices to display the processed electrical signal. This section also reviews different features that are available for diagnostic devices. The electrical characteristics of the recorded physiologic signal dictate the selection of electrodes, signal processor characteristics, and the display device, and these requirements are reviewed.

Applied Stimulus

An electrical response can be recorded following the application of an electrical stimulus. An electrical stimulus may be applied directly to a sensory nerve (i.e., when measuring sensory nerve conduction velocities) or to a mixed nerve [i.e., when measuring the motor response (M-wave response) or monosynaptic reflex (H reflex), or when recording the somatosensory evoked potential]. In each case, the parameters (amplitude, pulse duration, and frequency) of the stimulus must be appropriately selected to activate the excitable tissue (nerve, innervated muscle, or denervated muscle). The stimulus may also be optical (flashes of light to record the visual-evoked potential), auditory (clicks to monitor the auditory-evoked potential), or mechanical (a tendon tap will activate the stretch reflex, and the evoked muscle response can be recorded).

TYPES OF STIMULATING ELECTRODES

The electrical stimulation may be applied to the patient with *surface* (transcutaneous) or *invasive* electrodes. Surface stimulating electrodes may be made of canvas or felt, metal, silicon or rubber, sponge, a polymer, or a vacuum cup. Surface stimulating electrodes may require the use of a coupling medium, such as an electrolytic paste or gel.

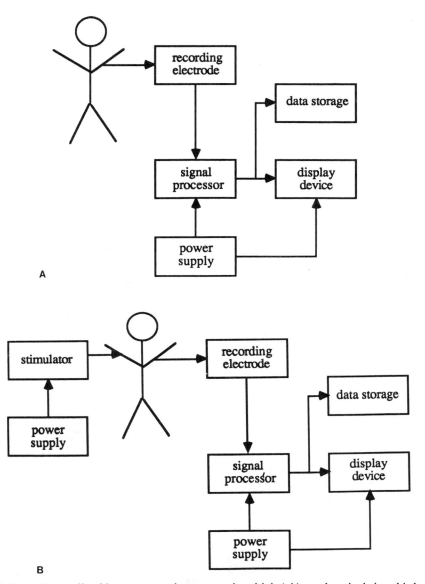

FIGURE 3-1. Generalized instrumentation system in which (*A*) an electrical signal inherent to the patient is recorded; (*B*) an electrical signal results from an externally applied electrical (or mechanical) stimulus.

The electrode shape and type of coupling medium are, in part, dictated by the tissue to be stimulated and the type and duration of the examination. For applications with a predetermined and relatively stable stimulation site (such as in the somatosensory evoked potential), an adhesive-backed silver-silver chloride electrode with a concave well for the electrolyte is preferred (Fig. 3-2). For some diagnostic purposes (as in a peripheral nerve injury), a handheld stimulating electrode is chosen in which the stimulation site and applied pressure can be easily changed (Fig. 3-2). In many in-

TABLE 3–1 Amplitude and Frequency Ranges of Electrical Signals of the Body

Electrical Event	Amplitude of Electrical Signal (Maximum Ranges, V)	Signal Frequency (Maximum Ranges, Hz)	Recording Electrode
EP (evoked potential: somatosensory, auditory, visual)	0.1–10 μV	DC—5 KHz	Platinum needle or gold cup
EEG (Electro-encephalo-gram)	1–5000 μV	DC—150 Hz	Platinum needle or gold cup
ENG (electro-neurogram)	0.01–3 mV	DC—10 KHz	Stainless steel needle or silver-silver chloride (surface)
EMG (electro-myogram)	0.1–10 mV	DC—10 KHz	Stainless steel needle or wire
		DC—1 KHz	Silver-silver chloride (surface)
ECG (electro-cardiogram)	0.5–4 mV	0.01–250 Hz	Silver-silver chloride (surface)

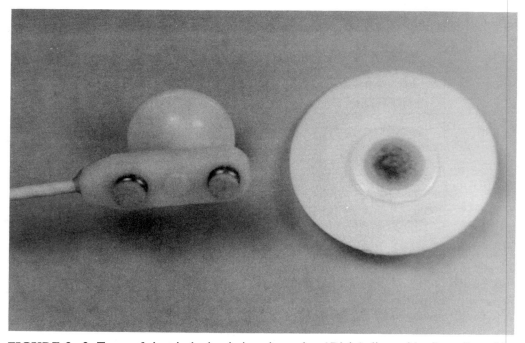

FIGURE 3–2. Types of electrical stimulating electrodes. (*Right*) disposable silver-silver chloride electrode with a "well" to retain electrode paste; the well is filled with a pre-gelled foam. (*Left*) handheld stainless steel stimulating electrode with felt covering.

stances (as in H reflex and nerve conduction studies), it is important that the stimulation site remain constant; in this case, the metal-stimulating electrode must be held in place with constant pressure.

SIZE OF STIMULATING ELECTRODES

The size of the stimulating electrode depends in part on the area of excitable tissue to be stimulated. It must also be remembered that electrodes of smaller size have higher impedance because electrode size is directly proportional to current flow. The smaller the electrode, the smaller the current flow for a given applied voltage to the stimulated area. Furthermore, with uniform electrode conductivity, current density is inversely proportional to the electrode size. Therefore, as electrode size decreases, current density increases. A small stimulating electrode will reduce the amount of current necessary to excite the tissue; however, the resulting high-current density may cause pain and/or tissue damage. A large stimulating electrode will distribute the area of the applied current, reducing the risk of tissue damage; however, an electrode which is too large may cause the current to spread to other excitable structures than the nerve or muscle of interest.

ORIENTATION OF STIMULATING ELECTRODES

Stimulating electrodes may be placed in a *monopolar* or *bipolar* configuration. In the monopolar orientation, the stimulating electrode is placed over the target area, where the greatest effect is desired. A second electrode is at *some distance* from the target area; this electrode is often called the *dispersive* electrode, because its larger size minimizes current density to the area to which it is applied (Fig. 3–3). The second electrode, also called the *reference* electrode, is not intended to be a ground connection.

In the bipolar technique, two stimulating electrodes are used; one is positive and the other is negative. Both stimulating electrodes are placed to affect the target area. In this

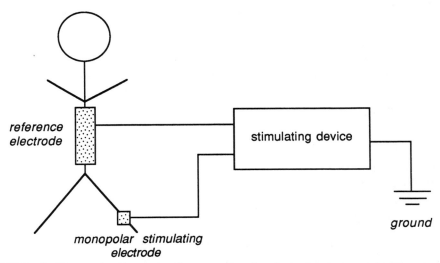

FIGURE 3–3. Monopolar electrode placement for electrical stimulation. (*A*) The stimulating electrode is placed over the "target area," (*B*) a second "reference" or "dispersive" electrode (not "earth ground") is placed at some distance from the stimulating electrode.

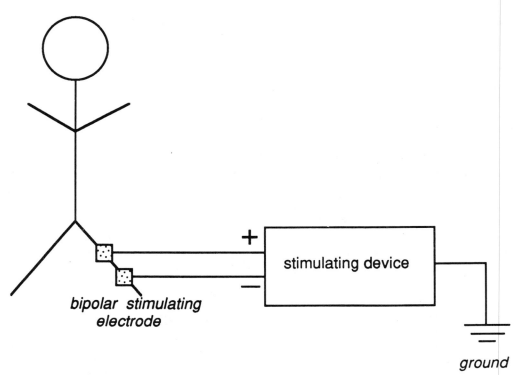

FIGURE 3–4. Bipolar electrode placement for electrical stimulation. Both stimulating electrodes (+) positive and (−) negative, are placed near each other at the "target area." A "reference" electrode is generally not required.

way, the current flow is limited to the excitable tissue of interest (Fig. 3–4). A reference connection is optional.

The use of the terms *bipolar* and *monopolar* has been somewhat obscured in clinical applications. The placement of a dispersive electrode *at a distance* from the stimulating electrode is ambiguous. The size of the dispersive electrode is *large* (that is, the dispersive electrode is larger than the stimulating electrode). Electrode size and placement is best determined by the efficacy of the stimulus to produce a physiologic response. For clarity in clinical applications, it is best to describe the placement of recording electrodes by exact location rather than use the terms bipolar and monopolar.

CONSTANT CURRENT VERSUS CONSTANT VOLTAGE

Constant (regulated) current stimulators provide a current which flows at a constant amplitude, within a specified impedance range, i.e., as the impedance changes, the voltage changes to maintain the current at a constant level. Constant voltage stimulators provide a constant voltage source, within a given range of impedances, i.e., the current changes in response to changes in impedance. It is the level of *current* which is responsible for the physiologic effect caused by electrical stimulation. Therefore, because impedances at the interface between the electrode and the body may vary during stimulation, constant current stimulators are preferred to constant voltage stimulators. With a constant current stimulator, the clinician has better control of the patient's physiologic response to electrical stimulation.

For most physiologic applications, a constant current source is preferable to a constant voltage source. The impedance of the electrodes, of the biological material, and of the electrode-body interface may change during stimulation; however, with constant current stimulation, the changes in impedance do not change the current flowing through the biological tissues. It is the level of current which is responsible for the resultant physiologic effects.

Recording Electrodes

With an appropriate device, signals of any type can be monitored whether they are electrical, optical, thermal, or radiant. When any type of signal is recorded, we prefer to display an electrical signal because of the advantages offered in further signal processing. A *transducer* is a device which converts energy from one form to another. In diagnostic systems in physical therapy, we generally work with the simplest case in which electrical signals are recorded from the body and the resulting voltage from the excitable tissue is monitored. The transducer is a conductive recording electrode, which is generally made of metal (Table 3–1).

PLACEMENT OF RECORDING ELECTRODES

The recording electrode (Fig. 3–5A to 3–5D) comes into direct contact with the patient, either on the skin (a *surface electrode*) or in a subcutaneous space.[1] A subcutaneous electrode may be *indwelling*, as in the case of an intramuscular electrode, or *implanted*, if it has been surgically placed on excitable tissue.

Surface recording electrodes are used when the excitable tissues encompass a fairly large surface area (Fig. 3–5A and 3–5B), for example, to record electromyogram signals from a large number of motor units, and gross signals from a large superficial nerve. Wire electrodes (Fig. 3–5C) are used to record EMG signals from deep small muscles whose potentials would be masked by overlying muscles when recording with surface electrodes. Needle electrodes are used for recording from small areas (Fig. 3–5D); for example, needles are chosen to monitor motor-unit recruitment patterns. Needles can be easily repositioned, and since they are indwelling electrodes which are in direct contact with body fluids, the impedance at the recording site is low. [When recording electrical signals from the body, it is important that the impedance of the amplifier (i.e., the signal processor) be much higher than the impedance of the electrodes. There are two ways to achieve this. One way is to make the impedance of the electrodes (i.e., the interface between the body and the electrodes) very small. The second method is to make the impedance of the recording amplifier very high]. For these reasons, needles are preferred for recording potentials in some applications. Unfortunately, however, they can cause pain on insertion.

MATERIALS OF RECORDING ELECTRODES

Surface electrodes are generally fabricated from bare and polished metals (e.g., silver or platinum) which conduct electricity well (i.e., the impedance or resistance to flow of

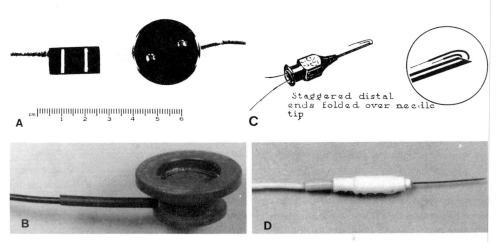

FIGURE 3–5. Types of recording electrodes: (*A* and *B*) surface electrodes and (*C* and *D*) indwelling electrodes. (*A*) An "active" surface electrode, in which electronics "condition" the signal (by amplification and filtering) are housed with the recording electrodes; these electronics in this electrode require external low voltage power of approximately 9 to 12 volts DC; a feature of the "active" electrodes is that they have a high input impedance that minimizes the amount of skin preparation and eliminates the use of an electrolyte; (*B*) concave silver–silver chloride electrode that holds the electrolyte; (*C*) fine wire indwelling electrode for recording EMGs; (*D*) platinum needle electrode for recording evoked potentials. ([*A–C*] From Basmajian, JV, De-Luca, CJ: Muscles Alive: Their Function Revealed by Electromyography (5th Edition). 1985, the Williams & Wilkins Co., Baltimore.)

electrons is low). However, because of the high impedance offered by the skin, these metals are much more effective conductors of electricity if the skin is properly prepared by abrasion and if an *electrolyte* medium is placed between the electrode and the patient. This electrolyte is usually a salt paste or cream. An effective electrode-electrolyte interface reduces impedance at the skin of the patient and the surface of the recording electrode, which makes it possible for the electrode to record smaller signals more accurately. Some recording discs are concave to retain the electrode paste or gel, and this increases the time the recording electrode can be used (Fig. 3–5B).

Recently, *active* surface electrodes have been designed which electronically incorporate a very high input impedance in the preamplifier (Fig. 3–5A). This improves the recording capabilities of the electrodes and reduces the need for skin preparation and a conducting medium.

Because subcutaneous electrodes come in direct contact with body fluids, which have a low resistance to the flow of electricity, an electrolyte is not required. Electrodes used for *indwelling* recordings are often made of platinum or stainless steel. Typical applications include the use of bipolar needle electrodes in EMG and electroneurography (ENG), and fine needle electrodes for recording potentials from the scalp in the somatosensory-evoked potential (Fig. 3–5D). Stiff wire electrodes of platinum or silver may be used for recording from deep muscles; these electrodes are insulated with Teflon or nylon, except at the tip. *Implanted* electrodes are generally fabricated of platinum, a soft and expensive metal. Platinum tolerates sterilization well, and tissue reactance to it is small.

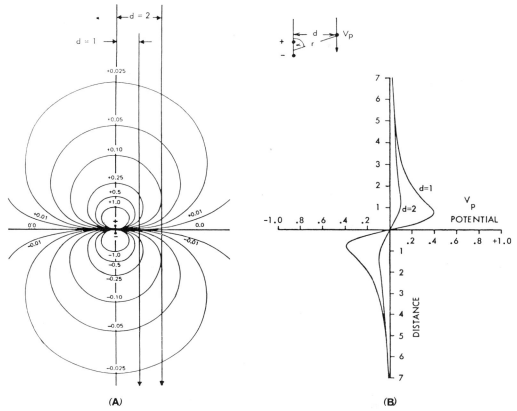

(A) **(B)**

FIGURE 3–6. The dipole and the distribution of the field potential. (*A*) There are an infinite number of isopotential lines that describe this field. (*B*) The electrical potential described by each line decreases as the distance from the source increases. (From Geddes, LA: Electrodes and the Measurement of Bioelectric Events. Wiley-Interscience, Division of John Wiley & Sons, Inc., New York, 1972.)

ORIENTATION OF RECORDING ELECTRODES

Surface and indwelling recording electrodes must be properly oriented with respect to the electrical signal of interest to ensure accurate recording of that signal. If a source of electrical potential (i.e., a dipole) is in a uniform-conducting medium which is infinite in its extent (i.e., a volume conductor), then current will flow and a potential field will be established.[2] This field is illustrated in Figure 3–6A and is described by an infinite number of lines of uniform potential (isopotential lines). These isopotential lines decrease in magnitude as the distance from the source increases (Fig. 3–6B). The reader should notice the isopotential line configuration, without concern for the assigned numerical values. When electrodes are placed close to the source of the electrical potential, a larger signal is recorded than when the electrodes are placed at a distance from the electrical source.

Recording electrodes may be placed in a *monopolar* or *bipolar* configuration. A monopolar electrode records electric potentials from a source when it is located anywhere near the source of the electric potential, and its measurements are referred to another electrode in a region of zero potential (i.e., the reference electrode is at an

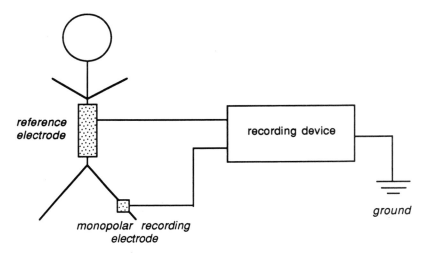

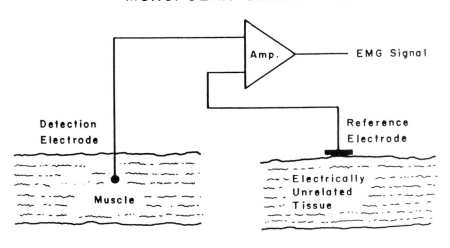

FIGURE 3–7. Monopolar recording electrode configuration. (*A*) example of a monopolar recording configuration, (*B*) schematic diagram of the monopolar recording technique. (From Basmajian, JV, DeLuca, CJ: Muscles Alive: Their Function Revealed by Electromyography (5th Edition). 1985, the Williams & Wilkins Co., Baltimore.)

infinite distance or *very far away* from the potential source) (Fig. 3–7). In the bipolar recording technique, two electrodes are placed *near* the source of the potential (i.e., excitable tissue) to detect the potentials with respect to a reference electrode (Fig. 3–8).

The advantage of monopolar recording is that the absolute potential is measured. However, if there are any other electrical signals in the vicinity that are not related to the signal of interest (e.g., electrical *noise*), these signals will also be recorded. Unfortunately, this noise may be a larger signal than the electrical event of interest. The

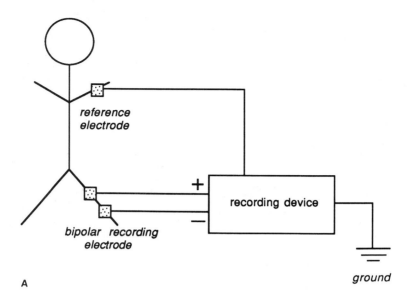

A

BIPOLAR DETECTION

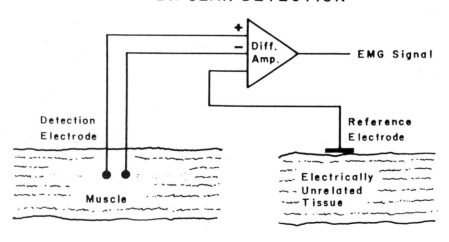

B

FIGURE 3-8. Bipolar recording electrode configuration. (*A*) Example of application of bipolar recording electrodes on the patient, a reference electrode is required for electrical stability of the differential amplifier, (*B*) schematic diagram of the bipolar recording technique. (From Basmajian, JV, DeLuca, CJ: Muscles Alive: Their Function Revealed by Electromyography (5th Edition), 1985, the Williams & Wilkins Co., Baltimore.)

advantage of the bipolar technique is that it gives better noise immunity, i.e., the electrical signal of the excitable tissue tends to be amplified, while the noise which is common to both electrodes tends to be rejected. However, the bipolar electrodes record an electrical signal which is a *spatial derivative* of the potential, which may be smaller than the actual potential produced by the source and smaller than the signal recorded by the monopolar technique (Fig. 3-9).

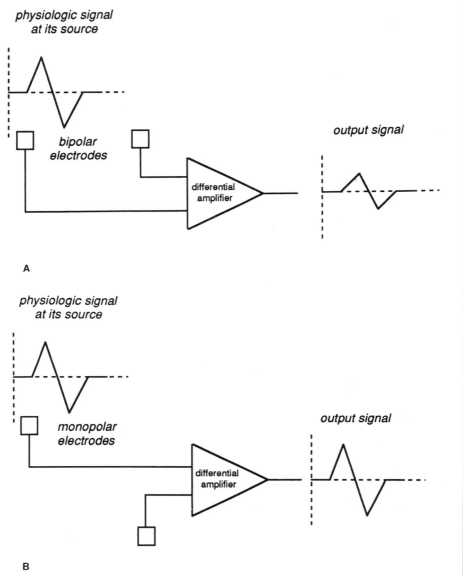

FIGURE 3–9. Comparison of the amplitude of a physiologic signal and the recording that may be displayed when (A) bipolar and (B) monopolar recording electrodes are used. Because bipolar electrodes record a spatial derivative of the electrical signal, the output signal may be smaller than that recorded from a monopolar electrode arrangement.

Unfortunately, ambiguous terms are used in these recording procedures. For example, the concentric needle electrode (Figure 3–10) can be used in either a monopolar or bipolar configuration. In monopolar recording, the reference electrode is placed at a distance *far* from the electrical event of interest. Bipolar electrodes are *close* to each other and yet *widely separated* with respect to the excitable tissue. While the terms bipolar and monopolar identify the general orientation of electrodes, it is best to describe the placement of recording electrodes by exact location for clarification.

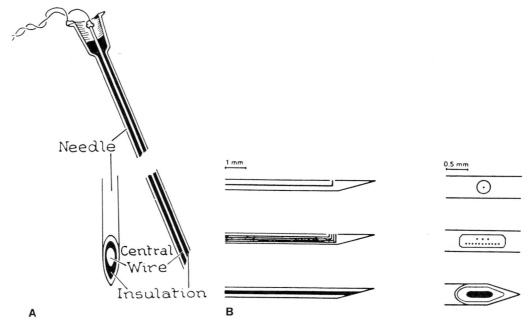

FIGURE 3–10. Concentric needle electrode design. (*A*) The construction of a concentric needle electrode in a monopolar configuration. A bipolar configuration would result from positioning two insulated wires in the cannula, as in Figure 5b. (*B*) Concentric needle electrodes, viewed from the tip, in a monopolar (*top*), multipolar (*middle*), and bipolar (*bottom*) orientation. (From Basmajian, JV, DeLuca, CJ: Muscles Alive: Their Function Revealed by Electromyography (5th Edition). 1985, the Williams & Wilkins Co., Baltimore.)

The recording of any electric signal is generally performed with respect to a reference electrode. In the bipolar technique (i.e., when the recording electrodes are closely placed), a reference electrode is generally also *nearby*. This reference electrode generally is *not* "earth" ground, but a "floating" ground, which is required by the differential amplifier for proper signal processing. When a monopolar recording technique is used, the reference electrode is far away. A second floating ground may also be used if the signals are sent to a differential amplifier.

The amplitude of a recorded signal must be reported with caution. To a great extent, the amplitude depends on the recording techniques used (i.e., the electrode type and orientation). For example, the magnitude of the EMG may have little meaning in surface recordings because of varied electrode-interface impedances and electrode placements from one recording procedure to the next.

Connecting the Patient to "Ground"

All hospital-approved medical devices which draw 60-Hz AC line power have ground connections which go to the earth (i.e., *earth ground*). If the medical instrument uses a *patient ground* connection and not the earth ground, this is usually a reference connection which is required for electrical stability in recording. In most cases, the patient is not connected to the earth ground, because of the risks from ground faults and leakage currents, which may risk the patient's safety as well as the safety of the clinician. While a patient may not be *directly* connected to the earth ground of a medical device, it is possible for the patient to be *indirectly* connected to earth ground. For example, if the clinician is touching both the grounded case of the medical device and the patient at the same time, the patient may become part of the pathway to ground. This may place the patient and the clinician at risk if the device has a large leakage current. These issues are discussed in more detail in the section on electrical safety.

Monopolar and bipolar *recording* techniques generally do not require the use of an earth ground, although a reference or floating ground may be part of the patient circuit. In some diagnostic applications, a true earth ground may be required for noise reduction. The use of true earth ground in the stimulation of a patient does not necessarily subject the patient to a greater risk of shock. When this technique is used, the clinician must be assured that *all* the equipment to which the patient is connected has the same ground potential and that the electrical system of the medical device is isolated from the power line. Furthermore, a ground-fault interrupter must be part of the circuit which supplies the equipment, the patient should be isolated from the power line, and the leakage current levels of all the medical devices should be verified to be at safe limits. External stimulation should not be applied to patients with demand-type cardiac pacemakers. These considerations are discussed more completely in the section entitled "Electrical Safety."

It is generally recommended that the *stimulus* outputs are not grounded. For bipolar stimulation, the patient leads are positive and negative, and the patient is not connected to earth ground through the stimulator. In monopolar stimulation, the patient leads *usually* are the active stimulus and a reference (*not* earth ground). However, in some medical instruments, the reference is indeed earth ground. The clinician should be aware of these situations, by verifying information provided in the operator's manual or by consulting a biomedical engineer.

Signal Processor

When a physiologic response is recorded from excitable tissue, the signal is generally too small to be immediately visualized on a display screen; electrical signals are in the range of several microvolts (e.g., somatosensory-evoked potential) to several millivolts [e.g., electrocardiogram (ECG) and EMG] (Table 3–1). Furthermore, the frequency ranges of signals include direct current (DC) to several thousand Hertz. Adequate display of the response requires some signal processing by amplifiers and filters.

SIGNAL AMPLIFICATION

When a low voltage and low frequency signal is recorded, simple amplification may be sufficient to make the response more visible (Fig. 3–11). The oscilloscope amplifier gain may be adequate to enhance the signal. As the gain of the amplifier (or the sensitivity control) is increased, a small signal is amplified and it appears larger on the display screen.

DIFFERENTIAL AMPLIFICATION

The signals recorded from either monopolar or bipolar electrodes may be fed to a *differential amplifier*. The differential amplifier amplifies the difference of two signals (Fig. 3–12). In the case of bipolar electrodes, the differential amplifier amplifies the

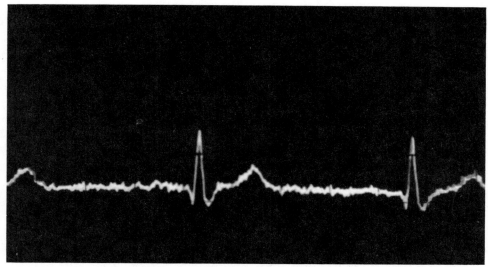

FIGURE 3–11. Sample display of the ECG on the oscilloscope using simple and differential amplification. The ECG signal was input to a differential amplifier (AC-coupled, with 100 Hz high frequency cutoff, a 60 Hz notch filter, and a gain of 100). This signal was put into an oscilloscope for display by simple amplification; the oscilloscope display settings are 2 V/div and 0.2 s/div. If the oscilloscope amplification were doubled by increasing the display gain to 1 V/div, the signal would appear to be twice as large on the display screen, but the actual measured amplitude would have been the same. That is, at 2 V/div (*shown*), this ECG waveform is 4 V, divided by differential amplifier gain of 100, or 4 mv. At 1 V/div display gain, the ECG waveform would appear twice as large on the display screen, but the actual measured amplitude is the same (4 mv).

differences of the signals from the two closely spaced recording electrodes. In monopolar recording, the differential amplifier amplifies the differences of the signals from the single recording electrode and the distant reference electrode.

Differential amplifiers are usually used with bipolar electrodes. The differential technique rejects signals common to both electrodes (i.e., common-mode rejection) and amplifies signals which are different. The two recording electrodes tend to see different potentials for a given localized electrochemical event (e.g., a nerve or muscle potential) when signals are *passed through* the amplifier. Any signals common to the two recording electrodes, such as 60-Hz noise from the power supply and DC noise, are rejected by the amplifier. In this way, the amplifier takes the signals recorded from bipolar electrodes, filters out noise, and improves the integrity of the electrical event of interest. The differential amplifier uses the reference electrode to compare the signals of the two recording electrodes. The amplifier actually subtracts the difference from one recording electrode and the reference electrode, and compares that with the difference from the second recording electrode and the reference.

Whether a particular source of noise is *common mode* depends on its location and orientation with respect to the recording electrodes (Fig. 3–13). Thus, for recording electrodes which are close together (bipolar), noise sources are far away from the recording site. This noise appears the same at both recording electrodes and will be rejected as common mode. Conversely, with electrodes which are far apart relative to

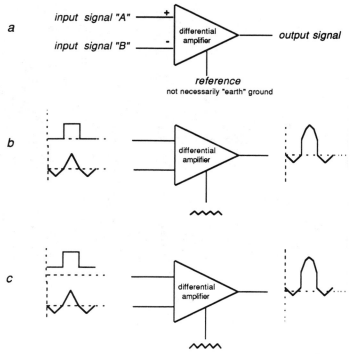

FIGURE 3–12. The differential amplifier. (*a*) Schematic diagram of a differential amplifier. In the standard configuration for the differential amplifier, there are two input signals, a reference (not necessarily "earth" ground), and a single output signal, (*b*) and (*c*) two illustrations dipict the way the differential amplifier processes an electrical signal. Note that the input signals are aligned in time. In (*b*), both signals are at the zero-baseline (*i.e.*, the signals have a zero "DC-offset"), in (*c*) the square wave is shifted above the zero-baseline (*i.e.*, it has a "DC-offset").

the noise, the noise may appear to be different at the two recording sites, and it will be passed through and amplified by the differential amplifier.

SIGNAL AVERAGING

If a single response to an electrical stimulus is very small and the noise in the environment is large with respect to the signal of interest, signal averaging may be performed. This technique is used to record nerve action potentials and evoked potentials. For example, the somatosensory evoked potential is normally about 1 to 10 μV (10^{-6} to 10^{-5} volts), but the background EEG is effectively 0.1 to 1 mV (10^{-4} to 10^{-3} volts). The somatosensory evoked potential is identified from the *noise of the EEG* by averaging the response to 100 to 200 electrical stimuli (Fig. 3–14).[3] That is, a weighted average is computed for 100 to 200 electrical stimulations.

INTEGRATION

Integration of an electrical signal applies to the calculation that is used to obtain the area under a signal waveform or curve (Fig. 3–15A), and is expressed in units of volts-seconds. An observed signal which has an average value of zero has a total

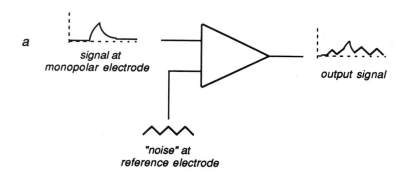

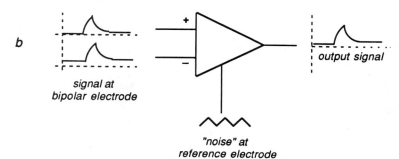

FIGURE 3–13. Differences between recording an electrical signal with differential amplification from (*a*) widely-spaced electrodes (with different noise at the two electrodes) and (*b*) bipolar electrodes.

integrated value of zero. Therefore, integration only applies to a full-wave rectified signal (Fig. 3–15B); the rectified value is always positive (Fig. 3–15C). The integrated value of a rectified signal increases as a function of time. Integration is frequently used to evaluate EMG responses, especially with recordings from surface electrodes. This technique simplifies the visual representation of the waveform, and it is a convenient method to quantify the magnitude of a response.

BANDPASS FILTERING

Physiologic responses of nerves and muscles have characteristic frequency ranges (Table 3–1). The noise of the external environment can be electronically filtered out of the recorded signal as long as the frequency ranges do not overlap. For example, DC and 60-Hz AC line noise can be eliminated from signals with a *bandpass filter*. This filter rejects signals at and above 60 Hz and passes (or keeps) a band of frequencies greater than DC and below 60 Hz (Fig. 3–16).

Some medical devices provide a frequency selection control as a switchable option for the clinician. Generally, this allows the examiner to choose between *low* frequency filters and *high* frequency filters, to help eliminate noise from the display. (Unfortunately, the use of the terms low and high frequency is somewhat arbitrary, and the

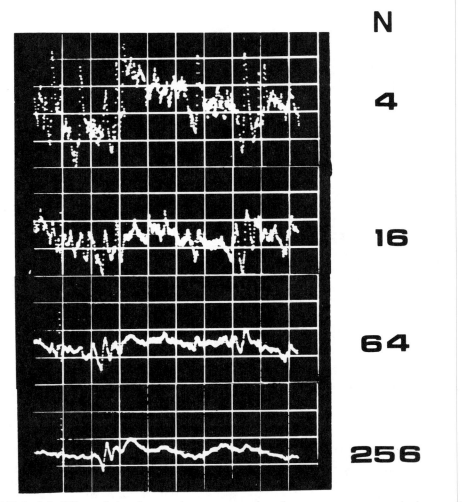

FIGURE 3–14. Effect of signal averaging on extracting the somatosensory evoked potential from "noise." Four "sweeps" of the averaging computer (n = 4) display a signal that is effectively unidentifiable in the presence of the "noise" of the EEG. After 256 averages (n = 256), the evoked potential waveform is easily identifiable. Scales are 2.5 μV/div and 12.5 ms/div. (From Myklebust, JB, et al,[3] with permission.)

operator's manual should be consulted for identification of the frequency ranges modulated by that filter.) For example, a 10-KHz (called a high frequency) filter will pass all signals below 10 KHz and filter out signals that are at or above 10 KHz. A 2-Hz (called a low frequency) filter will pass signals above 2 Hz.

The terms *high frequency* and *low frequency* filters on medical devices are *not* to be confused with *high-pass* and *low-pass* filters. A high-pass filter passes (keeps) the high frequency signals and filters out the low frequency signals. A low-pass filter passes the low frequency signal and rejects the higher frequencies. Therefore, a 10-KHz high frequency filter selection is *not* a high-pass filter; it is a low-pass filter with a cutoff frequency of 10 KHz (it passes frequencies below 10 KHz).

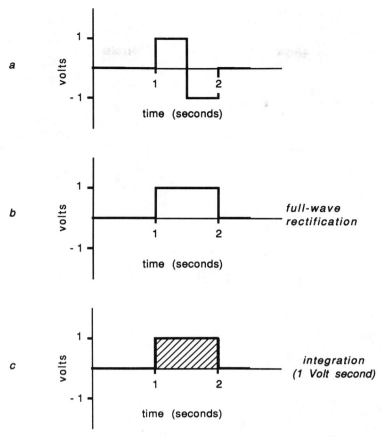

FIGURE 3–15. The process of integration of an electrical signal: (*a*) a biphasic pulse; (*b*) full-wave rectification of the signal, (*c*) computation of the integrated signal.

ANALOG-TO-DIGITAL (A/D) CONVERSION

For many clinical applications, the physiologic electrical responses from nerve or muscle are recorded, processed (amplified and filtered), and displayed as an *analog* output. This is the form of the output signal displayed on strip charts and many oscilloscopes (Fig. 3–11), and stored on FM tape recorders. However, for computer applications, the analog signal must be converted into a *digital* signal for precise data acquisition, storage, and later retrieval for analysis. The data are "digitized" by an analog-to-digital (A/D) converter, for which sampling rates and signal processing times are specified. The characteristics of the A/D converter are dictated by the frequency of the recorded signal and the number of channels of data which are being simultaneously sampled.

A/D converters fast enough to collect several (32 or more) channels of very-high-speed signals (several KHz) are available. However, high-speed data collection from multiple channels is very costly. Some A/D converters are specifically designed for a particular computer or microprocessor. They require that specialized computer software

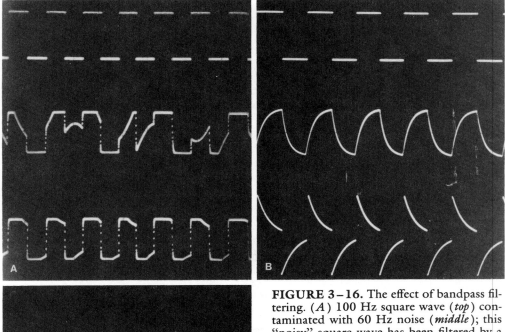

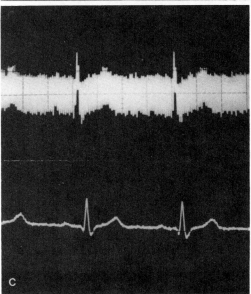

FIGURE 3–16. The effect of bandpass filtering. (*A*) 100 Hz square wave (*top*) contaminated with 60 Hz noise (*middle*); this "noisy" square wave has been filtered by a 60 Hz notch filter (*bottom*). (*B*) 100 Hz square wave (*top*) has been low-pass filtered (*middle*) (the high frequency cut off is 300 Hz); the 100 Hz square wave has been high-pass filtered (*bottom*) (the low frequency cut off is 30 Hz). Note that low-pass filtering rounds off the rapid changes to de-emphasize the high frequencies; this is comparable to integration. Also note that high pass filtering emphasized the rapid changes and eliminates the constant, flat part of the square wave; this is comparable to mathematical differentiation. (*C*) The ECG has been recorded from a single-ended input (*top*), in contrast to the ECG, which is then recorded from a differential amplifier (*bottom*). The 60 Hz noise contamination of the upper trace is eliminated by differential amplification; this is called *common mode rejection*.

be available to handle the data acquisition properly. The display of a digitized waveform on a computer monitor (or on a digital oscilloscope) does not necessarily appear different than an analog response to casual observation. Moreover, the presence of an A/D converter in a recording system may not be obvious in some commercially available data collection systems.

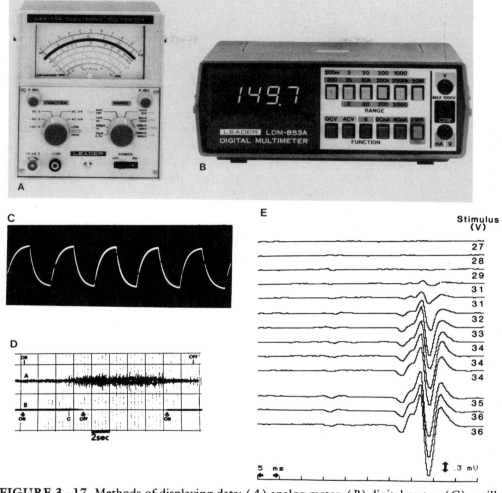

FIGURE 3–17. Methods of displaying data: (*A*) analog meter, (*B*) digital meter, (*C*) oscilloscope trace, (*D*) strip chart recording (From Barolat-Romana, G et al,[5] reprinted with permission.); (*E*) Digital display from a computer. (From Myklebust, BM, et al,[4] with permission.)

Data Output: Display and Storage Devices

An electrical physiologic response can be displayed as an analog or a digital signal. A meter display of an instantaneous voltage may be in analog or digital form (Fig. 3–17). A computer graphic display of data is a digital representation.[4] An entire waveform may be displayed on an oscilloscope (generally an analog device) or on a strip chart recorder (polygraph).[5] While a photograph may be taken of an oscilloscope display and measurements may be made from this and from the output of a strip chart recorder, neither of these methods allows further automated processing of the data. That is to say, the data cannot be reprocessed (filtered and amplified) or redisplayed in any other fashion.

An entire event or series of events may be preserved for future analysis on an FM tape recorder (analog data) or on a computer (digitized data). Both of these data-storage methods allow the electrical events to be analyzed by more complex strategies. Digitized data require less physical space than analog data on FM tape. Digitized data can be filtered and amplified with hardware or software, and can be subjected to further computer-signal analysis. However, the integrity of the recorded signal is only as good as the original data acquisition system permits.

Relationship between the Characteristics of the Recorded Signal and the Data Acquisition System

The time- and amplitude-dependent parameters of the physiologic signal which is recorded necessarily place constraints on the type of data acquisition system used. For example, very low amplitude signals will require amplification and/or averaging for proper display. Signals which are easily contaminated by movement artifact (low frequency noise) or 60-Hz power-line noise will require filtering. Some recording systems cannot reliably record very high frequency signals; for example, the movement of the ink pen of a strip-chart recorder may not be able to reliably follow the highest frequency EMG signals and the A/D converter of some computer systems may not be able to record very high frequency signals.

PHYSIOLOGIC SIGNAL CHARACTERISTICS

The first step in choosing the appropriate data acquisition system is to define the characteristics of the electrical signal of interest. The amplitude and frequency ranges of most normal physiologic signals are reported in Table 3–1. These parameters will often need to be revised when pathologic signals are being observed. In neuropathology, the amplitude and frequency of the electrical signal are often reduced (as in myopathy and neuropathy); however in some cases (such as anterior horn-cell disease with resultant collateral sprouting), the amplitude and/or frequency of signals may be increased.

CHARACTERISTICS OF THE RECORDING SYSTEM

When evaluating a recording system for the defined physiologic signal, the characteristics of the data acquisition system must be defined. The system's recording characteristics are also defined in terms of amplitude- and time-dependent parameters. All the components of the data acquisition system must be considered when evaluating its recording characteristics. These components may include the recording electrode, input amplifier, signal processor, A/D converter, and display device (monitor, analog or digital meter, oscilloscope, etc.). The system may implement very specific signal-processing features: simple signal amplification, differential amplification, signal averaging, integration, and bandpass filtering. The presence of these features and the associated parameters must be identified.

If the parameters of the physiologic signal exceed the capabilities of the recording system in *either* the time- or amplitude-dependent properties, then the output of the system will not be a true representation of the physiologic event. For example, if the amplitude of the input signal exceeds the capability of an amplifier, it may saturate the amplifier. That is, the full range of signal cannot be displayed, and the signal may appear to be "clipped" (or flattened on one end). (*It is also possible to damage an amplifier if the electrical signal is significantly greater than the rated maximum allowable input*.) The bandwidth (or frequency response) of the amplifier defines the range in which electrical signals are reliably reproduced; signals of frequencies outside of the rated frequency response of the system may be attenuated (reduced in amplitude) or may not be displayed.

Some other features of the recording system need to be identified to properly interface the patient with the equipment. The type of recording electrode configuration and electrode size will be dictated by the use of monopolar or bipolar recording techniques and the use of differential amplification. The ability to remove noise from the physiologic recording will also be affected by all of these conditions. The noise of the external environment can be electronically filtered out of the recorded signal as long as their frequency ranges do not overlap.

The relationship between the characteristics of the physiologic signal and the data-acquisition system can be illustrated in the following example in which the EMG signal of the biceps muscle is recorded. First, two surface recording electrodes are placed over the muscle belly. The distance which separates the electrodes is larger than any single myoneural junction. Different motor unit potentials are seen by the two electrodes, and these electrodes are, therefore, *widely spaced* with respect to the source. The EMG signals are amplified by a differential amplifier. The signals from the ECG, a distant noise source, are seen as the same noise by the two electrodes (which are *closely placed* with respect to the noise), and the ECG signal will be rejected by the differential amplifier. On the other hand, if one surface EMG electrode is placed over the biceps muscle and the second is placed on the soleus muscle of the leg, then the signals of the ECG will not be seen as the same noise to both recording electrodes (which are *widely spaced* with respect to the source), and the differential amplifier will pass the ECG along with the EMG signal.

Bandpass filtering can be used to improve the display of this EMG signal with respect to all the noise in the recording environment. Movement artifact (low frequency noise, i.e., DC to 10 Hz) and 60-Hz AC line noise can contaminate an EMG recording made with surface electrodes. The frequency range of interest for the EMG signal is about 60 to 1000 Hz. An amplifier for surface EMG signals usually includes a filter which *passes* signals above 60 Hz; this effectively eliminates contamination from signals at or less than 60 Hz, such as the ECG signal. Surface EMG signals are generally less than 1000 Hz, and signals greater than that can be filtered out. Thus, an amplifier for surface EMGs include a bandpass filter which passes (or keeps) a band of frequencies from 60 to 1000 Hz.

When the EMG signal is recorded from needle electrodes, the problem of noise is treated differently. Motor unit potentials are in a range from DC to 10,000 Hz. In this case, the bandpass filter passes signals from DC to 10,000 Hz, and a *60-Hz notch filter* can be used to eliminate the 60-Hz noise. In this case, a high-pass filter (which passes high frequencies and eliminates low frequency signals) cannot be used because the physiologic signal and the possible noise from movement are in the same frequency range. Greater skill on the part of the examiner is required to prevent contaminating the motor unit potential with movement artifacts.

THERAPEUTIC ELECTRICAL STIMULATION SYSTEMS

Electrical stimulation is applied to the body for therapeutic purposes for a variety of applications: pain control, muscle re-education of partially denervated muscle, rehabilitation of innervated muscle, control of edema, wound healing, bone healing, and the infusion of pharmacologic agents. These clinical applications are discussed in detail in subsequent chapters. This section describes features which are common to electrical stimulation instruments: a signal generator, stimulating electrodes, and controls for the modulation of the electrical stimulation. This section also reviews types of electrode designs and choices in stimulation parameters which are available. The effectiveness of therapeutic stimulation is dependent on the physiologic response of the stimulated tissues to the applied electricity. The physiologic response of excitable tissues following different types of electrical stimulation dictates the choice of therapeutic devices and stimulation parameters which are employed.

Signal Generator

The signal generator for therapeutic stimulators consists of a power supply, oscillator circuits, and output amplifier.

The *power supply* is either a *DC* source (direct current or unidirectional flow of electrons) or an *AC* source (alternating current or bidirectional flow of electrons) (Fig. 3–18). DC power supplies provide low voltages in the form of a battery (a source of chemically stored electrical charge). Conventional AC power supplies use 115-V, 60-Hz alternating current, or *line current.*

Most therapeutic stimulators deliver current (or voltage) at levels which are different than that provided by the power supply. A network of devices (transformer,

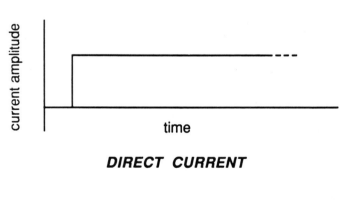

DIRECT CURRENT

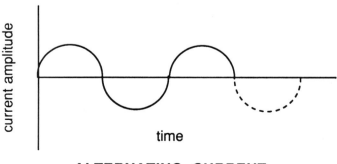

ALTERNATING CURRENT

FIGURE 3–18. Power supplies may provide either DC (direct current) or AC (alternating current). The waveforms of DC (*top*) and AC (*bottom*) currents are illustrated.

rectifier, filter, and regulator) converts the power to the proper form for clinical use. The *transformer* transforms DC to AC or AC to DC; transformers may also step up a voltage (or current) or step down a voltage (or current). The *rectifier* and *filter* are used together to convert AC to DC. The *regulator* ensures the output of the device is either constant current or constant voltage.

The *oscillator* circuits allow the frequency characteristics of therapeutic alternating current to be controlled or modulated by the clinician. Oscillators provide control over such parameters as the frequency, pulse duration, duty cycle, rise and decay (fall) times.

The *output amplifier* provides final regulation of the constant current (or constant voltage) to the patient, regardless of changing impedances (within a specified range) at the electrode site or skin-electrode interface.

Applied Stimulus

Electrical stimulation is therapeutically applied to the body by a controlled stimulus, which is either a constant current or constant voltage. The waveform of the stimulation (Fig. 3–19) and a range of time-dependent and amplitude-dependent parameters must be specified for patient safety and treatment efficacy.

CONSTANT CURRENT VERSUS CONSTANT VOLTAGE

As previously discussed, a constant current source is preferable to a constant voltage source for most physiologic applications. The impedance of the electrodes, of the biological material, and of the electrode-body interface may change during stimulation. However, with constant current stimulation, the changes in impedance do not change the current flowing through the biological tissues. It is the level of current which is responsible for the resultant physiologic effects.[6] Therefore, with constant current stimulation, changes in current are deliberate and not the result of impedance changes.

The physiologic effects of constant voltage and constant current pulses are modulated by the capacitance of the tissue, that is, the tissue's inherent tendency to store, rather than transmit, charge. This concept is particularly relevant to the therapeutic administration of electricity. When a *constant voltage* pulse is applied to the body, a large amount of current flows at the beginning of the pulse to charge the tissue capacitance (Fig. 3–20A). As the capacitor charges, the current declines, and it may reach a steady state if the pulse duration is long enough. Because of the large initial current flow at the onset of the pulses, the *effective* pulse duration may be less than the duration of the applied voltage pulse.

When a *constant current* pulse is applied to the body (Fig. 3–20B), the current which is transmitted to the tissue is unchanged over time. The voltage at the tissue rises rapidly because of current flow through the resistive portion of the electrode-tissue impedance; this is followed by a slow rise in voltage as the tissue capacitance is charged.

STIMULUS PARAMETERS

Electrical stimulation parameters for therapeutic applications are defined in terms of the stimulus waveform and its time-, frequency-, and amplitude-dependent properties. The stimulus *waveform* is the visual representation of the current or voltage. For therapeutic waveforms, clinicians frequently describe waveforms as either direct cur-

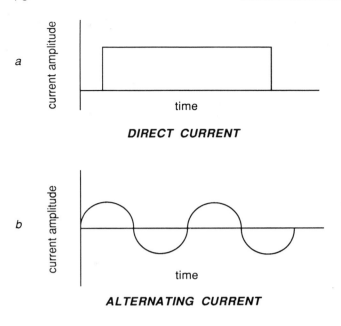

a

current amplitude

time

DIRECT CURRENT

b

current amplitude

time

ALTERNATING CURRENT

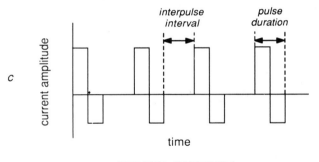

c

current amplitude

interpulse
interval

pulse
duration

time

PULSED CURRENT

FIGURE 3–19. Types of therapeutic waveforms: (*A*) DC (direct current) is the continuous unidirectional flow of charged particles with respect to baseline; (*B*) AC (alternating current) is the uninterrupted flow of charged particles which is bidirectional with respect to the baseline; (*C*) pulsed current is the uni- or bi-directional flow of charged particles that periodically ceases for a finite time before the next event.

rent, alternating current, or pulsed current (Fig. 3–19). In this context, DC is defined as the continuous unidirectional flow of charged particle in which the waveform characteristics do not change over time (Fig. 3–19A). The term *galvanic* has been used historically in the literature to describe an uninterrupted DC waveform.

AC is the uninterrupted bidirectional flow of charged particles (Fig. 3–19B). AC waveforms may be symmetrical (Fig. 3–21A) or asymmetrical (Figs. 3–21B and 3–21C) with reference to the baseline. The term *faradic* has been used historically to describe the unbalanced asymmetrical biphasic waveform (Fig. 3–21C). *Pulsed* (pulsatile or interrupted) current is the unidirectional or bidirectional flow of charged particles which periodically ceases for a finite period of time before the next event (Figs. 3–19C and 3–21A, 3–21B, and 3–21C). A *pulse* is an isolated electrical event separated by a finite period of time from the next event. The *interpulse interval* is the time between pulses (Fig. 3–22).

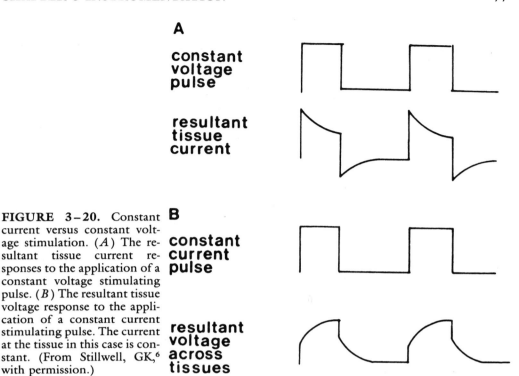

A

constant voltage pulse

resultant tissue current

B

constant current pulse

resultant voltage across tissues

FIGURE 3–20. Constant current versus constant voltage stimulation. (*A*) The resultant tissue current responses to the application of a constant voltage stimulating pulse. (*B*) The resultant tissue voltage response to the application of a constant current stimulating pulse. The current at the tissue in this case is constant. (From Stillwell, GK,[6] with permission.)

Time-Dependent Parameters

Pulsed current is described by special time-dependent properties of the pulse. (Because AC and DC waveforms are defined here as *continuous* events, these particular time-dependent terms do not apply.) The *phase* is the current flow in one direction for a finite period of time. The pulsed waveform may be *monophasic* or *biphasic*. In the monophasic waveform (Fig. 3–23), the pulse is equal to the phase, since the waveform deviates in one direction from the baseline and returns to the baseline after a finite time. The biphasic pulse (Fig. 3–22) is one that deviates in one direction from the baseline and then deviates in the opposite direction from the baseline before the pulse is complete. A biphasic waveform may be symmetrical (Fig. 3–21A) or asymmetrical (Figs. 3–21B and 3–21C). In the *symmetrical biphasic* waveform, all the waveform parameters (amplitude, duration, and rate of rise and of decay of the waveform) are identical with respect to the baseline (Figs. 3–21A and 3–24A). In the *asymmetrical biphasic* waveform, one or more of the waveform parameters is unequal with respect to the baseline. Asymmetrical biphasic waveforms may be *balanced* (Fig. 3–21B) or *unbalanced* (Figs. 3–21C and 3–24B). In a balanced asymmetrical waveform, the phase charges (that is, the areas under the curve above and below the baseline) are electrically equal. In an unbalanced asymmetrical waveform, the phase charges are electrically unequal.

The *phase duration* is the time elapsed from the beginning to the end of one phase (Fig. 3–25). The *interphase (intrapulse) interval* is the time between two successive components of a pulse when no electrical activity occurs (Fig. 3–25). *Pulse duration* (pulse width) is the time elapsed from the beginning to the end of *all* phases in one pulse (Fig. 3–25). The *interpulse interval* is the time between two successive pulses.

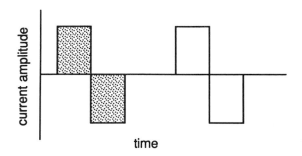

SYMMETRICAL BIPHASIC WAVEFORM
A

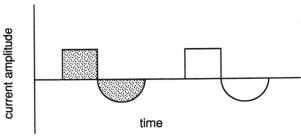

**BALANCED ASYMMETRICAL
BIPHASIC WAVEFORM**

B

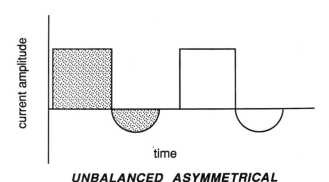

**UNBALANCED ASYMMETRICAL
BIPHASIC WAVEFORM**

C

FIGURE 3–21. Biphasic types of pulsed current. The biphasic waveform may be (*A*) symmetrical, or (*B, C*) asymmetrical with respect to the reference. The asymmetrical biphasic waveform may be (*B*) balanced (i.e., the phase charges are electrically equal), or (*C*) unbalanced (i.e., the phase charges are electrically unequal).

The *rise time* is the time for the leading edge of the phase to increase from the baseline to the peak amplitude of the phase (Fig. 3–26). The *decay (fall) time* is the time for the terminal edge of the phase to return to the zero baseline from the peak amplitude of the phase.

Frequency-Dependent Properties

Both alternating and pulsed currents are described by frequency-dependent properties. *Frequency* is the repetition rate of a waveform, expressed in pulses per second (pps)

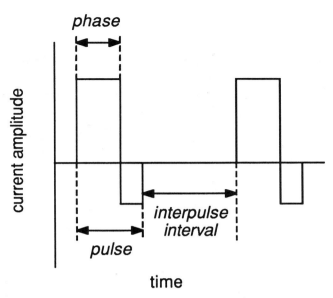

FIGURE 3–22. Time-dependent descriptions of biphasic pulses.

BIPHASIC WAVEFORM

or cycles per second (Hz). A *period* is the reciprocal of frequency (Fig. 3–24), that is, the time from a reference point of a pulse (or cycle) to the identical point of the next pulse (or cycle). In alternating currents, the waveform duration is equal to one period. In pulsed currents, the period equals the pulse duration *plus* the interpulse interval.

Amplitude-Dependent Properties

The amplitude-dependent property common to AC, DC, and pulsed current is *peak amplitude* (intensity), or the measure of the maximum value of current with reference to the baseline (Fig. 3–27A). For pulsed and alternating currents, the peak amplitude refers to the amplitude for each phase (Fig. 3–27B) and the *peak-to-peak amplitude* is the maximum amplitude between the two phases (Fig. 3–27C).

Pulsed and alternating currents can be further described in terms of a combination of time- and amplitude-dependent properties. *Phase charge* is the charge within each phase, this is, the integrated sum of intensity times time or the area which can be

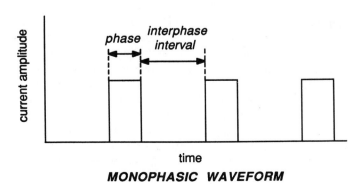

FIGURE 3–23. Monophasic type of pulsed current.

MONOPHASIC WAVEFORM

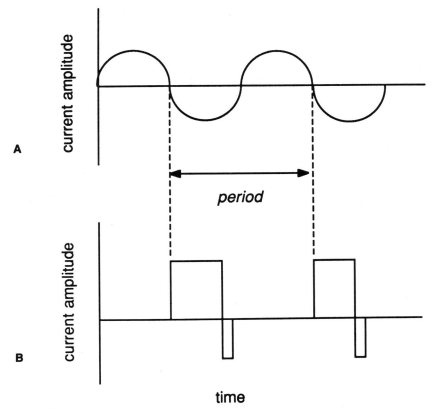

FIGURE 3–24. Period of a waveform is the time from a reference point of a cycle or pulse to the identical point of the next cycle or pulse. The period is shown for (*A*) a continuous alternating, or (*B*) pulsed current waveform.

measured under the curve of the waveform. The *pulse charge* is the sum of charges of the component phases of the pulse.

CURRENT MODULATIONS

Pulsed and alternating currents can be modulated, that is, varied within a specific time frame. These modulations may be used alone or in combination, and they may be sequential or varied with respect to pulse per cycle or a series of pulses per cycle. *Amplitude* modulations are variations in the peak intensity in a series of pulses or cycles. *Phase duration, pulse duration,* and the *frequency* may also be modulated. *Ramp* (surge) modulations are increases or decreases in the phase charges over time. Ramp modulations may be accomplished by changing either the phase/pulse duration or the amplitude of the phase/pulse (Fig. 3–28). The time period of the ramp should be specified for a complete description of the waveform.

The pattern of a series of pulses may be described in forms of time-dependent parameters. A *train* is a continuous repetitive sequence of pulses or cycles of pulsed current (Fig. 3–29A). A *burst* (interrupted train) is a finite series of pulses or an

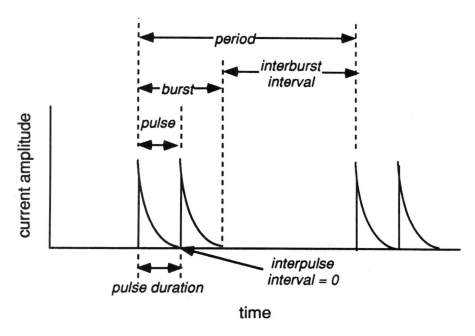

HIGH VOLTAGE PULSED CURRENT (HVPC)
MONOPHASIC ("TWIN-PULSE") WAVEFORM

FIGURE 3–25. Summary of time-dependent parameters illustrated in special type of monophasic waveform, the "twin-peak" waveform of high voltage pulsed current (HVPC).

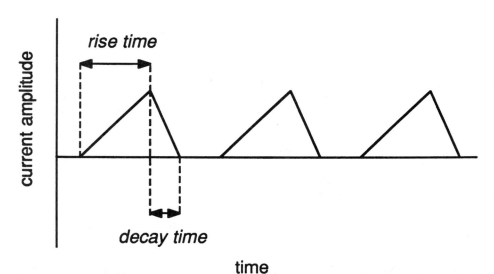

FIGURE 3–26. Rise and decay times of pulse waveform.

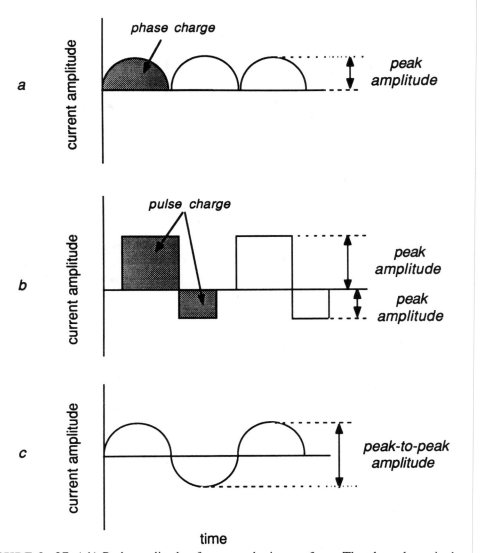

FIGURE 3–27. (*A*) Peak amplitude of a monophasic waveform. The *phase charge* is the area under the curve of the monophasic waveform. (*B*) Peak of each phase of a biphasic waveform. The *pulse charge* is the area under the curves of the biphasic waveform. (*C*) Peak-to-peak amplitude of alternating current.

"envelope" of pulsed current, delivered at an identified frequency, amplitude, or duration (Fig. 3–29*B*). The bursts are separated by an interburst interval; burst duration is the elapsed time from the beginning to end of one burst. The mixing of alternating current at different frequencies that are *out of phase* with each other is referred to as "beat" (Fig. 3–30) and is often used in the *interferential* technique. This particular electrotherapeutic technique is presented in detail in Chapter 6. The clinical significance of current modulation is discussed in the chapters which follow, specific to each electrotherapeutic application.

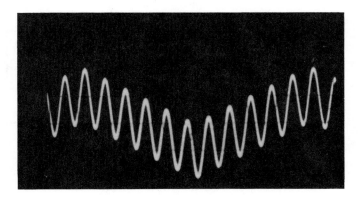

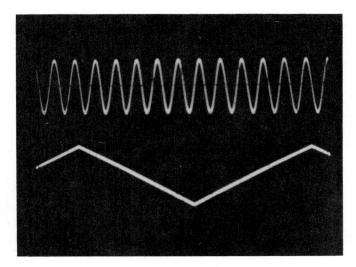

FIGURE 3–28. Ramp modulation of a waveform (*top*). The 250 Hz sine wave (*middle*) is modulated by a 25 Hz ramp (*bottom*) to produce the waveform at the top.

COMPUTATION METHODS FOR DESCRIBING CURRENT FLOW

Duty cycle is the ratio of on-time to *total*-time of trains or bursts of pulses (Fig. 3–31). The duty cycle is generally expressed as a percentage. That is, if the pulse duration of a waveform is 25 ms, and the period is 100 ms, then the duty cycle is 25 ms/100 ms or 25 percent. The clinical implications of duty cycle are presented in Chapter 7 relative to the physiologic phenomenon of neuromuscular fatigue in response to electrical stimulation.

Electrode Systems

TYPES OF STIMULATING ELECTRODES

Electrodes are fabricated of an electrically conductive material that is used to transfer electric charge to biologic tissue (see Fig. 3–2). As in recording-electrode systems, therapeutic stimulating electrodes may be used on the skin's surface (i.e., transcutaneous) or percutaneous (i.e., invasive and penetrating the skin). Surface elec-

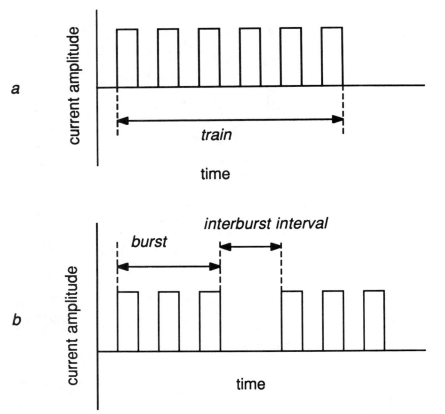

FIGURE 3–29. (*A*) Train of pulses and (*B*) bursts of pulses.

trodes generally require skin preparation to reduce skin impedance and the use of an electrolyte-coupling medium. Surface electrodes may be made of metal, silicon, or a polymer. Percutaneous electrodes come into direct contact with body fluids and tend to have a lower impedance than surface electrodes; percutaneous electrodes may be needles that are inserted or fine wires that are introduced onto nerves or muscles either surgically or with a syringe.

SIZE OF STIMULATING ELECTRODES

As previously described for electrodiagnostic systems, with uniform electrode conductivity, current density is inversely proportional to the electrode size (surface contact area). As the contact area of the stimulating electrode decreases for a specified current intensity, current density increases. This phenomenon explains why the smaller electrode in a monopolar configuration is selected to be the *active* electrode while the larger electrode serves as the dispersive or reference electrode. Because electrode size is directly proportional to current flow, larger electrodes have lower impedance; that is, for a given voltage, a larger electrode provides a greater current flow.

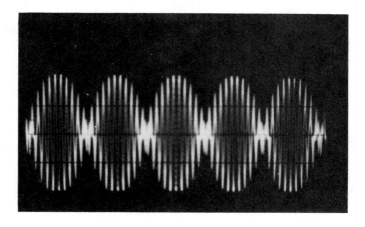

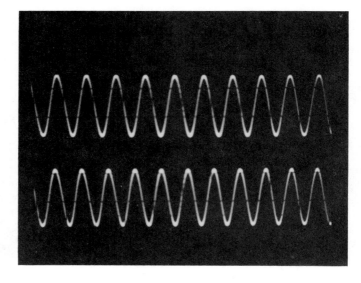

FIGURE 3–30. The waveform at the beat frequency of 120 Hz (*top*) results from adding two sinusoidal waveforms, one at 1000 Hz (*middle*) and the second at 1120 Hz (*bottom*). Display scales are 5 ms/div (*top*) and 1 ms/div (*middle and bottom*).

ORIENTATION OF STIMULATING ELECTRODES

Electrodes in therapeutic electrical stimulating systems can be oriented in a monopolar, bipolar, or quadripolar configuration. As previously discussed, in the *monopolar* orientation, the electrode of the stimulating circuit is placed over the target tissue (active electrode), where the greatest effect is desired. A second, larger reference or dispersive electrode is placed at some distance from the active electrode (Fig. 3–3).

In the bipolar configuration, two electrodes from one circuit are placed over the target tissue (Fig. 3–4). One electrode is positive, and the other is negative. A reference electrode is not required. In the *quadripolar* design, electrodes from two or more circuits are positioned so that currents geometrically intersect (Fig. 3–32). This type of electrode placement may be used for the interferential stimulation technique. *Interferential stimulation technique* describes the presumed paths of current flow when quadripolar electrode orientation allows the currents from more than one circuit to intersect geometrically. That is, *quadripolar* refers to the position of the electrodes; the term *interferential*

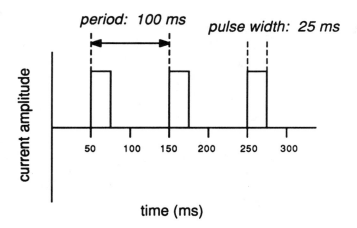

period (T) = 100 ms

pulse width (PW) = 25 ms

duty cycle = PW / T = 25 ms / 100 ms = 25 %

FIGURE 3–31. Duty cycle of a waveform.

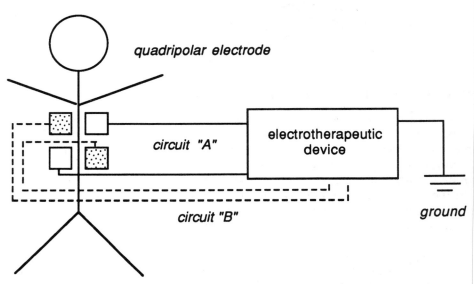

FIGURE 3–32. Quadripolar orientation of electrodes. The electrodes of two or more circuits are positioned so the currents intersect geometrically.

refers to a stimulation technique that uses the quadripolar orientation of the electrodes. This technique is described in detail in Chapter 6.

Relationship between the Physiologic Properties of Excitable Tissue and the Properties of the Stimulation System

To ensure that the desired physiologic effect is caused by the application of electrical stimulation of excitable tissue, it is imperative that proper stimulation parameters be chosen. When an electrical stimulation is chosen for a particular therapeutic application, the decision about the desired and preferred features of the electrical stimulation system is dictated by the excitable tissue to be stimulated and the type of effect that is desired. Electrical stimulation can cause a range of chemical and thermal alterations in the body, either directly or indirectly, and a range of neural and muscular responses can result. Furthermore, the parameters of electrical stimulation that effect changes in the intact neuromuscular system are different for the neuropathologic state. Clinical applications of electrical currents are discussed in detail in the chapters that follow.

When choosing an electrical stimulation system for a therapeutic application, careful consideration must be given to the parameters of the electrical signal, the site(s) for stimulation, as well as the relationships among dimensions and types of electrodes. The application of therapeutic currents have been described in the clinical literature in terms of modulations of AC, DC, or pulsatile current. Furthermore, various labels have been applied to stimulus levels (e.g., low and high voltage; low intensity current; and low, medium, and high frequency current). These terms are meaningful only within a specified context. For purposes of clarity in a physiologic application, it is necessary to state the *exact properties of the stimulus waveform* rather than use the name of a technique or other label that may not fully describe all the time- and amplitude-dependent properties of the waveform. The Standards Committee of the Section on Clinical Electrophysiology of the American Physical Therapy Association has summarized the signal parameters of electrical stimulation according to therapeutic goals.[7]

ELECTRICAL SAFETY

The annual incidence of electrical shock injuries and deaths from electrical devices in the home and work environments is steadily increasing. New instruments and advanced techniques for clinical practice, as well as the use of older equipment, mean that the physical therapist routinely must pay great attention to electrical safety hazards in the work setting.

A biomedical instrument is designed to meet *minimum* safety requirements. With age, protective components of the device may deteriorate. When a safety fault develops, the equipment can be a hazard to the patient and the staff. Periodic inspection and testing of grounding and safety systems are vital for the prevention of accident and injury. Preventive maintenance must be performed to avoid equipment hazards.

There are many hazardous sources of current. The most obvious is direct contact with a live conductor. However, any line-powered electric device may be a hazardous current source if there is a direct connection between the power source and the metal case, or by means of other accessible conductive parts of the device: a direct short circuit, conduction of current through biological fluids, indirect capacitive or inductive coup-

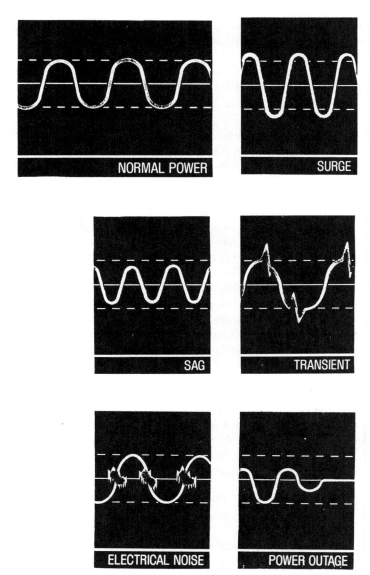

FIGURE 3–33. (*A*) Normal 60 Hz AC power, (*B*) power surge, (*C*) power sag, (*D*) electrical transient, (*E*) electrical noise, (*F*) power outage. (Courtesy of Wisconsin Electric Power Company, Milwaukee, Wisconsin.)

ling, or incorrect connections (such as improperly wired electrical outlets or probes plugged into the wrong jacks). Electrical hazards may also result from the misapplication of therapeutic currents. Explosive gases (oxygen or anesthetic agents) can be ignited by static electricity or direct or alternating currents. Instruments should be isolated from surges (Fig. 3–33) and other electrical transients that may be found on electrical power lines during everyday use and during a conversion from normal to emergency power.[8] These surges and transients may be injurious to solid-state (electronic) equipment and computers, and they may compromise the safety of the patient and the clinician. For this

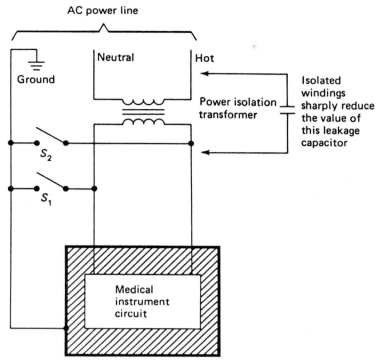

AC power line

Ground

Neutral

Hot

Power isolation transformer

Isolated windings sharply reduce the value of this leakage capacitor

S_2

S_1

Medical instrument circuit

FIGURE 3–34. A power isolation transformer in the medical device protects the patient from macroshock and microshock hazards, because there is no direct connection between the circuitry and the patient and the line-powered circuitry. Power for the circuit to the patient is transferred by transformer links that have low coupling capacitance. Switches S_1 and S_2 represent a short circuit between either side of the AC line and the grounded instrument case. Only a few milliamperes of current flow through either short circuit, which protects the patient from hazardous shocks.

reason, power-isolation transformers and surge-protection devices are frequently used (Fig. 3–34).[9]

Whether there is an electrical hazard depends on the magnitude of the available current and the presence of a complete circuit, often provided by a pathway to ground. Recall that *ground* (earth) refers to a return path for a source of current. (For a current to flow, it must leave the source, pass through objects which conduct electricity, and return to a source; this is a complete circuit.)

Definition of Electrical Hazards[10]

For a physiologic effect to occur, the body must become part of an electric circuit: Current must enter the body at one point and leave at some other point. According to Ohm's law, the greater the voltage (potential), the more current flowing through a wire; greater resistance limits the current flow. Three general effects can occur when an electric current flows through biological tissues: resistive heating of tissue, electrical stimulation of excitable tissue, and electrochemical burns (from direct current). In

TABLE 3–2 Hazardous Physiologic Effects of Increasing Levels of Current in the Adult Human Subject*

Perception of Current Flow† (The effects of being startled by the pain of electricity are not included here.)

DC: 3.5 mA (female) — 5.2 mA (male)
   60-Hz AC: 0.7 mA (female) — 1.1 mA (male)

Microshock AC Curents

10–20 μA at the myocardium (less than the level of perception)
If the current enters the heart by a transvenous catheter of the myocardial electrode, a minute current can produce a fatal shock without the patient perceiving anything.

Macroshock AC Currents

5 mA in subcutaneous tissue
If the current flow is from the body surface through the skin, a relatively large amount of current is needed to produce a harmful shock.

(Cannot) "Let-Go" AC Current

10.5 mA (female) — 16 mA (male)

Respiratory Effects of AC Current

18–22 mA across the chest

Ventricular Fibrillation with AC Current‡

During cardiac catheterization: 180 μA may cause fibrillation
From arm-to-leg: 215 mA may cause fibrillation
Across the chest of 150-lb man: 320 mA may cause fibrillation§

Electrical Burns

More than 250 mA, more than 1000 V (A small current (several amps) can cause burns if it is sustained, due to power dissipation.)

   *Adapted from Geddes,[11] Dalziel,[12] and Sances and associates.[13]
   †Current levels for the perception of pain depend on the type of electrode with which the current is applied to the body, the waveform of the applied current, the region of the body to which the current is applied, the skin resistance, and the resistance offered by subcutaneous fat.
   ‡For defibrillation, required as a treatment for ventricular fibrillation, 6–10 A is applied across the chest.
   §The amount of current that causes fibrillation increases with frequency of stimulation and body size; the DC threshold for fibrillation is higher than for AC current.

physiologic systems, it is high *current* levels that cause physiologic damage. Some physiologic effects of increasing levels of current in the adult human subject are listed in Table 3–2.

HAZARDS OF ALTERNATING CURRENT

In *macroshock*, the body is exposed to perceptible levels of electric current. Currents as low as 1 mA (at 60-Hz AC) are perceived as a tingling sensation; 16-mA current causes muscles to contract so the individual cannot let go. Higher levels of electricity can cause tissue damage, respiratory arrest, and cardiac arrest. More than 80 mA of current can cause ventricular fibrillation as well as skeletal muscle contractions that are so rapid and forceful that involuntary jerking can pull the person away from the contact with the electrical source or break bones. A startling reaction caused by macroshock currents can result in secondary accidents (falling, etc.). *Microshock* occurs with exposure to currents below the threshold of perception which, when applied directly to the myocardium with sufficient density (i.e., with cardiac catheter tips), can produce ventricular fibrillation. Currents in this range generally are not regulated by building codes because they are usually not a threat to life, except under unusual circumstances.

HAZARDS OF HIGH FREQUENCY AC

While high frequency AC was formerly thought to be innocuous, this type of current can cause hemorrhagic lesions of the heart and ventricular fibrillation at high current densities. High frequency AC currents can pass by radiation, capacitive coupling, or inductive coupling, and can produce effects at sites remote from the point of intended application. For this reason, patients with pacemakers must be protected from exposure to some types of electric and magnetic fields, such as those found in some motors, cautery devices, diathermy and microwave units, and magnetic resonance imaging (MRI) devices. It is particularly noteworthy that external fields created by these devices may turn off demand-type cardiac pacemakers.

HAZARDS OF DIRECT CURRENT

Injury can be caused by direct current, even at low amplitudes. For example, cutaneous burns can result from electrolytic effects. The fibrillation threshold for DC currents is higher than for AC currents; the extent of this difference has not been explicitly defined.

Grounding and Ground Faults

Wall receptacles are fed by a conduit with a black wire to a 115-V transformer. This is the *hot* wire through the circuit breaker. The *neutral* or white wire goes to the joint terminal of two 115-V circuits: it goes to ground (earth) and the transformer casing. Therefore, because the neutral wire is grounded, a power voltage exists between the hot (black) wire and any other metal object that is also grounded (Fig. 3–35). If the wire insulation is defective in an instrument, and the case of the instrument is *hot*, a current can pass through a person if he or she simultaneously is touching the hot case and providing a path to ground. This generally is not a problem if the third *ground* (green) wire is intact and provides a low impedance path for the current flow.

However, *ground faults* can develop. In a ground fault, a current pathway exists from the hot wire directly to ground as shown by the arrows, indicating current flow through the person in Figure 3–36A.[19] The problem of a ground fault exists if a person of low resistance is in contact with a *hot* device and is grounded; in this way the person becomes the path of least resistance for current flow from the device to ground (Fig. 3–37A). Caution should be exercised when using equipment with metal casings. If an active current is shorted to the casing, a person (patient or clinician) touching the metal case could get a shock. *Ground fault interrupters* (GFIs) sense these abnormal conditions and cut the power to the device; thus, the person no longer serves as a path for the current to flow to ground (Fig. 3–36B).

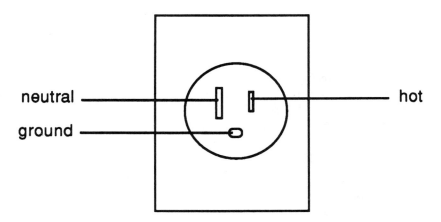

hot: ungrounded circuit conductor
     black wire

neutral: grounded circuit conductor
        white wire

ground: equipment grounding conductor
        green wire

FIGURE 3–35. Wiring diagram of a "polarized" electrical outlet; the slots for the neutral (*larger*) and hot (*smaller*) are identified.

The use of GFIs is based on the principle that all the current in a hot wire returns through the neutral wire. GFIs compare the currents of the hot (black) and neutral (white) wires. If the GFI detects more than 3 mA current difference between the hot and neutral, it interrupts all power to the equipment (see Fig. 3–37B). The GFI is installed on the wall receptacle. Once tripped (i.e., it terminates current flow to all equipment on that same electrical circuit), the GFI can be reset manually with the reset switch on the receptacle. A tripped GFI does not trip the circuit breaker.

Special care should be taken when the patient is connected to two pieces of equipment. If the ground connections are separate in these two devices, current can flow from the higher to the lower voltage machine by way of the patient.

In some new medical instruments (such as evoked-potential averaging computers and electrical stimulators for EMG examinations) in which the patient is intentionally grounded, the device is equipped with a special circuit to stop the current flow to the patient in the event of a fault. The operator's manual or a biomedical engineer should be consulted to determine if this feature exists on a piece of equipment.

Leakage Current

Leakage currents exist in all AC instruments. Insulated conductors have *stray* capacitance, and wire insulation can fail. Usually, the instrument case is at ground

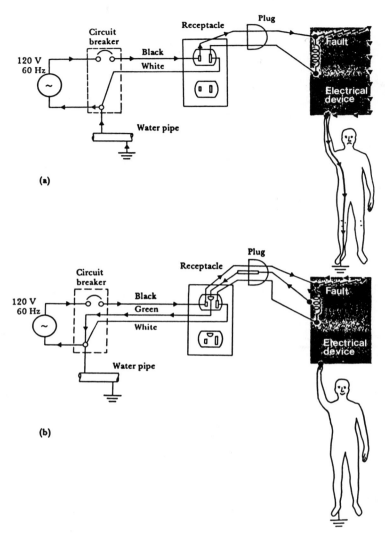

FIGURE 3–36. The condition called *macroshock* occurs when there is a ground fault from the hot line to the equipment case. This may occur, (*A*) when the case is not grounded, and (*B*) when the case is grounded. (From Webster, JE,[9] with permission.)

potential. However, a broken ground connection may permit a voltage to be carried on the case. A person touching the case and ground will provide a path for the leakage current to pass through (Fig. 3–38).

An additional hazard may occur when an electrical device which is carrying a leakage current is touched by the clinician (who is high resistance but not grounded), who in turns touches the patient (who is grounded). In this case, the leakage current may be passed onto the patient, who may get a shock. A short circuit may cause a fault current to take the path of least resistance to ground. This may trip the circuit breaker, but only *after* the hazard has occurred.

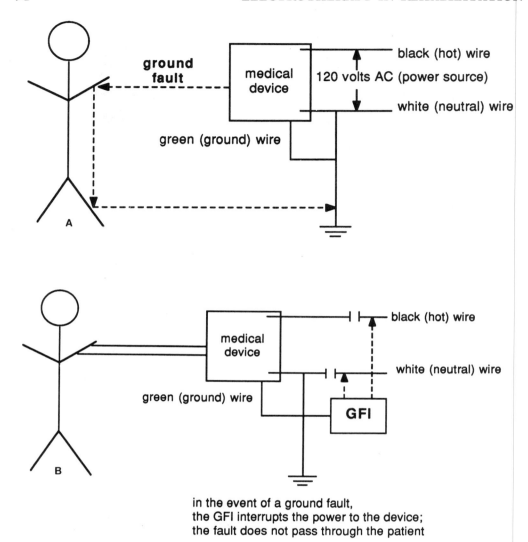

FIGURE 3–37. Schematic diagrams of (*A*) the path of current in a ground fault and (*B*) the effect of a ground fault interrupter (GFI) in a patient circuit.

Methods of Patient Isolation

In the ideal world, *isolated circuits* connect directly to the patient to eliminate current paths through the patient. It is best to prevent the existence of a conductive path from isolated and ground circuits; the current flowing by leakage or in a fault should be limited to less than 1 mA. Perfect isolation is achieved if this current is infinitely small or if it is separated by an infinite distance from other parts of the device.

In the real world, a small capacitance exists between isolated and grounded circuits. However, the problems this presents can be minimized with high isolation impedance

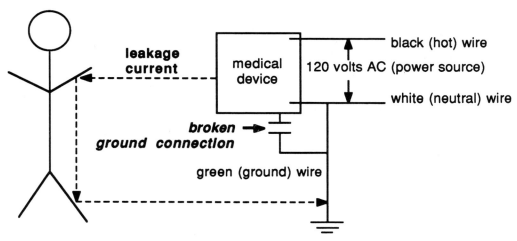

FIGURE 3-38. Schematic diagram of the pathway of leakage current.

(10 MΩ = 1 × 10^7 ohms), optical isolation of the patient from electrical devices, and the use of line isolation monitors and ground-fault interrupters.

Optical isolation prohibits the direct passage of current to the patient. Electrically recorded signals from the patient are preamplified and converted to light waves by an optical transmitter (Fig. 3-39). For example, a light-emitting diode (LED) converts the output of an amplifier to a low-intensity light; an optical receiver receives the light impulses and outputs that information to another amplifier. Optical isolation protects the patient against leakage currents, insulation breakdown, and short circuits by eliminating the direct physical connection between the patient and the source of stray voltages from the medical instrument.

A *line isolation monitor* is a detector that trips an alarm if the impedance between the power line and ground drops below a specified level (e.g., 60 KΩ), which in turn trips the circuit (Fig. 3-40).[14] Isolation techniques reduce the hazards of electrically powered equipment, but the patient is *not* protected if a grounding connection fails.

Recommendations for a safe work environment are presented in Table 3-3.

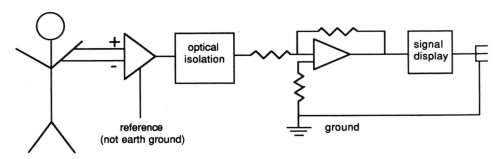

FIGURE 3-39. Schematic diagram of the use of optical isolation to protect the patient.

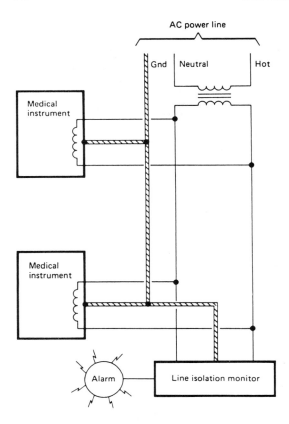

FIGURE 3–40. Line isolation monitor. When the impedance of either leg of the AC line drops below 60,000 Ω above ground, the line isolation monitor detector is activated. The detector then trips the alarm to its left. (From DuBovy, J: INTRODUCTION TO BIOMEDICAL ELECTRONICS, 1978. Reproduced with permission of McGraw-Hill/Gregg Division.)

Guidelines for Evaluation of the Safety of Electrodiagnostic and Electrotherapeutic Devices

CLINICIAN'S RESPONSIBILITIES

It is important that the clinician understand the techniques for proper operation of medical instruments as well as the potential hazards associated with the use of electric current. Responsible use of medical devices minimizes the risks to the patient and clinician of accidental electrical injury or death. While designers and manufacturers of medical devices have a responsibility to produce safe instruments, users of the equipment should take proper care of the equipment, arrange regular maintenance checks, and be alert to hazards that could occur in the lifetime of the machine.

Routine Maintenance

The clinician has a responsibility to perform routine safety checks of medical equipment to ensure that it is in proper working order. It is important to verify that electrical stimulators in diagnostic and therapeutic devices are providing the appropriate electrical signal to the patient and that use of the applied current or voltage will not put the patient or therapist at risk for injury. In many cases, the oscilloscope can be used to verify the stimulus characteristics of the equipment. This verification procedure is discussed below.

TABLE 3–3 Recommendations for a Safe Work Environment

The following specific techniques are suggested to minimize the risk to the patient and the clinician when electrical equipment is in use:

Use hospital grade 3-prong plugs.

Make sure power switches for instruments are well marked, and use power switches to turn the power on and off.

Never disconnect a machine from the wall power outlet with the power turned on.

Always check the power controls and other monitoring devices for perfect working order before applying the treatment to a patient.

Use UL-listed equipment: UL listing ensures that in a new piece of equipment, the leakage current is less than 5 mA at 60 Hz for most applications. (The UL listing is for the equipment design, not the individual piece of equipment, and it does not provide for changes that occur with age and use of equipment.)

Use ground fault interrupters (GFIs): If a fault current goes to ground, the GFI opens and interrupts the current flow to protect the patient.

Use optical isolation units: Optical isolation isolates the patient from the equipment ground.

There should be no metal in the pathway of low-, medium-, or high-frequency currents, fields, or waves.

Do not place electrical equipment next to radiator pipes or water pipes within reach of the patient or clinician.

Do not use cheater plugs, frayed plugs or cords, or extension cords.

Never pull the plug from the socket by pulling on the power cord.

Have repairs made to pilot lights or control functions which do not operate or which function sporadically or partially.

If water gets into any electrical equipment, have it serviced before use.

Perform routine safety checks of outlets, power plugs, and equipment performance; check power plugs and outlets for loose connections.

Call on the department of clinical or biomedical engineering: They use equipment safety testers to test leakage currents, evaluate the integrity of line cords, instrument filters, equipment front ends, and transformers in new and existing equipment.

Think twice about grounding the patient.

Technique for the use of ultrasound equipment:

Use rubber gloves to protect yourself when administering ultrasound under water.

Do not pull the cable connection of the movable angled ultrasound transducer head.

For shortwave and microwave diathermy and interferential units:

Prevent disruption of frequencies by not using interferential machines near short-wave diathermy, microwave, and ECG machines, and within 10 m of patients with pacemakers.

Do not treat patients with pacemakers with shortwave diathermy, microwave diathermy, or interferential therapy.

Provide treatment couches and chairs for shortwave diathermy and microwave diathermy that are made of wood or plastic, not metal.

Direct the antenna of microwave units against a wall to prevent leakage of radiation to the patient or clinician; patients and clinicians with metal-rimmed glasses can have microwaves reflected to their eyes.

Never drag diathermy or microwave machines by their "arms."

Oscilloscope Verification of Signal Characteristics

The oscilloscope is an instrument which can be used to identify and verify the characteristics of electrical signals that are produced by standard electrodiagnostic and electrotherapeutic devices used by physical therapists. The oscilloscope is useful in identifying signal characteristics because it can reliably display a wide band of frequency ranges (usually 0.2 Hz to 1 MHz) and a large range of amplitudes (usually 0.1 mV to 50 V).

The oscilloscope can be used to verify that the voltages and frequencies that a stimulator applies to the patient are in the expected ranges. Unfortunately, this voltage output is not always easily obtained for many medical devices used by physical therapists. Furthermore, the current that the patient receives is not represented in the oscilloscope display, nor are the properties of the electrode and the patient-electrode interface represented. The impedance which determines how the voltage is translated into a current stimulus cannot be measured or represented in this kind of output; however, the ranges of applied voltages and their associated pulse durations and frequencies can be identified.

The accuracy of recording devices can also be verified with the oscilloscope. The output of a generic stimulator can be simultaneously inputted into the recorder and the oscilloscope, and the signal characteristics can be compared.

OTHER SAFETY MEASURES

Always check power controls, current or voltage-intensity and frequency controls, pilot lights, current meters, and other monitoring devices for perfect working order. Have repairs made to controls which do not operate consistently.

The integrity of power plugs, and the secure fit of the plug in the wall outlet, should be assured. The ground of power plugs must *never* be removed. Do not use cheater plugs or extension cords. If the wall outlet is not adequate (e.g., the outlet is not grounded, it is too far away from the treatment room, or too many electrical devices are being served by the same circuit, causing the power to drop or the circuit breaker to trip) then an electrical engineer should correct the problem.

Remember that any fluid (e.g., saline, water, coffee, or baby's formula) in an electrical instrument can cause a short circuit; *the equipment must be serviced after an accident involving liquids.*

Use of Operator's Manuals

Operator's manuals are always provided with new pieces of equipment; when in doubt about the function of control switches and knobs, the manual should be consulted. If a manual is missing from older equipment, the manufacturer should be requested to provide a replacement copy. *The operator's manual should be kept with the device or should be easily accessible.* It is a valuable tool that documents the function of the device and its components. The manual can also be used to document the age of the equipment and repairs which have been made.

MANUFACTURER'S RESPONSIBILITIES

The manufacturer has a responsibility to produce safe instruments. Most reliable manufacturers will provide for the clinician and the clinical engineer basic performance characteristics of the device. This information, as well as specific techniques for safe operation are generally contained in the operator's manual. The clinician needs to be apprised of these performance characteristics for the equipment in standard terminology. This information is necessary to make appropriate choices about which devices to purchase, to identify failure of the device, and to follow appropriate methods for maintaining the equipment. Some manufacturers supply service contracts for instruments, which prohibit alterations or repairs from being made except by the manufacturer. Other vendors make schematic diagrams available to clinical engineers for maintenance and repair purposes. Finally, many manufacturers also provide customer support in the event that the equipment does not operate as expected.

THE ROLE OF BIOMEDICAL ENGINEERING

The department of biomedical engineering provides an extremely valuable service in safety testing of new and used medical equipment, repair, and the evaluation of performance standards of diagnostic and therapeutic devices. In some clinical settings, each piece of equipment which interfaces with a patient is subjected to safety inspections on a regular basis by the department of clinical engineering.

Biomedical engineers can evaluate the safety of individual pieces of equipment: they can test leakage currents, and monitor the integrity of line cords, instrument filters, transformers, and the *front ends* of instruments. Furthermore, engineers can monitor the safety of devices that are used in combination; they can provide necessary information about the role of patient grounding when the patient is connected to one or more devices.

Biomedical engineers can evaluate the electrical safety of the clinical environment in terms of total delivery of current; that is, they can evaluate the number of circuits in an area and present and potential power requirements. Engineers can also make recommendations about the accessibility of power outlets in a treatment area. The role of the clinical engineer in ensuring an electrically safe work environment should not be overlooked.

SUMMARY

The ability to effectively perform an electrodiagnostic or electrotherapeutic treatment procedure requires that the physical therapist understand the underlying physiologic or pathophysiologic mechanisms, as well as have a clear idea about how medical instrumentation can best be used in a particular patient setting. The information in this chapter is intended to serve as a general reference for devices which are presently available as well as equipment which will be used in the future. This chapter has reviewed general principles of instrumentation design for diagnostic and therapeutic equipment used by physical therapists, and general principles of electrical safety. It is hoped that this information will be used to make the process of selecting the appropriate device for a particular clinical application easier and to make the transition from using one device to another less complicated.

Determining the preferred therapeutic or diagnostic instrument for purchase can be a formidable task. The cost of devices which are intended for similar applications may vary. The cost-benefit trade-offs must be identified. The user must consider safety, portability, durability, ease of use, power demands, and the ability to upgrade functions and features and/or incorporate the device with other equipment which is currently in the clinical setting or which will be purchased. Are all the functions which are necessary for a particular application available to the clinician? Are all the functions available on the device necessary? What technical support is offered by the manufacturer or clinical engineer? Are the performance characteristics clearly available and appropriate for the clinical application?

During the last 15 to 20 years, there have been tremendous changes in the types of electrical instruments which are routinely found in physical therapy departments. Physical therapists are asking more questions about how a device works, how it can best be used in a particular clinical setting, whether a particular instrument or type of instrument is necessary, and what role it should play in evaluation and treatment.

The changing demands by third-party payers means that therapists are using hard-copy output to document the results from therapeutic and diagnostic systems. The use of computer systems by physical therapists in evaluation and treatment is becoming routine. Familiarity with general instrumentation such as oscilloscopes is no less a part of the clinician's skills.

Our rapidly changing technology makes solid-state devices more available. This means that newer equipment may have lower power requirements and may be more portable. Solid-state equipment may (or may not) be cheaper, quieter, and may (or may not) be less susceptible to contaminating noise from the outside world. It is also more sensitive to alterations in power supplied by AC power lines.

Choosing the preferred device for a particular application is an important task. The faces of instruments vary considerably between and among manufacturers. While these differences in outward appearance are easily identified, they do not necessarily translate into differences in function or performance. It is the *performance characteristics* (not the outward appearance of the device) that are critical and are more difficult to identify and characterize. Physical therapists are asking manufacturers of medical devices to standardize and clarify the electrical parameters of therapeutic and diagnostic stimulators. Therapists are consulting with clinical engineers to make sure that new and older devices are performing as expected. Biomedical engineers are also being asked to evaluate the safety of an instrument and of the entire clinical environment.

To facilitate and clarify communication among different professions, the Section on Clinical Electrophysiology of the American Physical Therapy Association has recently compiled *Electrotherapeutic Terminology in Physical Therapy*[7] and *Standard Terminology of Electrodiagnosis*. These documents enable physical therapists, engineers, and manufacturers to speak the same language about medical instrumentation. Our patients will benefit from this interdisciplinary sharing of information and our ability to adapt our skills in the face of ever-changing technology.

REFERENCES

 1. Basmajian, JV and DeLuca, CJ: Muscles Alive: Their Functions Revealed by Electromyography, ed 5. Williams & Wilkins, Baltimore, 1985.
 2. Geddes, LA: Electrodes and the Measurement of Bioelectric Events. Wiley Interscience, New York, 1972.
 3. Myklebust, JB, Cohen, BA, Sances, A, Jr, and Cusick, JF: Review of acquisition and analysis of somatosensory evoked potentials. J Clin Eng 5:33, 1980.
 4. Myklebust, BM, Gottlieb, GL, and Agarwal, GC: Orientation-induced artifacts in the measurement of monosynaptic reflexes. Neurosci Lett 48:223, 1984.
 5. Barolat-Romana, G, Myklebust, JB, Hemmy, DC, Myklebust, B, and Wenninger, W: Immediate effects of spinal cord stimulation in spinal spasticity. J Neurosurg 62:558, 1985.
 6. Stillwell, GK (ed): Therapeutic Electricity and Ultraviolet Radiation, ed 3. RML Library Series. Williams & Wilkins, Baltimore, 1983.
 7. Electrotherapeutic Terminology in Physical Therapy. Section on Clinical Electrophysiology of the American Physical Therapy Association, Alexandria, VA, 1990.
 8. Wisconsin Electric Power Company: Understanding Power Disturbances. Consumer Brochure, 1987.
 9. Webster, JE (ed): Medical Instrumentation: Application and Design. Houghton-Mifflin, Dallas, 1978.
10. Roth, HH, Teltscher, ES, and Kane, IM: Electrical Safety in Health Care Facilities. Academic Press, New York, 1975.
11. Geddes, LA and Baker, LE: Principles of Applied Biomedical Instrumentation, ed 2. Wiley Interscience, New York, 1975.
12. Dalziel, CF: Electric shock hazard. IEEE Spectrum 9:41, 1972.
13. Sances, A, Larson, SJ, Myklebust, J and Cusick, JF: Electrical injuries. Surg Gynecol Obstet 149:97, 1979.
14. DuBovy, J: Introduction to Biomedical Electronics. McGraw-Hill, New York, 1978.

CHAPTER 4

Electrical Evaluation of Nerve and Muscle Excitability

Charlene Nelson, M.A., P.T., E.C.S.

The skilled clinician will acknowledge that thorough evaluation of the patient may require electrophysiologic assessment of the integrity of the neuromuscular system. For example in a patient with diminished quadriceps function following a total knee arthroplasty, electrical testing can help to differentiate the presence of femoral nerve involvement versus inhibition of muscle contraction because of pain or apprehension. The physical therapist must know the indications for and appropriate selection of electrical tests, and the implications or significance of the test results.

Electrical tests used for clinical evaluation of the excitability and integrity of the neuromuscular system are divided into traditional tests and contemporary tests in this chapter. This classification is based primarily on the historical time periods over which the procedures were developed and have been used and is not intended to imply a value measure of the tests. The indications for and usefulness of each procedure will be discussed in their respective sections.

HISTORICAL REVIEW

Electrodiagnostic testing had its beginning in the mid- to late-1800s. An excellent historical review of traditional electrical evaluation techniques may be found in Sidney Licht's *Electrodiagnosis and Electromyography*.[1] The early recognition of motor points by Duchenne[2] and the later mapping of these points by other scientists, were major steps in the development of electrical testing. As instrumentation and understanding of electrophysiology developed during these early years, the strength-duration curve procedure and measurement of chronaxie were described and used on laboratory animals. Adrian reported using these electrodiagnostic techniques in humans in 1916.[3] Strength-duration curves, chronaxie measurements, and other electrical tests gained importance with their frequent use in evaluating peripheral nerve injuries during the two world wars. The tests are valuable when performed by skilled and experienced professionals. Their clinical use diminished, however, as newer technology provided electromyography and nerve-conduction testing. An understanding of the electrophysiologic rationale of traditional tests is basic to understanding contemporary electrical testing and to intelligent and effective application of electrotherapeutic techniques.

NEUROPHYSIOLOGIC PRINCIPLES OF ELECTRICAL EVALUATION

Neurophysiology of nerve and muscle is discussed in Chapter 1. Three important concepts underlie electrical stimulation for evaluation of neuromuscular function: (1) the intensity or strength of an electrical stimulus required to elicit a response must be sufficient to depolarize the nerve or muscle-cell membrane to the critical excitatory level (threshold); (2) the stimulus pulse duration, that is, the length of time the current is flowing in a single stimulus pulse, must be long enough to allow the membrane electropotential to reach threshold; and (3) the rise time of the stimulus pulse must be short enough for the stimulus intensity to reach the membrane's critical excitatory level before accommodation can occur. *Accommodation* is further described as a phenomenon in which the threshold of membrane excitability automatically rises when the membrane is stimulated with a stimulus of slowly increasing intensity. Nerve fibers accommodate at a much more rapid rate than muscle fibers.[4] Stimulators used for most of the traditional electrical tests and for nerve conduction tests utilize a square-waveform pulse, and therefore, accommodation is avoided.

For the purpose of this discussion of electrical testing, the concept of motor point needs clarification.[2,5] *Motor point* is defined as a small area overlying a muscle where a slight visible contraction is most easily elicited with a minimal-amplitude (intensity) electrical stimulus. This "normal" motor point is usually located near the proximal portion of the muscle belly. This area is more responsive because here the stimulus is activating the muscle through the motor nerve fibers, which enter the muscle near this site. When denervation occurs, the normal motor point site is no longer present and the most responsive area over the muscle fibers must be located and stimulated directly. This "muscle" motor point is usually found distal to the normal motor point. Diagrams of motor points are shown in the Appendix on page 400.

Contraindications and Precautions

All traditional electrical evaluation tests require similar safety precautions and are contraindicated in the same circumstances. For this reason the information presented in this section should be considered applicable to each of the traditional tests described in this chapter.

Electrical stimulation may interfere with the sensitivity of the demand pacemaker and should not be used with patients depending upon this cardiac-regulating device. Electrical stimulation should not be used over the carotid sinus because the stimulation may induce cardiac arrhythmia. To avoid the possibility of cardiac arrhythmia or fibrillation, electrodes should not be placed so the path of electrical current passes across the heart.[6] The effect of electrical stimulation on the developing fetus and on the pregnant uterus have not been determined; therefore, stimulation should not be applied over the abdominal area during pregnancy.

TABLE 4–1 Electrical Test for Reaction of Degeneration[5,10]

Status of Muscle Innervation	I Muscle Response Elicited with a Series of Short-Duration Pulses (<1 ms) Applied Continuously at Frequency ≥ 20–50 Hz (Usually Biphasic or AC Pulses)	II Muscle Response Elicited with Individual 100-ms Pulses (Usually Monophasic or Interrupted DC Pulses)
Normal peripheral nerve innervation	Smooth, continuous isotonic (tetanic) contraction	Brisk, individual twitch contraction
Partial RD: degeneration of part of nerve fibers	Partial or diminished tetanic contraction	Partial or diminished, sluggish individual contraction
Complete RD: degeneration of all nerve fibers; muscle tissue retains contractile elements	No contraction	Very slow, sluggish individual contraction
Absolute RD: degeneration of all nerve fibers; muscle tissue severely atrophic, fibrotic, or noncontractile	No contraction	No contraction

TRADITIONAL CLINICAL ELECTRICAL EVALUATION TESTS

Reaction of Degeneration Test

The reaction of degeneration (RD) test is a useful screening procedure for assessment of problems that may involve lower motor neurons. Normally innervated muscle will respond with a brisk twitch when stimulated with a short-duration pulse lasting less than 1 ms and also when stimulated with longer pulse durations, for example, 100 ms (Table 4–1). If these pulses are applied in rapid succession, the muscle will respond with a sustained or tetanic contraction. In contrast, a muscle that has lost its peripheral innervation will not respond to a stimulus of 1 ms or shorter but will contract in a sluggish manner when the longer pulse duration stimulus is applied.

When performing the classical RD test, also referred to as the faradic and galvanic test, a small, hand-held electrode is used to search as precisely as possible for the motor point of the muscle of interest. If a larger electrode is used, current will spread by volume conduction to other muscles, making the test less accurate. Figure 4–1 shows a sample setup for RD testing. The motor point area is first stimulated with a series of short-duration (less than 1 ms) pulses.[5] (See Table 4–1, part I.) The stimulus is applied at a frequency greater than 20 Hz which would be expected to produce a tetanic or sustained contraction; either a monophasic or biphasic waveform may be used. If a monophasic or asymmetrical biphasic waveform is used, the negative (cathode) electrode is used as the active stimulating electrode over the motor point, in keeping with the polar formula,[5] which states that an action potential is generated with the least

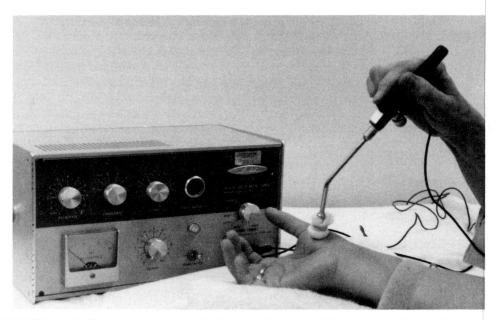

FIGURE 4–1. Setup for reaction of degeneration test (RD) using small handheld active electrode overlying abductor pollicis brevis muscle.

intensity of current using a cathodal stimulus. The rationale for this occurrence is described in Chapter 1. If a tetanic response occurs, the muscle has intact peripheral innervation. If no response or a sluggish response is seen, peripheral denervation is likely. The second part of the classical RD test (Table 4–1, part II) is stimulation of the involved muscle with a long-duration pulse (formerly termed *galvanic current*). This may be done with a make and break key of the pencil-type electrode, using a direct current stimulator or using a stimulator that will automatically provide a monophasic pulse of at least 100-ms duration and preferably longer. A slow or sluggish response to this part of the test indicates that contractile muscle tissue is present but that the muscle is either partially or completely denervated (see Table 4–1). Results of the RD test are reported as either normal innervation, that is, no reaction of degeneration, or as in varying states of degeneration. The reader is referred to Shriber for a more thorough explanation of the RD test.[5]

INDICATIONS FOR REACTION OF DEGENERATION TESTING

The RD test is usually not done until at least 10 days after onset of the problem, so that the process of neural degeneration can progress to a stage in which electrical changes would appear. An abbreviated form of the test for reaction of degeneration may be used as a quick screening test for differentiating a muscle with normal peripheral innervation from a muscle with peripheral denervation. Usually, only the first part of the test is necessary to establish the presence of normal innervation. Many small, portable, neuromuscular electrical stimulators deliver suitable stimuli for this test. If an abnormal response is seen, signifying the presence of a reaction of degeneration, more sophisticated electrical testing would be indicated to clarify the problem. The RD test is only a gross screening procedure and should not be expected to differentiate or precisely identify the location of pathology. The RD test may be indicated in conditions of unexplained paralysis. If there is a question of differentiating functional or psychogenic paralysis from an organic or physical pathology, a normal RD would be consistent with intact peripheral innervation. The clinician will realize that an abnormal response to the RD test only signifies a problem in some part of the peripheral motor nervous system. A normal response does not eliminate the possibility of pathology in the central nervous system or in the muscular system, and, of course, multisystem problems could be present. The following case report illustrates an application of the RD test.

CASE STUDY

1

JL is a 66-year-old male who is referred for rehabilitation following a surgical procedure for total hip replacement on the right lower extremity. He has been followed postoperatively for 2 weeks and was noted shortly after surgery to have paralysis of ankle dorsiflexors on the operated right lower extremity. The tibialis anterior, extensor digitorum, and peroneus longus muscle strength grades are zero. Plantar flexion and strength of muscles about the knee have good strength grades. Sensation over the dorsal great toe web space is diminished; deep tendon reflexes are normal except for ankle dorsiflexion. Dorsiflexion and sensation on the left, nonoperated extremity are normal.

RD TEST REPORT

A test for RD was performed 2 weeks after surgery, resulting in an absent response (presence of RD) in the tibialis anterior and extensor digitorum muscles, and normal response (no RD) in the gastrocnemius muscle of the involved extremity. The tibialis anterior muscle of the contralateral extremity also shows a normal response.

The presence of denervation (RD) in the two muscles of the involved extremity is consistent with degeneration of the peroneal nerve. This test does not clarify the anatomic site of the lesion, for example, at the fibular head, peroneal component of the sciatic nerve in the thigh, or at a more proximal location. Furthermore, the test does not completely rule out the additional possibility of an upper motor neuron problem. Follow-up strength-duration, chronaxie, or nerve conduction testing and electromyography would be indicated for this patient, and simulated reports of these tests on this patient are given in their respective sections of this chapter.

Strength-Duration Curve and Chronaxie Test

Strength-duration curves and chronaxie measurements were widely used for electrodiagnosis of peripheral nervous system disorders from the 1930s to the 1960s. Their frequency of use sharply declined with the development of nerve conduction testing and electromyography. When performed by the clinician experienced in strength-duration (S-D) curve and chronaxie measurements, these tests provide a reliable means of assessing the location, severity, and progress of peripheral motor-nerve degeneration and regeneration.[7] The S-D curve has the limitation of providing data to evaluate neuromuscular integrity only in the local fibers responding to the stimulus. This limitation can only be overcome by testing several muscles in the distribution of the nerve(s) of interest. Because of the current emphasis on nerve conduction tests and electromyography, new instrumentation for performing S-D curves and chronaxie testing has been nearly absent from the market. Clinicians have demonstrated a preference for the contemporary electrical testing techniques, and a revival of the traditional testing techniques is not anticipated. An understanding of the electrophysiologic concepts of chronaxie and the strength-duration relationship is essential, however, for effective selection and utilization of clinical electrotherapeutic procedures such as neuromuscular electrical stimulation and transcutaneous electrical nerve stimulation (TENS), and for effective application of both traditional and contemporary electrical evaluation techniques.

The three concepts of intensity, pulse duration, and rise time of the electrical stimulus described in the preceding section on neurophysiologic principles of electrical evaluation are emphasized here and now take on quantitative values. Excitable tissue will respond by discharging an action potential only if an applied electrical stimulus meets certain criteria of both intensity (amplitude) or strength, and pulse duration or time. The *intensity* of the stimulus must be strong enough to depolarize the membrane to its threshold level for excitability, and, in addition, the stimulus must be of sufficient *duration* to overcome the capacitance of the membrane. *Rheobase* refers to a minimal intensity of stimulus amplitude (strength) required to elicit a minimal visually perceptible muscle contraction, and *chronaxie* relates to a specific stimulus duration. A stimulus of a very long (infinite) pulse duration and of amplitude just strong enough (minimal intensity) to depolarize the cell membrane to its threshold level of excitability, causing an action potential, is called a *rheobase* strength stimulus. Chronaxie is the minimal pulse *duration* of a stimulus of twice rheobase strength that will cause the excitable cell membrane to discharge. The chronaxie for nerve is short, usually a pulse duration less than 1 ms, while the chronaxie for muscle is much longer, usually longer than 10 ms.[8] Chronaxies for several muscles and for different types of nerve fibers have been determined.[8,9]

Plotting an S-D curve and determining chronaxie values require an electrical-stimulation instrument capable of producing square-wave monophasic pulse stimuli of at least 10 selectable, precise pulse durations ranging from 0.01 to 100 ms. The instrument must also have a meter for accurate measurement of stimulus intensity. Wynn Parry's[7] discussion of S-D curves proposes using a constant voltage stimulator rather than a constant current stimulator. He relates that although the output of the constant current stimulator is more stable (because it compensates for changes in tissue impedance), both types of stimulators give equally accurate results, and the constant voltage stimulator is preferred in the interest of patient comfort and tolerance. He further reports that chronaxie values measured with a constant voltage stimulator are different from values measured with a constant current stimulator and therefore the data should not be used interchangeably. (The reader is referred also to Shriber[5] for thorough descriptions of the S-D procedure.)

When collecting data for an S-D curve, the motor point or area of greatest electrical sensitivity must be precisely located with the negative (cathode) stimulating electrode. Using progressively shorter pulse durations, the values of stimulus amplitude which produce a minimal muscle contraction are recorded and then plotted on the graph.

STRENGTH-DURATION / CHRONAXIE TEST

PULSE DURATION (msec.)	Muscle _abd. dig. min._ L_R✓ Date _6/1_ stim. amp. (mA)	Muscle _abd. dig. min._ L✓R_ Date _6/1_ stim. amp. (mA)	Muscle _abd. dig. min._ L✓R_ Date _7/16_ stim.amp.(mA)
100	2	4	3.5
30	2	5	3.5
20✻	2	8	6
10✻✻	2	13	7
3	2	20	9
1	2	No response	10
0.5	3		18
0.3	4		No response
0.1	5		
0.05	12		

A	B	C

FIGURE 4–2. Data recorded from strength duration/chronaxie test. (*A*) Stimulus amplitude values (in milliamperes) measured from right normal abductor digiti minimi muscle, (*B*) left denervated abductor digiti minimi muscle 2 weeks after injury, and (*C*) partially reinnervated muscle on left recorded 6 weeks later. Normal chronaxie on right is 0.3 ms at 4 mA (two times the rheobase value of 2 mA). Chronaxie of left abductor digiti minimi muscle is 20 ms (as noted by *) following injury of the ulnar nerve at 8 mA (two times the rheobase value of 4 mA). Six weeks following initial test chronaxie has improved to 10 ms as indicated by **.

Figure 4–2 illustrates such a record. Figure 4–3 shows the plotted values of the S-D curve recorded at the motor point of a normally innervated muscle (*A*), a curve of a severely denervated muscle (*B*), and a curve indicating partial regeneration (*C*). The curve of regeneration (*C*) shows discontinuities (kinks) which represent different nerve fibers in different stages of regeneration. In wallerian degeneration, alterations in the myelin sheath and axon distal to the lesion occur in 2 to 3 weeks; therefore, the S-D test will not reveal an accurate picture of denervation if it is performed earlier than 14 days after injury.[10] Axonal regeneration time varies over the course of recovery and in different nerves, but progresses at an average of 1 mm per day. Follow-up S-D curves should not be scheduled too frequently, keeping this neural growth rate in mind. Serial S-D curve tests must be recorded over several weeks, and dated, so that progress of the pathology can be evaluated. The clinician needs to keep in mind that in the normal S-D curve, the *motor* nerve to the muscle is being stimulated and evaluated. When denervation has occurred, the nerve is degenerated or partially degenerated, and, therefore, the stimulus is now applied directly to the muscle, usually at a site distal to the original motor point. In this situation, the curve of denervation (Fig. 4–3*B*) represents the response of the muscle itself, rather than the motor nerve.

Chronaxie and rheobase can be determined from the S-D curve. For the normal curve, *A* in Figure 4–3, twice the rheobase current of 2.0 mA = 4.0 mA. A chronaxie of 0.3 ms (on abcissa) was required to get the response at this stimulus amplitude.

Clinical reports of S-D curves include copies of the curves and a subjective interpretation of changes seen in the series of curves over time. Shifts in the curves to the left or right of the graph and any other changes in the curve (e.g., its shape) and their

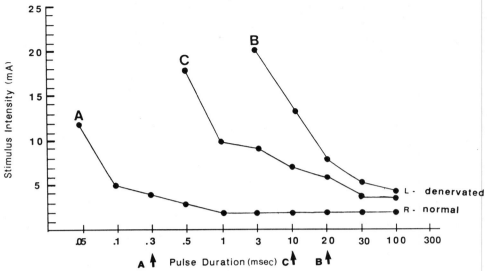

FIGURE 4–3. Plot of strength duration test values recorded in Figure 4–2 with chronaxies marked by arrows. (*A*) Normal abductor digiti minimi muscle on right hand, chronaxie 0.3 ms; (*B*) denervated muscle on left hand 2 weeks after injury, chronaxie 20 ms; and (*C*) partially reinnervated muscle on left hand 6 weeks after injury, chronaxie 10 ms.

significance are described. The chronaxie values for each muscle tested are included in the report. Normal chronaxies are less than 1.0 ms and usually are 0.1 ms or less. Chronaxie for fully denervated muscle may be 30 to 50 ms. Wynn Parry cautions against using only chronaxie values for neuromuscular assessment, because the chronaxie represents only one point on the curve and would fail to show the variations in pathology that may exist in different nerve fibers.[7]

At birth, the chronaxies of infant human nerve and muscle are high compared with those of adults.[11] Nerve chronaxie reduces to adult values within the first 3 months of life; muscle chronaxie gradually approaches adult value during the first 8 months. After 18 months, chronaxie remains constant without changing in the later years of life.

INDICATIONS FOR S-D CURVE AND CHRONAXIE TESTING

Strength-duration curves and chronaxie measurement have been used for evaluation of a variety of lower-motor-neuron pathologies. Their greatest value is for assessment of peripheral nerve injuries. Good judgment is required to plan the examination so that possible neuroanatomic sites of lesions in a peripheral nerve plexus can be differentiated. When skillfully performed, these tests can provide reliable and accurate information on the status of peripheral innervation and denervation. S-D curve and chronaxie testing are as objective as nerve-conduction testing and electromyography, are noninvasive, and can provide valuable information on the status and progress of peripheral nerve injuries. Other applications of the S-D curve and chronaxie tests are for evaluation of peripheral neuritis, other peripheral nerve diseases that may involve axonal degeneration, and motor-neuron disease conditions.[7] The tests may be used to complement other evaluative procedures in differentiating between normal nerve tissue and neuropathology.

STRENGTH−DURATION/CHRONAXIE TEST

Patient ___JL___ Unit No. _36-27-89_ Referred by _____

Birthdate _4/7/28_ Sex M _X_ F _____

Problem _Weakness right lower extremity_____

Date	Nerve/Muscle Tested	S−D Curve	Chronaxie (normal<1 msec)
2/10	rt. deep peroneal/tibialis anterior	markedly shifted to right; smooth curve	20 msec
	rt. deep peroneal/ext. dig. brevis	same	30 msec
	rt. common peroneal/biceps femoris (short head)	normal	.2 msec
	rt. tibial/gastrocnemius	normal	.1 msec
	lt. deep peroneal/tibialis anterior	normal	.05 msec

Impression: Chronaxies and strength-duration curves are consistent with severe degeneration of rt. deep peroneal nerve at level of fibular head. Values for rt. peroneal nerve above knee, rt. tibial and lt. peroneal nerves are within normal limits. Follow-up test in 6-8 weeks may be helpful.

Signature _____

FIGURE 4−4. Strength-duration/chronaxie test report of 2/10 on Case Study 1, JL.

CASE STUDY

1 (continued from p. 105)

In Case Study 1 concerning JL, the RD test indicated denervation of the peroneal nerve but did not provide quantitative data. A report of a strength-duration test and chronaxie determination of this patient on 2/10 (2 weeks after surgery) is shown in Figure 4−4, and a follow-up test 6 weeks later (3/30) is shown in Figure 4−5. The original S-D test shows increased chronaxie in the tibialis anterior and extensor digitorum muscle, substantiating the RD test. If the compromise had been at the ankle or in the course of the nerve in the lower leg, chronaxie of the tibialis anterior muscle would be normal. If the peroneal division of the sciatic nerve in the thigh had been compromised, chronaxie of the short head of the biceps femoris

---

STRENGTH–DURATION/CHRONAXIE TEST

Patient ___JL___   Unit No. _36-27-89_ Referred by _____

Birthdate _4/7/28_   Sex M _X_   F _____

Problem   _Weakness right lower extremity_____

Date	Nerve/Muscle Tested	S–D Curve	Chronaxie (normal<1 msec)
3/30	rt. deep peroneal/tibialis anterior	moderately shifted to right; irregular	10 msec
	rt. deep peroneal/ext. dig. brevis	markedly shifted to right; smooth	30 msec

Impression: Chronaxies and strength-duration curve of rt. deep peroneal nerve to tibialis anterior shows improvement compared with test of 2/10, compatible with early regeneration.   No change is noted in distal segment of nerve, to ext. dig. brevis, in which test values continue to indicate severe denervation. Follow-up testing in 6-8 weeks is suggested.

Signature   _____

FIGURE 4–5. Strength duration chronaxie test report of 3/30 (see Case Study 1, JL).

muscle would be increased. Thus, the site of the compromise is most likely in the area of the fibular head. The S-D test of 3/30 shows that chronaxie of the tibialis anterior muscle has decreased to 10 ms, indicating that some regeneration may have occurred during the 8 weeks since onset. A subsequent test 6 to 8 weeks later will show if regeneration is continuing and following the usual rate of neural regeneration. These test results can contribute to decisions on treatment, including surgical intervention.

Galvanic Twitch-Tetanus Ratio Test

The galvanic twitch-tetanus ratio test determines the relationship between the intensity of a direct or continuous (galvanic) current required to obtain a single minimal-twitch contraction (rheobase or threshold current) and the intensity of direct current needed to elicit a sustained or tetanic contraction.[10] A negative current is conducted through a small electrode (active electrode) applied to the motor point of the muscle, and a dispersive electrode is placed a short distance away from the active electrode. In the normally innervated muscle, the ratio of these two current intensities, that is, the rheobase intensity (twitch intensity) to the sustained contraction intensity (tetanus intensity), is usually 1:3.5 to 6.5. Therefore, if the threshold-twitch response can be obtained with a 1.0 mA current, then a sustained contraction requires 3.5 to 6.5 mA of current. In a denervated muscle, the ratio approaches unity, meaning both the minimal and sustained contraction can be obtained with about the same intensity of current. The test is highly subjective, painful, and probably no longer useful as a clinical evaluation procedure.

Nerve Excitability Test

A test of the response of a peripheral nerve to an electrical stimulus, called the nerve excitability test, has been used extensively for serial evaluation of facial nerve palsy (Bell's palsy).[12,13,14] The physiologic basis of the test is that the amplitude of a stimulus required to elicit a minimal response increases as the process of degeneration progresses.

The instrument used for the test must produce a square wave monophasic pulsed (very short rise time) electrical stimulus of 0.3- or 1.0-ms duration and an interpulse interval (rest interval) of 1 s and provide a variable intensity current that can be accurately measured from a meter or other display device.

In the case of a facial nerve paralysis, the nerve is stimulated as closely as possible to the site at which it emerges from the stylomastoid foramen above the angle of the mandible, using the negative pole as the active electrode. A dispersive electrode is placed nearby, for example, at the posterior aspect of the cervical spine. The threshold-amplitude stimulus of the facial nerve is measured on the involved side and compared with that of the patient's normal side. A difference of greater than 2 mA between the normal and involved side when using a 1.0-ms duration stimulus,[13] or greater than 3.5 mA when using a 0.3-ms stimulus[14] is considered significant and consistent with a denervation process. The test can be performed 1 or 2 days after the onset of paralysis to establish baseline values and then repeated periodically to detect a change in excitability. A significant change due to denervation usually appears between the 4th and the 21st day after onset; the test results are useful to the physician in making decisions regarding surgical decompression or other interventions. The unique contribution of this test is that, if it is done early enough, it can provide important information on the status of the nerve before total degeneration occurs. Although the determination of minimal muscle response is subjective, with a little practice this simple test can be accurately performed and may provide valuable information.

CONTEMPORARY ELECTRICAL EVALUATION TECHNIQUES

Evaluation of animal muscle electrical action potentials has been of interest to researchers since the 1800s.[1] Contemporary clinical electromyography (EMG) and nerve-conduction evaluation in humans emerged after Gasser and Erlanger's report, in 1922, of the application of the cathode-ray oscillograph for monitoring electromyograms.[15] Another landmark in the development of human EMG was Adrian and Bronk's introduction of the coaxial needle electrode in 1929.[16]

Clinical applications of motor-nerve-conduction compound-action potential (CAP) amplitude measurements were published by Harvey and Masland in 1941,[17] followed by reports of nerve-conduction velocity measurements by Hodes, Larrabee, and German in 1948.[18] Credit for publication of the earliest sensory-nerve-conduction studies is given to Dawson and Scott who, in 1949, reported using needle and surface electrodes to record the small sensory potentials.[19] Dawson's work is also of historical importance because he reported in 1947 recording small cortical potentials through the skull and scalp, evoked by stimulating peripheral nerves.[20] Excellent bibliography tracing the history of electrophysiologic evaluation was compiled by Licht[1,21,22] and Kimura.[23]

Nerve Conduction Tests

The purpose of nerve conduction testing is to assess the time and quality of the conduction of neural impulses in peripheral motor and sensory nerves. The technical aspects of measuring transmission of nerve impulses and the characteristics of the response are essentially similar for motor and sensory conduction tests and evoked-potential tests. A controlled monophasic pulsed electrical stimulus is applied to the skin overlying a nerve. When the threshold for excitation of the nerve membrane is attained, an action potential occurs and is propagated along the nerve *in both directions* (Fig. 4–6). Time for nerve impulse transmission in the axon is measured (latency of nerve conduction), velocities of impulse conduction within segments of the axon are calculated, and the amplitude and shape of the response are evaluated.

Because the rate of neural transmission is proportional to the thickness of myelin surrounding the nerve fibers and the length of nerve segments between the nodes of Ranvier, nerve conduction velocity becomes slower in conditions with a decreased amount of myelin.[24,25] The results of a nerve conduction test in a patient with a suspected neuropathic condition can be compared with normal conduction values. Analysis of specific features of conduction, such as amplitude, duration, and shape of the response waveform, is useful in differentiating demyelinating degeneration processes from axonal degeneration processes.

Instrumentation needed for nerve conduction testing includes a differential amplifier capable of detecting and accurately amplifying signals in a range from 2 μV to 50 mV, an electrical stimulator that provides square wave monophasic pulsed stimuli of durations from 0.05 to 1.0 ms, and output amplitude up to 500 V or 100 mA, synchronized with the sweep of a storage oscilloscope (see Chapter 3). The stimulus frequency

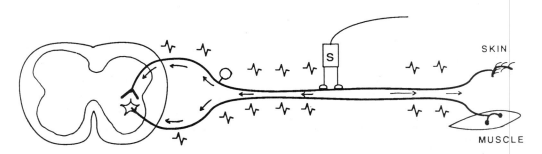

Mixed Motor and Sensory Nerve

FIGURE 4–6. Application of electrical stimulus (S) to peripheral nerve with resulting conduction of nerve action potentials in both proximal and distal directions in motor and sensory neurons.

capability should be variable from single stimuli to pulse trains of 50 Hz. Several appropriately designed commercial nerve-conduction instruments are available.

The responses from the specific sites of interest, which may be from muscle in motor nerve conduction tests, from peripheral sensory nerves, or from the scalp in evoked potential studies, are recorded. The clinician will recognize that the distinction among these techniques is the precise location of the stimulating and recording electrodes and, of course, the selection of appropriate instrumentation and parameters for applying the stimulus and monitoring the response. In addition, education, experience, and judgment are major factors in the clinician's ability to formulate a plan for electrical evaluation of the patient's condition, which would include selection of appropriate nerves, sites of stimulation, and modification of the plan as the results of each part of the test are interpreted.

MOTOR NERVE CONDUCTION

Clinical motor nerve conduction tests are used to quantitatively measure certain characteristics of impulse transmission in peripheral motor neurons, specifically in alpha motor neurons, and of the muscle response. To evaluate motor nerve conduction, bipolar recording electrodes are securely attached to the skin over one of the more distal muscles innervated by the nerve of interest. Surface recording and stimulating electrodes are usually used; however, on occasion, needle electrodes may be needed for recording or stimulating. One of the recording electrodes is placed over the motor point of the muscle being examined, and its wire lead is connected to the negative (cathode) input terminal of the preamplifier (Fig. 4–7). This electrode is usually called the active recording electrode. The second of the bipolar recording electrodes (reference electrode) is placed 2 cm or more distal to the active electrode and connected to the positive (anode) input terminal of the preamplifier. Better recording can be obtained if the arrangement of the recording electrodes is parallel to the direction of the muscle fibers and the reference electrode is placed over the insertion of the tendon or more distally.

The polarity configuration of the recording electrodes must be maintained if the initial phase of the muscle response seen on the oscilloscope is to have an upward (negative) direction. If these electrodes are inadvertently reversed, the response on the oscilloscope will begin in a downward direction. This can be confusing to the clinician, and, although the actual response latency would be identical in either configuration, a measurement error may occur because of misinterpretation of the response. A third surface electrode, the ground electrode, must be used with nerve conduction testing for the purpose of minimizing extraneous external electrical interference in the recorded response. This electrode is placed near the recording electrode and is connected to the preamplifier ground terminal input (Fig. 4–7).

A bipolar surface electrode is used for stimulation. The negative (cathode) stimulating electrode is applied distal to the stimulating positive (anode) electrode (Fig. 4–7). The sites of stimulation depend on the particular problem being evaluated; usually the nerve is stimulated at a distal location, such as at the wrist or ankle, and at a second, more proximal site, for example, at the elbow or knee. The stimulus amplitude is gradually increased until a muscle twitch contraction is seen and a response appears on the oscilloscope screen. Because different nerve fibers have different thresholds of excitation, a *supramaximal* stimulus is necessary to be certain that all of the fastest conducting nerve fibers are being monitored. As the maximum amplitude responses

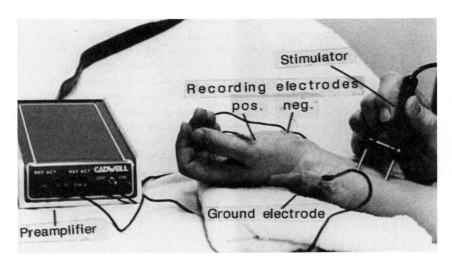

FIGURE 4–7. Setup for median motor nerve conduction test. Stimulating electrodes on median nerve at wrist; recording active (negative) electrode is over motor point of abductor pollicis brevis muscle; the reference (positive) electrode is distal and the ground electrode is on dorsum of hand. Recording and ground electrodes are connected to preamplifier.

appear, they are stored on the oscilloscope screen (Fig. 4–8). From the image on the oscilloscope, the latency time measurements are taken between the stimulus artifact and the beginning of the upward (negative) deflection of the muscle response. Amplitude of the response is measured, and the waveform shape is assessed by observation. These features should be similar when evoked by stimulation at different sites along the same nerve. The electrical response recorded at the muscle by this procedure is often referred to as the *M wave* or *M response*. This distinguishes this form of response from *F waves* and other responses described later in this chapter. Skin temperature in the area being tested must be warm, approximately 30°C or higher, in order to avoid inaccurate readings of decreased conduction velocity, which can occur with cooling.

For motor conduction testing, the nerve is electrically stimulated and time latencies are recorded for various nerve segments. Latencies in motor nerve conduction are measures of the time (in ms) for conduction of impulses in the axon, but they also include the time needed for neuromuscular transmission across the motor endplate synapse and the time needed for excitation and contraction of the muscle fibers. To determine conduction time in motor nerve fibers exclusively, two sites are stimulated and the latency from the more distal site is subtracted from the more proximal latency, leaving a difference that is the time of conduction between the two sites of stimulation. For these conduction times to have meaning when compared with normal values, a conduction velocity is calculated. The distance over which the time is measured must be known; this distance is measured between the location of the most distal stimulating electrode at each of the two stimulation sites. A velocity of conduction for the segment is therefore calculated using the formula:

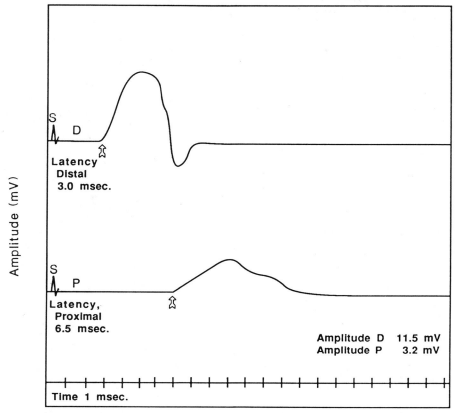

FIGURE 4–8. Simulated motor conduction response. Top trace is normal response from stimulus at a distal site. Lower trace is abnormal, with low amplitude and temporal dispersion of waveform.

$$NCV \ (m/s) = \frac{D(mm)}{\Delta T(ms)}$$

where

$$\text{Nerve conduction velocity} = \frac{\text{distance between two stimulus sites}}{\begin{array}{c}\text{time difference between latencies}\\ \text{from two stimulus sites}\end{array}}$$

The measurements of importance for comparison with normal values are the latencies recorded from the most distal site, amplitude of the response recorded from the distal site (and other amplitudes if they are markedly reduced), and velocities calculated from every segment of interest. A nerve conduction test report should give all of these values. The examiner should then compare the data with normal values, analyze the significance of any variations from normal, and include a summary impression or assessment of the results in the report. Each clinic should maintain a list of normal nerve

TABLE 4–2 Normal Motor-Conduction Values of Commonly Tested Nerves in Adults*

Nerve	Distal Latency (ms)	Velocity m/s (meters/second)
Median		
Wrist-muscle (8 cm)	<4.2	
Elbow-wrist		≧ 45
Ulnar		
Wrist-muscle (8 cm)	<4.0	
Elbow-wrist		≧ 45
Radial		
Forearm-muscle (8 cm)	<3.5	
Mid-humerus-forearm		≧ 45
Peroneal (deep) (7 cm)		
Ankle-muscle	<5.5	
Above fibular head-ankle		≧ 40
Tibial (10 cm)		
Ankle-muscle	<5.5	
Knee-ankle		≧ 40

*Based on data from references 100 to 104 and on data from our laboratory.

conduction values as a standard for comparison with test results, making certain that the test procedures used by the examiner are the same as in the procedure used in the established standards. As an example, the procedure description should specify the distance to be used between the distal cathode stimulation site and the placement of the negative recording electrode. Comparisons between test results and normal standards, and comparison of results from serial tests, are valid only if standardized procedures are used. Normal adult conduction values for some of the more frequently tested motor nerves are shown in Table 4–2. In infants, motor nerve conduction velocity is about half that of adults, reaching lower adult values by age 3.[26-30] In older aged subjects, motor nerve conduction becomes slower but continues to fall within lower limits of normal. Most studies report that the slowing becomes more evident after age 65 but varies among individuals of older age.

When analyzing nerve conduction test results, the clinician must consider whether any of the data are abnormal, then determine whether the abnormal conduction findings are limited to a single nerve or a nerve plexus, and if so, at what site or level. If the abnormal conduction is not clearly limited to a nerve or plexus, the clinician assesses the extent of the dysfunction and determines whether the abnormalities are consistent with a generalized, systemic neuropathy. If sequential tests are done on a patient, comparisons of results are interpreted cautiously, because small differences in latencies and velocities may occur because of technical variables such as slight errors in measurement of body surface distances and skin temperature variations.

Indications for Motor Nerve Conduction Testing

Motor nerve conduction testing is useful in establishing or ruling out the presence of a peripheral neuropathy, and in determining and localizing a peripheral nerve entrapment or a plexopathy. Another feature of the assessment of nerve conduction test results is differentiation, when possible, between nerve conduction changes consistent with a demyelinating process and those seen with an axonal disorder. Peripheral nerve demyelination will cause slowing of nerve conduction. If all of the motor fibers in a nerve have some degree of demyelination, the latencies will be long and conduction velocities slow. If, however, a portion of the nerve fibers are partially demyelinated while others are not, the latencies, and therefore the velocities, may be normal, while more subtle changes may be detected, such as reduced amplitudes and temporal dispersions of responses (see Fig. 4–8). Slowing of nerve conduction is clearly consistent with some degree of demyelination. Absence of conduction, or conduction block, can occur in a markedly demyelinated nerve.[25] A block may occur across a limited segment of the nerve, such as in a neurapraxia; whereas stimulation of the nerve distal to the demyelinated region may show normal conduction.[31] In a demyelinating peripheral nerve disease, conduction may be slow in those areas of the nerve that are more susceptible to the degenerative process. Guillain-Barré syndrome, tends to cause greater slowing of nerve conduction in the proximal (radicular) segments of the nerves, although slowing may also occur in the more distal segments.[32]

In disorders that primarily or initially involve axonal degeneration, the major conduction change is a decrease in amplitude of the motor conduction response.[24] Nerve conduction velocity may be slightly slowed or even remain normal. If conduction velocity is slow, this change may appear in the distal segments of the nerve, correlating with the centripetal pattern of axonal degeneration and a predominance of terminal neuron pathology. Many peripheral neuropathies are first manifested by either primarily axonal or demyelinating degeneration, and then the pathology progresses to include both the axis cylinder and myelin. The type of nerve conduction abnormalities found can be correlated, therefore, with the type of pathology, and these distinctions must be made in the analysis and assessment of the test data.

CASE STUDY

1 (*continued from p. 110*)

The continued report of Case Study 1 illustrates the application of the motor nerve conduction test and how it relates to other electrical tests. The absence of a response of the right deep peroneal nerve on 2/10, in the presence of normal conduction in other tested nerves (Fig. 4–9), is consistent with a compromise or entrapment of the peroneal nerve, although other problems such as a mononeuropathy multiplex should be considered. The follow-up test report on 4/10 shows that a response is now recorded from stimulation of the peroneal nerve, indicating improvement (see Fig. 4–10). Peripheral nerve conduction is not slowed with a central nervous system lesion, so the observed conduction changes do not indicate a central lesion. Careful correlation of electrical test findings with patient history and clinical signs and symptoms is essential. As reported, the exact site of the lesion cannot be determined by this test. The problem could be in the course of the nerve at the ankle, in the leg, or more proximal. When stimulation of the nerve at the ankle does not elicit a response in the muscle, stimulation at a more proximal

```
                    MOTOR NERVE CONDUCTION TEST REPORT


    Patient    JL         Unit No.  36-27-89   Referred by _____

    Birthdate  4/7/28     Sex M  X    F _____

    Problem    Weakness right lower extremity _____
```

Date	Nerve	Distal Latency	Amplitude	Conduction Velocity
2/10	rt. deep peroneal: ankle to muscle fibular head to ankle	no response no response	- -	- -
	rt. tibial: ankle to muscle knee to ankle	5.2 msec	7mV	48m/sec
	lt. deep peroneal: ankle to muscle fibular head to ankle	4.6 msec	6mV	46m/sec

```
    Impression:  Absence of conduction in right deep peroneal motor nerve
    with normal conduction in right tibial and left peroneal motor nerve
    is consistent with a lesion of the right deep peroneal nerve.  The
    level of the lesion cannot be determined from this test.  EMG testing
    is suggested.  Follow-up nerve conduction testing in 6-8 weeks may be
    helpful.


                        Signature    _____
```

FIGURE 4–9. Motor nerve conduction test report of 2/10 (see Case Study 1, JL).

site will not produce a response. The reason for testing at the head of the fibula is to be certain that the nerve is actually located and stimulated, and to look for a response which could occur because of an anomalous route of innervation such as an accessory deep peroneal nerve.[33,34] Results of sensory nerve conduction in this patient will be discussed later in this chapter.

F-WAVE NERVE CONDUCTION

In contrast with the conventional motor nerve conduction test in which conduction of the M-wave response is used to evaluate parts of the nerve peripheral to the point of stimulation, the F-wave measurement is useful for evaluating the more proximal segments of the peripheral motor nerves, particularly the nerve root and plexus regions. Whereas the F-wave response is easy to obtain, it is inconsistent in occurrence and

```
┌─────────────────────────────────────────────────────────────────────────┐
│                    MOTOR NERVE CONDUCTION TEST REPORT                     │
│                                                                           │
│   Patient ___JL___    Unit No. 36-27-89  Referred by _____      │
│                                                                           │
│   Birthdate 4/7/28   Sex M _X_  F _____                                  │
│                                                                           │
│   Problem   Weakness right lower extremity _____   │
│                                                                           │
├─────────┬───────────────────┬──────────┬──────────────┬──────────────────┤
│         │                   │ Distal   │              │ Conduction       │
│  Date   │      Nerve        │ Latency  │  Amplitude   │ Velocity         │
├─────────┼───────────────────┼──────────┼──────────────┼──────────────────┤
│  4/10   │ rt. deep peroneal:│          │              │                  │
│         │ ankle to muscle   │ 7.2 msec │   0.5mV      │                  │
│         │ fibular head to   │          │              │                  │
│         │ ankle             │          │              │   22m/sec        │
├─────────┴───────────────────┴──────────┴──────────────┴──────────────────┤
│     Impression:  Conduction in right deep peroneal motor nerve is         │
│     markedly slow and amplitude is low.  Results indicate improvement      │
│     compared with test of 2/10, in which there was no response.  Follow-   │
│     up testing in 6-8 weeks is suggested to monitor progress.             │
│                                                                           │
│                                                                           │
│                        Signature     _____      │
└─────────────────────────────────────────────────────────────────────────┘
```

FIGURE 4–10. Motor nerve conduction test report of 4/10 (see Case Study 1, JL).

variable in latency, and therefore its clinical usefulness is thought by some authors to be questionable.[35]

When a peripheral motor neuron is electrically stimulated, the impulse not only travels along the axon toward the periphery in an orthodromic direction to evoke a response in muscle fiber, that is, the M-wave response, but an action potential is also transmitted centrally along the axon in an antidromic direction.[36] When the impulse reaches the cell body, if certain conditions of electrical potential exist at the somadendritic membrane, the axon will be reactivated. A recurrent impulse is then transmitted peripherally over the efferent axon in the orthodromic direction, and another response is evoked in the muscle fiber (Fig. 4–11). This second, later response (F-wave response) has a much longer latency than the first response because in this response the action potential traverses a much longer distance before the muscle fiber is activated. These late responses were first described by Magladery and McDougal in 1950, who labeled them F waves.[37] Trontelj in 1973[38] and Shiller and Stålberg in 1978[39] reported that when the ulnar nerve is stimulated at the elbow or wrist, recordings made from single-fiber electromyographic needle electrodes produce an F wave in fewer than 55 percent of the neurons stimulated. The F-wave response obtained was constant in shape and consistent in latency, indicating that the response is recorded from a muscle fiber innervated by the same motor neuron that was stimulated to produce the M-wave response. When an F wave is recorded with surface electrodes, both the waveform shape and the latency are variable. Shiller and Stålberg proposed that this occurs because the surface electrode is recording F waves, which arise from (several) different motor neurons.[39] Although the

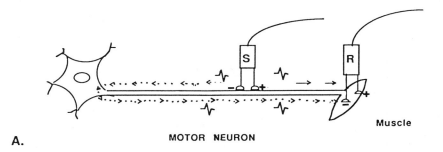

A.   MOTOR NEURON   Muscle

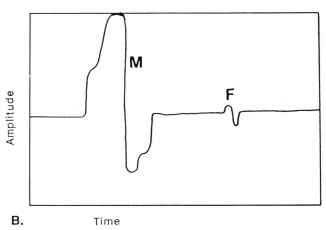

B.   Time

FIGURE 4–11. (*A*) Stimulus is applied to motor neuron. Impulse is propagated distally (*solid arrows*), resulting in M-wave motor nerve conduction response (*B*). Impulse also travels proximally to anterior horn cell, (*B*) motor neuron is reactivated and impulse travels distally, resulting in later F wave.

exact electrophysiologic mechanism of the F wave is inconclusive at this time, the response does not involve a central synapse or an afferent or intermediary neuron, and apparently reactivates the alpha motor neuron that is initially electrically stimulated. Therefore, the F wave is *not* a reflex phenomenon and is known to involve only motor neuron conduction.

When the F-wave test is used clinically, surface recording electrodes are placed over the muscle in the same arrangement as when recording the M-wave response and the nerve is stimulated, usually at a distal site. The stimulating cathode is usually placed in the proximal direction, in contrast to the distal placement when performing the standard motor conduction test. A supramaximal stimulus is used at a rate of 1 Hz or slower. More proximal stimulation sites can be used, but the F wave will not be visible or may be blocked if the latency of the F-wave response becomes too similar in time to the latency of the M-wave response. Because the F wave does not appear every time the nerve is stimulated, several stimuli are required to obtain a sufficient number of responses for accurate assessment of pathology. A method often used is to stimulate the nerve until 5

TABLE 4–3 Normal F-Wave Distal Latencies for Commonly Tested Nerves in Adults*

Nerve	Latency Range (ms)
Median	22–34
Ulnar	23–32
Peroneal	40–56
Tibial	38–58

*Based on references 40, 41, 43, and 105 and on data from our laboratory.

to 10 F-wave responses are obtained and then measure and record the latency to the beginning of the shortest F-wave response.[40] The F wave can be recorded from most peripheral nerves and can be identified if it has the following characteristics: (1) requires a supramaximal stimulus; (2) is inconsistent in occurance; (3) is inconsistent in waveform, usually less than 500 μV in amplitude;[31] (4) is slightly variable in latency each time it appears; and (5) falls within the range of normal values of latency for F waves (see Table 4–3). Most clinical studies of F waves report only F-wave latency. Several investigators have proposed methods of calculating F-wave conduction velocity and F-wave: M-wave ratios, but these calculations require measurement of distances over uneven body surfaces and other factors that introduce considerable error.[35] The most direct and reliable measure is that of latency.

F-wave latencies are positively correlated with arm length. Weber and Piero[41] published a useful nomogram and formula for predicting ulnar-nerve F-wave latency. Using their formula,

$$\text{F-wave latency (ms)} = [\text{arm length (cm)} \times 0.31] - [0.123 \times \text{forearm velocity (m/s)}] + [11.05]$$

The arm-length distance they used was measured from C-7 (seventh cervical vertebra) to the tip of the ulnar styloid process. It is common practice to compare test results with data on tables of normal values. Dorfman and Bosley found a significant increase in F-wave latency with increased age,[42] and their findings have been corroborated in our own studies. In a sample of 51 normal subjects 67 to 89 years of age, we found a mean F-wave latency of 27.4 ± 2.6 ms for the median nerve compared with a mean F-wave latency of 24.5 ± 2.2 ms in 20 subjects 18 to 34 years of age.[43]

Indications for F-Wave Response Evaluation

Measurements of the F-wave response are indicated in assessing conduction in disorders known to have predominantly proximal neuropathology. Examples of this are Guillain-Barré syndrome, Charcot-Marie-Tooth disease, and thoracic outlet syndrome. The test is also useful in differentiating a more proximal lesion from a distal problem, such as localizing a possible nerve entrapment.

NEUROMUSCULAR JUNCTION TRANSMISSION: REPETITIVE STIMULATION TEST

A variation of motor nerve conduction testing, called repetitive stimulation (RS), is useful for evaluation of problems of impulse transmission across the synapse at the neuromuscular junction. The RS was first reported by Jolly in 1895[44] and later modified by Harvey and Masland[45] for clinical studies of myasthenia gravis. The test is based on physiologic processes that occur at the synapse.

Normally a small amount of acetylcholine (ACh) is continuously and spontaneously released across the neuromuscular synapse at rest, contributing to the miniature endplate potentials (MEPP) that can be recorded by electromyography. When the motor neuron is activated, a larger, predetermined quantity of ACh is released from the axon terminal and moves across the synaptic cleft to the postsynaptic muscle end plate. Details of this physiologic action can be found elsewhere.[46,47] When a supramaximal electrical stimulus is repeatedly applied to the normal motor neuron at a rate of 3 to 5 per second, the amplitude of the recorded muscle response is rather constant. Responses to a series of 10 stimuli, recorded before and after resistive exercise, do not decrease more than 10 percent from the initial response in the series. If a physiologic defect is present at the postsynaptic receptor site, such as in myasthenia gravis, the amplitude of the fifth or sixth response may be decreased, compared to the initial response. A decrement of greater than 10 percent is considered to be abnormal.[48]

When electrical stimuli are applied to the normal nerve at a faster rate, usually 10 to 20 per second for a series of stimuli lasting up to 10 seconds, there can be a decrease of up to 40 percent between the amplitudes of the initial and later responses.[47] With certain defects at the presynaptic region, a decreased response may occur initially with a slow rate of stimulation, while a significantly increased response may result with faster stimulus rates. An increment to greater than 100 percent of the initial response is regarded as significantly abnormal. With certain defects at the presynaptic region, the amount of ACh stored is apparently normal, although the amount released at the presynaptic motor axon terminal is decreased, resulting in a low-amplitude motor response at slow-stimulation rates. At higher stimulation rates the *total* quantity of ACh released is increased, providing an amount sufficient to produce responses with *normal* or *near normal* amplitudes.[47,48] This increased response can occur in conditions, such as small-cell bronchogenic carcinoma and in botulism, and was reported as a *myasthenic syndrome* by Eaton and Lambert in 1957.[49]

In performing the RS test, recording electrodes are attached over the motor point of the muscle, and the nerve is stimulated at a distal site, as in motor nerve conduction testing. Several precise details must be adhered to in administering this test, including complete immobilization of the body part being tested and firm strapping of both the recording and stimulating electrodes to prevent the slightest electrode displacement. Medications must be withheld before the test, and skin temperature must be measured and controlled, because the amplitude alteration may not occur at skin temperatures below 35°C. If a positive test is not obtained from a peripheral muscle, such as stimulation of the ulnar nerve and recording from the abductor digiti minimi muscle, more proximal muscles (for example, upper trapezius, deltoid, or orbicularis oculi muscles) need to be examined.

In a variation of the RS, called the double-step repetitive-stimulation test,[50,51] change in amplitudes of responses to electrical stimulation is measured before and after a temporarily induced ischemia of the extremity. In a small series of patients, Gilchrist and Sanders[51] found that the double-step RS of the upper trapezius muscle was slightly more sensitive than the routine RS test (non-double-step) of the trapezius in revealing an amplitude decrement. These authors, further, found the double-step test to be only 60 percent as sensitive as the *single-fiber electromyograph* (SFEMG) technique. In the latter test, which requires a special single-fiber-needle electrode recording of the responses from two muscle fibers innervated by a single motor unit, *jitter* was considered abnormal if it exceeded 60 ms. Jitter is the variability in conduction time or latency required to elicit a response in different muscle fibers innervated by terminal axons of the same motor unit.[52] The increased jitter is compatible with dysfunction in transmission at the neuromuscular junction. Increased jitter alone, is not pathognomonic of myasthenia gravis, because increased jitter and also conduction blocking can be found in other neurogenic and muscle diseases.[53] When SFEMG is not available, RS testing is a good alternative, but it must be meticulously performed and the results must be carefully interpreted relative to other clinical findings.

SENSORY NERVE CONDUCTION

Nerve impulses transmitted over the portion of peripheral sensory (afferent) neurons distal to the dorsal root ganglion or cell body are evaluated by sensory nerve conduction tests. Latency and velocity of impulse transmission, and amplitude of the sensory response recorded from the nerve are analyzed to assess the status of sensory nerve conduction. Peripheral nerve injuries and neuropathies involving demyelination may produce changes in sensory nerve conduction.

As stated earlier in this chapter, action potentials resulting from threshold-level electrical stimuli applied to a nerve are propagated in both directions, that is, distally and centrally (toward the spinal cord). Amplitudes of sensory response are considerably smaller than motor responses and technically more difficult to measure. Two techniques of measuring sensory conduction are commonly used, the antidromic and the orthodromic. In the antidromic technique, mixed motor and sensory nerves are stimulated, for example, the median nerve at the wrist. Impulses propagated distally are recorded from a branch of the sensory nerve, as in the example in Figure 4–12, which uses ring

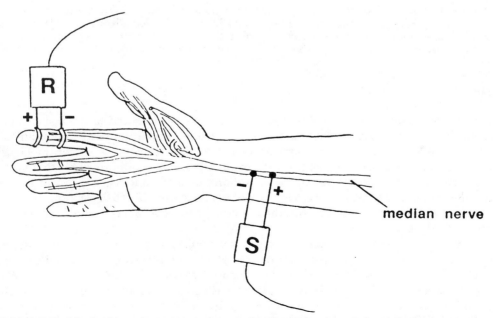

FIGURE 4–12. Antidromic sensory nerve conduction. Stimulus (S) is applied to median nerve at wrist, and sensory nerve impulse is recorded (R) from index finger.

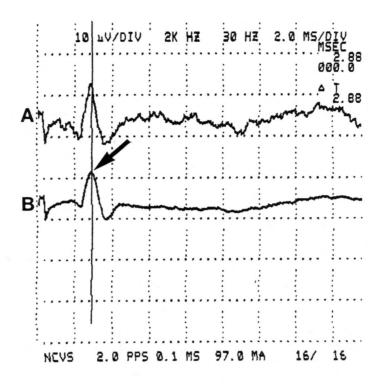

FIGURE 4–13. Ulnar sensory nerve conduction response recorded at wrist using orthodromic technique. (*A*) Response from single stimulus. (*B*) Averaged response from 16 single, repeated stimuli. Arrow in (*B*) indicates point where vertical time marker line has been placed at peak of negative phase to measure latency, which is 2.8 ms. Parameters of instrument setting appear on grid.

electrodes to encircle the index finger. Latency is usually measured to the peak amplitude of the response because the exact initial deflection of the response is often difficult to determine.[54] A diagram of sensory nerve conduction response is shown in Figure 4–13. Measurements can also be taken from stimulation at more proximal stimulation sites, such as at the elbow and axilla. The antidromic technique has a disadvantage in that both motor and sensory nerves are stimulated, resulting in muscle contraction and movement artifact, and possibly introducing error if these artifacts are included in the measured response.

In the orthodromic technique the stimulus is applied at a distal point, for example, with ring electrodes encircling a digit or disc electrodes placed over a distal sensory branch of the nerve, so that sensory-nerve impulses are recorded as the impulse is transmitted centrally (Fig. 4–14). Again, latency is usually measured to the peak amplitude of the response. Latencies recorded using the orthodromic technique are not significantly different from latencies recorded by the antidromic procedure.[55]

Sensory velocities can be calculated from the distal-response latencies, without the

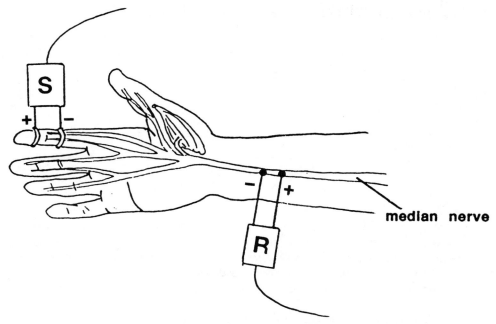

FIGURE 4–14. Orthodromic sensory nerve conduction. Stimulus (S) is applied to index finger and sensory nerve impulse is recorded (R) from median nerve at wrist.

necessity of using two stimulus sites, because the distal latency represents only time of sensory nerve impulse transmission, without the additional factor of neuromuscular synaptic-transmission time. For example, calculation of orthodromic median sensory nerve conduction velocity (SNCV) when stimulating at the index finger, recording at a distance 14 cm proximally at the wrist (see Fig. 4–14) and measuring a latency of 2.8 ms from finger to wrist, would be as follows:

$$\text{SNCV} = \frac{\text{distance (mm)}}{\text{time (ms)}} \qquad \text{SNCV} = \frac{140 \text{ mm}}{2.8 \text{ ms}} \qquad \text{SNCV} = 50 \text{ m/s}$$

Velocities can be calculated for any accessible segment of interest, and peak-to-peak response amplitudes are measured. Although response amplitudes from orthodromic recording are smaller than antidromically recorded responses, because they are recorded through a greater thickness of subcutaneous tissue, the orthodromic response is a more specific measure of sensory nerve conduction. Normal values for more frequently tested sensory nerves are listed in Table 4–4. As with motor nerve conduction, sensory conduction has been shown to be slower in infants, reaching low-normal adult values at age 3.[56,57] Slowing of sensory conduction also can occur in normal humans over age 65.[57,58]

A report of a sensory nerve conduction test should include all distal latencies, all velocities calculated, and amplitudes. The procedure should be standardized and documented in each clinic. For example, if testing is usually done using the orthodromic technique, and a standard distance of 14 cm is used between stimulating cathode and the recording electrode, these details should be outlined in a procedure manual. Any

TABLE 4–4 Normal Sensory Nerve Conduction Values of Commonly Tested Nerves in Adults*

Nerve		Distal Latency (ms)	Velocity m/s
Median digit II-wrist	(14 cm)	<3.6	≥ 38
Ulnar digit V-wrist	(14 cm)	<3.6	≥ 38
Radial thumb-wrist	(14 cm)	<3.5	≥ 40
Superficial peroneal foot-leg	(14 cm)	<3.6	≥ 40
Sural lateral malleolus-leg	(14 cm)	<4.2	≥ 38

*Based on data from references 103, and 106 to 109 and on data from our laboratory.

procedural variations used in a test should be noted, for example, in some instances a distance longer or shorter than the routine procedure is necessary, or the antidromic technique may be needed to detect a sensory response with a markedly reduced amplitude. Several excellent manuals and texts describe details of sensory nerve conduction techniques for many nerves and discuss analysis or interpretation of the results.[59,60,61]

Indications for Sensory Nerve Conduction Testing

Sensory nerve conduction testing is indicated in many of the same conditions as is motor nerve conduction testing. Sensory testing should be particularly important, however, in evaluating conditions in which there are clinically demonstrable sensory changes. Sensory conduction findings will be normal in patients with avulsion of the dorsal spinal nerve roots, in spite of diminished sensation, and therefore, the skilled examiner carefully interprets all data.

CASE STUDY

1 (*continued from p. 118*)

Figure 4–15 illustrates the results of sensory-nerve-conduction testing on this patient. The technique for testing the sensory branch of the deep peroneal nerve has not been standardized. The sensory branch of the superficial peroneal nerve is a division of the superficial peroneal which is formed as the common peroneal nerve divides, usually just below the fibular head. If conduction had been normal in the superficial peroneal nerve and absent in the deep peroneal nerve, the lesion would clearly be distal to the common peroneal nerve. Absence of conduction in the superficial personal sensory nerve in this case, in addition to the loss of deep peroneal motor nerve conduction (p. 117 and Fig. 4–9) indicates a lesion *above* the division of the common peroneal nerve. The sural nerve (a purely sensory nerve of the leg) was tested to establish the status of sensory conduction in this patient. If sural conduction had been abnormal, a peripheral neuropathy would need to be ruled out by further testing.

H-REFLEX RESPONSE

The H-reflex response is primarily of value in assessing the continuity and function of the sensory and motor monosynaptic pathways of the first sacral nerve roots (S-1),

SENSORY NERVE CONDUCTION TEST

Patient ___JL_____ Unit No. 36-27-89 Referred by _____

Birthdate _4/7/28_ Sex M _X_   F _____

Problem   Weakness right lower extremity _____

Date	Nerve	Distal Latency	Amplitude	Conduction Velocity
2/10	rt. superficial peroneal: foot to ankle (12 cm)	no response	-	-
	rt. sural (14 cm)	3.6 msec	8uV	39m/sec

Impression: Absence of response in right superficial peroneal nerve. Normal sural nerve conduction.

Signature _____

FIGURE 4–15. Sensory nerve conduction test report of 2/10 (see Case Study 1, JL).

although the response can be elicited in some of the other nerve roots under specific circumstances as described later in this section. This response is frequently used in assessment of S_1 radiculopathy from herniated disc or other pathology in this region.

As described earlier in this chapter, when an electrical stimulus is applied to a mixed motor and sensory peripheral nerve, impulses travel both distally and proximally along the nerve fibers (Fig. 4–6). Action potentials from the distal parts of IA afferent neurons are propagated centrally to the spinal cord and are transmitted across the synapse to alpha-motor neurons within the anterior horn of the spinal cord. The motor neuron is then activated, resulting in action potentials that travel peripherally to the muscle, causing a muscle contraction. The response was first described by Hoffman in 1922[62] and was later named the H wave by Magladery and McDougal in 1950.[37]

Clinical measurement of the H-wave response is performed with the same equipment as is used for conventional motor and sensory nerve conduction testing. The gain or sensitivity of the amplifier is set at a more sensitive level because the response is usually low in amplitude. The latency of the H-wave response is long because the distance over which the impulses travel is long. The response can most consistently be elicited by stimulating the tibial nerve at the popliteal fossa, with the stimulating cathode proximal to the anode and the recording electrode overlying the medial portion of the soleus muscle. The H-wave response can be recognized by the following characteristics: As the stimulus is gradually increased, the H-wave response appears either at a lower stimulus intensity or at about the same stimulus intensity than is needed to elicit the M-wave response. As the stimulus is further increased to a supramaximal level for the M-wave response, the H-wave response decreases and disappears; the latency is quite constant each time the response occurs, and the waveform is consistent, although the amplitude increases and then decreases, as the stimulus amplitude increases.

An excellent description of the technique and a method of predicting the H-reflex-response latency for the tibial nerve was reported by Braddom and Johnson.[63] The latency was found by those authors to be highly correlated with leg length and age; therefore, these factors are included in their predictive formula and nomogram. Using their formula, H-wave-response latency of the tibial nerve may be calculated as follows:

$$\text{H-wave-response latency} = [0.46 \times \text{leg length (cm)}] + 9.14 + [0.1 \times \text{age (years)}]$$

Leg length is measured from the stimulus site at the popliteal fossa to the prominence of the medial malleolus. Latency is considered within normal range if it falls within ± 5.5 ms (2 standard deviations) of the calculated latency. According to Braddom and Johnson,[63] the difference in H-wave-response latency between the right- and left-tibial nerves should not be greater than 1.2 ms, providing the leg lengths are not markedly different. In 100 normal subjects they found a mean latency of 29.8 ms (± 2.74 ms) for the tibial nerve. A technique for recording the H-reflex response from the flexor carpi radialis when stimulating the median nerve has been reported by Sabbahi and Khalil.[64]

H-wave responses can be elicited from several nerves of the upper and lower extremities in infants, gradually appearing with less consistency up to 1 year of age.[28] The H-wave response can also be elicited in selected peripheral nerves of patients with central nervous system disorders;[65] here the amplitude of the response may be higher than normal. Because the H-wave responses in these conditions are inconsistent, we have used them infrequently in our clinic, except for differential testing for first sacral nerve root (S-1) radiculopathy, in which they are quite helpful. The greatest advantage of the H-wave response in testing for radiculopathy is that this test provides information about function of the dorsal spinal root, which is often compromised by herniated discs and foraminal-impingement problems. Conduction abnormalities would not be revealed by conventional peripheral motor and sensory nerve conduction tests. A further advantage is that an H-wave response change occurs concomitant with the root compression, while electromyographic evidence of denervation may take up to 3 weeks to develop.

Clinical Evoked Potentials

Evoked potential (EP) tests discussed in this chapter are clinical tests that measure voltage changes recorded from the brain and nerve pathways leading to the brain as a result of application of various types of external stimuli to sense organs or peripheral nerves.[66] These tests are valuable in that they can be used to measure function of both the peripheral and central nervous system pathways, including the sequential transmission of orthodromic impulses across sensory axodendritic synapses. The tests are most frequently used to evaluate propagation of sensory potentials, although in some procedures, potentials evoked in motor nerves or mixed motor and sensory nerves are measured.[67] Evoked potential tests are useful in evaluating neurologic function in the spinal cord, brain stem, and specific regions of the sensory cerebral cortex. This discussion of evoked potential tests is presented as introductory information only, with the intention of enlightening the clinician who is not currently knowledgeable in these procedures and the interpretation of their results.

Observation of spinal evoked potentials in animals was reported by Barron and Matthews[68] in 1938, and Dawson[20] published studies of cerebral evoked responses in humans in 1947. With more recent improvements in instrumentation and technology, which make it possible to average characteristics of a large number of repeated responses, clinical studies of evoked potentials have become an important tool for evaluating electrophysiologic function.

The more commonly used clinical evoked potential tests may be divided into three categories named according to the responses of the system being evaluated, namely, *somatosensory* (SSEP), *visual* (VEP) and *brainstem auditory evoked potentials* (BAEP). The techniques used for these tests have certain common features. For each of the evoked potential tests, a suitable stimulus is applied repeatedly at a repetition rate appropriate for the particular response, and all of the recorded responses are electronically averaged. The purpose of averaging is to sort out the desired response, which is rather constant in latency and waveform, from the random interference signals. The type of stimulus, and the stimulation and recording sites, depend on the neuronal pathways being studied. Surface recording electrodes are placed on specific areas of the scalp overlying sites of electrical activity in the brain elicited by the peripheral sensory stimulus. A standard system of recording electrode placement, called the *Ten Twenty Electrode System of the International Federation (10–20 System)*, specifies sites for scalp-electrode locations to record responses of electroencephalographic activity (EEG).[69] This electrode placement system has been adopted by many laboratories for recording electrode placement in evoked potential testing. The three types of evoked potential tests are briefly described.

SOMATOSENSORY EVOKED POTENTIALS

Of the three EP tests, the SSEP is the procedure most frequently used by physical therapists, as it is an extension of motor and sensory peripheral nerve conduction tests. The test is also administered by other qualified evoked potential technologists.

The same type of electrical stimulus used in conventional nerve conduction tests is applied over a peripheral nerve. The median, tibial, and peroneal nerves are more commonly tested. The stimulus is applied with the cathode placed proximal to the anode, and intensity is increased to slightly above motor threshold, that is, the point at which a mild to moderate muscle contraction is seen.[70] The stimulus is applied repeatedly from 250 to 1000 times or more as indicated by the quality of the response. A stimulus rate of 2 to 10 per second is used. An active surface recording electrode is placed on the contralateral scalp, over the cortical area representing the body area being stimulated. Evoked potentials may also be recorded from areas over the spinal cord, for example, C5 (fifth cervical vertebra spinous process) and other peripheral sites such as Erb's point in the study of the median nerve. Amplitude and latencies of the responses are measured and compared with normal values. Slowing of SSEP conduction has been reported in infants; adult values are usually attained by age 5. Slowing occurs after age 65, with values falling within the low-normal range for younger adults.[42,71]

Evoked potential responses are named according to their polarity, that is, N for negative peak or P for positive peak; latency is measured to peak amplitude of the response as seen in Figure 4–16. Thus, a response with a negative peak occurring at a latency of 13 ms from time of stimulus application would be labeled N13. Evoked

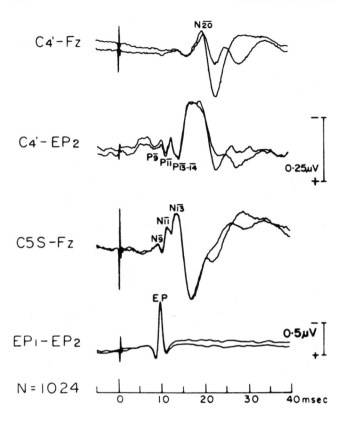

FIGURE 4–16. Somatosensory evoked potentials (*SSEP*) elicited by electric stimulation of median nerve at wrist. Recordings were taken from Erb's point (*EP*) and scalp and noncephalic sites using the 10–20 System.[69] $C_{4'}$ is a scalp-recording electrode located 2 cm posterior to C4 in the 10–20 System; F_z is a recording site at midline of frontal scalp region; C5S is the site of the fifth cervical vertebra spinous process. *P* and *N* designate positive or negative direction of the signal, respectively. Bars over numbers signify latency values (in ms) and are theoretical rather than observed responses. The zero in the time calibration corresponds to stimulus onset. (From Chatrian,[72] p 43, with permission.)

responses are usually reported in terms of these latencies, but for some conditions nerve conduction velocities are calculated by subtracting latencies obtained between two sites and dividing the difference into the distance measured between the two sites. Latency and polarity for each recorded point will depend on the location of both the active and reference recording electrodes. Examples of normal adult SSEP latencies for the median and tibial nerves are shown in Table 4–5, which illustrates the type of data that may be reported. No attempt is made here to provide normal values for data comparison in testing because standard normal data will vary somewhat among clinics. Abnormal

TABLE 4–5 Example of More Commonly Recorded Somatosensory Evoked Potentials[72]

| Nerve | Recording Site | | Evoked-Response Latency (ms) |
	Active	Reference	
Median	Erb's point	Contralateral Erb's point	N9
	C5S cervical spine	Scalp (Fz)	N13
	$C_{3'}$ and $C_{4'}$ scalp	Contralateral Erb's point	P9, P13–14
	$C_{3'}$ or $C_{4'}$ scalp	Scalp (Fz)	N20
Tibial	L3 lumbar spine	4 cm rostral to L3	N20
	Cz' scalp	Fpz' scalp	P37, N45

responses include absence of responses, delayed (increased) latencies, and decreased amplitudes recorded at various sites; these may indicate pathology at certain locations along the somatosensory pathway.

VISUAL EVOKED POTENTIALS

Because of the ophthalmologic implications and the uniqueness of the techniques, special training is necessary for technologists performing visual evoked potential tests. Integrity of the visual system can be assessed in two parts. The electroretinogram (ERG) evaluates responses of the retina to a visual stimulus applied to the eye; the cerebral visual evoked potential test records responses at the scalp overlying the occipital or temporal lobes.

In the ERG procedure, recording electrodes are applied to the retina, either using topical or general anesthesia. Flashes of variable luminance stimuli are presented to one or both eyes, and latency and amplitude of the evoked responses are measured. Pathology of the retinal photoreceptors is evaluated by the ERG.[72]

For the cerebral VEP procedure, visual stimuli, such as a contrasting light stimulus in a reversing black-and-white checkerboard pattern, are presented to one or both eyes. The term recommended by the American Electroencephalographic Society for this test is pattern reversal evoked potentials (PREP).[72] Characteristics of the stimulus, including pattern reversal speed, size of the overall pattern or field, luminance, and check-square size are taken into consideration. A series of unpatterned visual stimuli is also used in VEP testing. The montage of scalp recording electrode placement is specified in the protocol. Peak latency and amplitude of the electronically averaged responses are measured, and in some procedures, the difference between latencies of the responses to the left and right eyes is calculated. Partial absence of the response also has specific clinical significance.[73] Data are compared to standard normal values. Cooperation and attention of the patient are necessary for measurement of cerebral VEPs.

Pathology of the optic nerve, chiasma, and postchiasmal pathway can be detected using VEP tests. In demyelinating disorders, for example, optic neuritis or multiple sclerosis, changes in VEP may be manifested by slowed conduction time and therefore increased latency, reduced response to high frequency stimuli because of prolonged refractory times, or even complete conduction block resulting in an absence of the evoked response. According to Halliday,[73] the VEP is particularly helpful in evaluating patients in whom a diagnosis of multiple sclerosis is not clinically definite. This test is probably more useful in these cases than the BAEP or the SSEP tests. Disorders with axonal degeneration may result in reduced amplitudes of the VEP responses, either with or without changes in latency. Examples reported are Huntington's chorea[74] and Friedreich's ataxia.[75]

AUDITORY EVOKED POTENTIALS

This brief discussion of auditory evoked potentials is limited to neurologic applications of the procedure. Use of auditory evoked potentials for the specific evaluation of hearing dysfunction is of particular interest to clinicians with special training in audiology but is outside the scope of this text.

Studies of the short latency auditory evoked potentials occurring within 10 to 15 ms of the application of a series of high-intensity click sounds are termed brainstem auditory evoked potentials (BAEP).[72] The responses elicited occur as impulses pass along the cochlear division of the eighth cranial nerve (auditory nerve) and along the central auditory pathway through various synapses in the brainstem, and are ultimately recorded with surface electrodes located on the vertex (C_Z in the 10–20 System) and on one or both ear lobes or the mastoid processes. The normal BAEP response consists of up to seven potentials, called components I–VII, each thought to represent a response elicited from a specific neural site along the auditory pathway to the cerebral cortex.[76] The appearance or absence of the components and the amplitude and latency of each are evaluated and compared with normal values. Several other auditory evoked potential techniques are in use, and longer latency components are sometimes measured; however, the BAEP appears to be more frequently used to evaluate neurologic function of the auditory nerve and the central auditory pathways.

The BAEP has been useful in evaluation of acoustic neuromas and other space-occupying lesions in the area of the cerebellopontine angle.[77] Abnormalities of BAEP in patients with multiple sclerosis have also been reported by several investigators,[77–79] but the significance of the findings varies considerably among the authors. Absence of auditory evoked potentials has been used in the assessment of brain damage resulting in coma and in brain death.[80] Robinson and Rudge advise caution and further evaluation in this application of the test, however, because other factors such as damaged sensory end organs can also produce BAEP abnormalities.[81] Changes in the BAEP recorded more than 12 hours after injury in patients with head trauma have been shown to be a reasonable guide to prognosis.[80]

Clinical Electromyography (EMG)

While the tests discussed earlier in this chapter describe evaluation of the neuromuscular system by monitoring responses of the muscles or nerves to the application of external electrical stimuli to the nerve, EMG provides a means of monitoring and evaluating electrical activity of muscle directly, that is, without artificial stimulation. In this chapter, basic information about EMG is offered to help the reader understand the concept of the procedure, meaning of data obtained, and clinical significance of the findings. Detailed texts on clinical EMG are available for those interested in achieving a greater understanding of or performing EMG. A list of suggested books is provided at the end of the chapter.

An advantage of EMG over the other procedures is that characteristics of muscle during relaxation and voluntary contraction can be studied. Such features may reveal, to varying extents, the electrophysiologic status of the central nervous system, peripheral nervous system, neuromuscular junction, and muscle tissue per se. The most valuable contribution of EMG is its usefulness in evaluating electrical activity of lower motor neurons and muscle fibers, as EMG is helping in identifying electrical changes consistent with pathologic processes in these anatomic areas. In no condition is EMG alone pathognomonic. Each finding in the EMG examination is interpreted by the examiner and used in a continual process of planning and modifying the ongoing examination according to the results found at each examined site. The final summary or impression of the interpreted EMG examination is then carefully correlated with other diagnostic test information and clinical findings, and used by the referring practitioner in formulating a diagnosis and/or determining a plan of treatment. The EMG examiner must have detailed knowledge of anatomy, especially neuroanatomy, and be competent in integrating this knowledge with pertinent aspects of pathology relative to neurologic, orthopedic, and other system dysfunction in all age groups. Skills in muscle testing and other neuromuscular evaluation techniques are essential qualifications of the practitioner administering electrophysiologic tests. The education and laboratory training required of physical therapists provide these practitioners with an excellent background prerequisite to performing effective clinical electromyography.

The instrumentation required for EMG is basically similar to that used in nerve conduction testing, but an electrical stimulator is not needed. A sterile needle electrode is inserted directly into the muscle, and endogenous electrophysiologic activity produced by depolarization and repolarization of the muscle cell membrane is transduced from the electrode through a preamplifier to an amplifier, as in Figure 4–17. The electrical signals are then transmitted to a variety of processing, display, and storage components, which include an audio amplifier for studying the sound characteristics and a storage oscilloscope for reviewing the raw electromyographic signals. These components are reviewed in detail in Chapter 3. Monopolar and concentric needle electrodes are most commonly used in routine clinical EMG. Detailed descriptions of these electrodes, instrumentation, and the technique can be found in other texts.[82,83] Other types of electrodes such as the single-fiber EMG needle electrode used in studies of muscle fibers innervated by a single motor unit[84] are used for special evaluation procedures.

The quality and sharpness of each monitored muscle potential is highly dependent on the proximity of the electrode tip to the muscle fibers. When the needle electrode is in the muscle, the electromyographer carefully monitors the feel of the needle tip within the muscle, and the interplay of the needle tip with the sound of responses heard on the

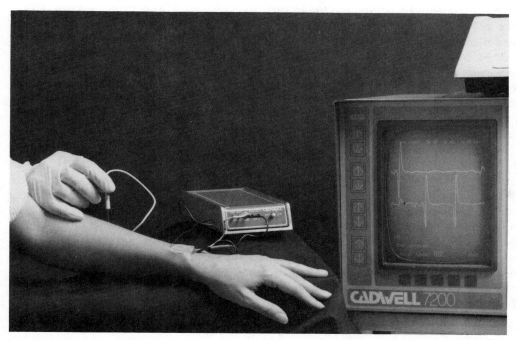

FIGURE 4–17. Clinical electromyography (EMG) using a concentric needle electrode in extensor digitorum muscle. Normal muscle action potentials are displayed on oscilloscope.

speaker and the shape of the electrical signal observed on the oscilloscope. Discrete true motor unit action potentials cannot usually be monitored by conventional EMG techniques because the muscle fibers in proximity to the needle recording surface are innervated by axons of several different motor units.[85] Even so, the term motor unit potential (MUP) is commonly used in routine EMG when referring to the electrical activity detected from the needle recording area. Many different areas of the muscle are examined by repositioning the needle within each cutaneous insertion site. More than one insertion site may be needed to fully study a muscle. Accurate and thorough EMG requires cooperation of the patient; therefore, rapport and communication between patient and examiner are critical aspects of the procedure. Electromyographic activity is studied under three conditions: (1) while the muscle is at rest, that is, completely relaxed; (2) during a mild contraction, just strong enough to produce individual motor unit action potentials; and (3) during a very strong contraction, held with enough force to recruit as many motor units as possible.

NORMAL EMG

Normal muscle which is completely at rest is described as electrically silent, that is, no muscle action potentials are seen. Miniature endplate potentials (MEPPs) can be encountered in the motor endplate region, and although they appear spontaneously, they are a normal response. As the needle is moved about in the relaxed muscle with short but brisk movements, brief, abrupt bursts of electrical activity will be observed. This is normal insertion activity.

When a slight voluntary muscle contraction is performed, individual muscle action potentials are observed. These potentials normally have four phases or less and are usually biphasic or triphasic,[86] although approximately 10 percent of the potentials seen in a muscle may be polyphasic (more than four phases).[87] Amplitude and duration of the potentials of each muscle are evaluated. Normal values for different age groups, recorded from several different muscles using concentric needle electrodes, were reported by Buchthal, Guld, and Rosenfalck in 1954,[88] and later by Kimura.[86] Chu-Andrews and Johnson[89] have published parameters of motor unit potentials of several muscles recorded with monopolar needle electrodes. With increasing age, mean motor unit action-potential duration is increased.[88,90]

In normal recruitment, first one or two motor unit potentials discharge, gradually increasing in discharge frequency. As the strength of voluntary contraction increases, additional units are recruited and rapidly increase in frequency, until, at maximal effort, individual action potentials can no longer be discerned, the baseline trace of the oscilloscope is almost completely obliterated, and a full or complete *interference pattern* occurs. When a maximum or very strong voluntary contraction is obtained, the examiner monitors the pattern of muscle action potential recruitment, discharge frequency, and amplitude. A true maximal contraction cannot usually be attained because of discomfort or other reasons, and therefore, in our clinic, the pattern is considered normal if recruitment occurs in the normal manner and approximately 75 percent of the baseline is obliterated by muscle action potential activity. Characteristics of normal EMG during rest and minimal and strong contractions are listed in Table 4–6 and are illustrated in Figure 4–18.

ABNORMAL EMG

Abnormal EMG may be observed under all three conditions in which normal electrical activity is studied: at rest, during minimal contraction, and during strong

TABLE 4–6 Characteristics of Normal and Abnormal Electromyographic Potentials

Neuro-muscular Status	At Rest		Minimum Contraction			Strong Contraction	
	Insertion Activity	Spontaneous Activity	Muscle Action Potentials			Recruitment Pattern	Amplitude
			Amplitude	Duration	Waveform		
Normal	Brief discharges	None	100–2000 μV	3–15 ms	Diphasic and triphasic	Full or complete interference (>75%)	Concentric: 2000–5000 μV
		End-plate potentials			10% polyphasic		Monopolar: 2000–8000 μV
Abnormal	Absent response	Fibrillation	Absent	Less than 3 ms	Polyphasic	Decreased (<75%)	<2000 μV
	Increased or prolonged	Positive sharp waves	Low or over 5 mV			Discrete potentials Single unit	Concentric: >5000 μV
		Fasciculation		Longer than 15 ms			Monopolar: >8000 μV
		Complex repetitive discharges				Early recruitment	
		Myotonic potentials on percussion			Myotonic potentials		

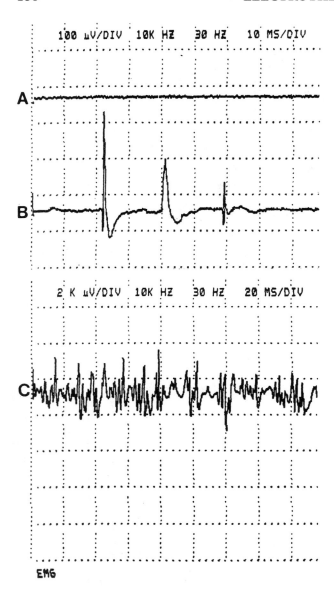

FIGURE 4–18. Normal electromyographic activity recorded with monopolar needle electrode in biceps brachii muscle during three conditions of muscle contraction: (*A*) at rest, no electrical activity (electrical silence); (*B*) minimal voluntary contraction, discrete motor unit potentials recorded from muscle fibers near electrode; and (*C*) strong voluntary contraction, many motor unit action potentials discharge so that the baseline of the tracing is almost completely disrupted — therefore, a full or complete interference pattern is produced.

contraction. Abnormal EMG characteristics are listed in Table 4–6; examples of abnormal EMG potentials are illustrated in Figure 4–19.

During rest, spontaneous activity, that is, fibrillations, positive sharp waves, fasciculation potentials, and complex repetitive discharges[91,92] can be found. The source of this abnormal spontaneous EMG activity is not known. Hypersensitivity of muscle fibers to acetylcholine[92] and alterations in muscle fiber membrane stability have been postulated but studies are inconclusive. Fibrillation potentials and positive sharp waves are thought to be spontaneous discharges of single muscle fibers, while fasciculations and complex discharges represent electrical activity from groups of muscle fibers. For

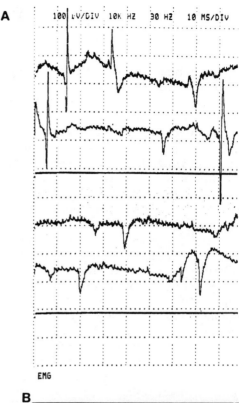

FIGURE 4-19. Abnormal electromyographic activity recorded with monopolar needle electrode: (*A*) spontaneous fibrillations and positive sharp waves, and (*B*) polyphasic potentials — may occur spontaneously (fasciculation) or during voluntary contraction.

detailed descriptions of these and other abnormal EMG characteristics the reader is referred to the suggested books at the end of this chapter.

Spontaneous activity is commonly graded on a scale of 1 to 4, with greatest abnormality rated 4, or it may be reported in qualitative terms such as moderate spontaneous activity. Insertion activity may be increased (sometimes termed *irritable*), decreased, or absent.

When minimal voluntary effort is performed by the patient, the elicited muscle action potentials may be polyphasic, the duration and amplitude of the individual potentials may be increased or decreased, or action potentials may be absent. Parameters of duration, amplitude, and the extent of polyphasia are reported. With maximal contraction, the interference pattern may be reduced so that several individual muscle-action potentials may be identified. With a greater loss of muscle electrical activity, only discrete potentials or even isolated single motor units alone will be seen with maximal effort of contraction by the patient. Another abnormality that can be observed is an alteration of the recruitment pattern, in that many motor units discharge at a rapid frequency early in the contraction when the patient is using considerably less than maximum effort.

An interesting type of abnormal EMG activity which may occur when the muscle is mechanically stimulated, such as with needle movement or manual percussion of the muscle, or when the muscle is contracting is the myotonic discharge. The true myotonic discharge waxes and wanes because the potentials vary both in amplitude and frequency.[89,90] Myotonic discharges are sometimes confused with the complex repetitive discharges that occur spontaneously (at rest), are constant in frequency, and can stop abruptly.[91,92]

For many years, and even currently, the analog EMG signal has been analyzed by visually observing and manually measuring the parameters of action potentials, and subjectively judging the fullness of the interference pattern. Methods of electronic analysis were proposed in earlier years but were not readily available. In more recent years, instrumentation and technology have been designed to make electronic analysis feasible in clinical settings. Stålberg and Antoni,[93] Stålberg and associates,[94] and Chu-Andrews and Johnson[89] have described methods of objective analysis of EMG using special instrumentation. Their methods include the conventional measurement of motor unit potential peak-to-peak amplitude and duration. In addition, *area*, defined as the integral or total voltage of the rectified signal, the number of *turns* or polarity reversals within a motor unit potential, and *muscle fiber density*, the number of muscle fibers within the recording area of the needle electrode, are also measured. Stålberg and associates,[94] propose a procedure of plotting the number of turns per second against the mean amplitude per turn at various levels of muscle contraction. From this X–Y plot, those authors define a frequency distribution pattern as a cluster or "cloud" in which the data are normally concentrated. They have applied their methods to study the EMG of patients with neuromuscular disorders, using monopolar and concentric needle electrodes. They report predictable shifts of the data pattern, for example, with myogenic disorders, the cloud shifts to the right-lower quadrant of the plot, representing an increased number of turns and small amplitudes. These changes are consistent with the increased frequency and decreased duration and amplitude of action potentials seen in myopathies.

To determine the total electrical activity in a majority of muscle fibers in a motor unit, a *macro-EMG* technique has been used.[94] Two recording channels are used, and recordings are made of the signal between a modified single fiber EMG needle electrode in one channel and a subcutaneous concentric needle recorded on a second channel. While methods of automatic analysis of EMG signals are highly desirable, they have not as yet been standardized and are not, at this time, widely used in clinical EMG.

Clinical significance of the EMG can only be determined by careful correlation of the EMG findings with specific pathologic changes and the anatomic sites of these changes. Although EMG findings cannot be accurately and distinctly categorized into a simplified list of changes indicative of diseases and dysfunctions, alignment of EMG abnormalities with general categories of pathologic conditions is helpful to the clinician in understanding the meaning of the EMG report and are discussed later in this chapter.

INDICATIONS FOR ELECTROMYOGRAPHIC EVALUATION

Certain EMG abnormalities are usually characteristic of neuropathy, whereas other EMG changes are characteristic of myopathy. Neuropathy can be differentiated into peripheral neuropathy, or lower motor neuron pathology, and myelopathy for the purpose of clarification of EMG findings. Peripheral neuropathy includes dysfunction of cranial and spinal nerves, nerve roots, nerve plexuses, and peripheral nerves and generalized systemic peripheral polyneuropathy. Myelopathy includes involvement of structures within the spinal cord, including upper motor neurons, neural tracts, as well as the lower motor neurons (anterior horn cells). The term motor neuron disease is often applied to disorders involving more than just the cell body of the alpha motor neuron.[95]

Electromyographic abnormalities most characteristic of peripheral neuropathy include increased action potential durations and an incomplete interference pattern.[96] Additional changes frequently seen, in peripheral neuropathies but which may also be found in other conditions, are fibrillations, positive sharp waves, complex repetitive discharges, and an increased number of polyphasic potentials. The distinction between the type of neuropathy, for example, a systemic polyneuropathy versus a mononeuropathy, must be determined by analyzing the anatomic distribution of the EMG changes. With radiculopathies (such as may occur with a herniated disc), these same EMG changes can be seen; however, the most common early findings are positive sharp waves and polyphasic potentials in the peripheral and paraspinal muscles supplied by the compromised spinal nerve root or roots.[97] If the disc is avulsed primarily in the posterior direction toward the dorsal (sensory) root, little or no EMG abnormalities may be found in spite of pain in a dermatomal distribution.

With myelopathy or diseases affecting the motor neurons, the characteristic findings are action potentials of increased amplitude (giant potentials) and duration, a reduced interference pattern, and fasciculation potentials.[49] In addition, complex repetitive discharges and other spontaneous activity described under peripheral neuropathy may be seen.

Myopathies characteristically exhibit potentials with decreased duration and amplitude, and an interference pattern with an increased number of action potentials relative to the strength of contraction,[49,83] producing a pattern sometimes called early recruitment. With infectious or acute myopathies, spontaneous activity may be prominent.

With myotonic conditions, characteristic EMG myotonic discharges can be found. The type of EMG abnormalities will depend on the variety of the myotonic disorder and the clinical signs and symptoms, and in some of the myotonias, the EMG changes may be temperature dependent.[98,99]

CASE STUDY

1 (continued from p. 126)

An EMG report of Case Study 1, JL, is presented in Figure 4–20, to illustrate how this test can help in identifying and localizing a peripheral nerve lesion.

Spontaneous activity does not usually appear before 2 weeks after onset of a peripheral nerve lesion.[92] Earlier testing would show decreased or absent voluntary motor unit activity, but probably no spontaneous EMG activity. Testing 3 to 4 weeks after the onset may show a marked increase in spontaneous activity in those muscles that are denervated. The rare single units seen in the peroneus longus

ELECTROMYOGRAPHY REPORT

Patient ___JL___ Unit No. _36-27-89_ Referred by _____

Birthdate _4/7/28_ Sex M _X_ F _____

Problem _Weakness right lower extremity_____

Date	Muscle	Insertional Activity	Spontaneous Activity	Muscle Action Potentials	Interference Pattern
2/10	rt. tibialis anterior	decreased	fibrillation +1 positive sharps +1	none	none
	rt. peroneus longus	decreased	fibrillation +1 positive sharps +1	rare, low amplitude	rare single units
	rt. gastroc-nemius	normal	none	normal	75%; normal recruitment
	rt. biceps femoris (short head)	normal	none	normal	100%; normal recruitment

Impression: EMG shows occasional spontaneous activity and loss of muscle action potentials in peroneal nerve distribution, compatible with severe denervation below the knee. Rare action potentials in peroneus longus indicate that degeneration of superficial peroneal nerve may be incomplete. EMG in tibial nerve distribution and peroneal nerve distribution above knee is normal. Follow-up EMG in 3-4 weeks may be helpful in clarifying the problem.

Signature _____

FIGURE 4-20. Electromyography report of 2/10 (see Case Study 1, JL).

muscle indicate that at least a small portion of this muscle's innervation may be preserved. Again, the follow-up test should help to clarify whether this activity is preserved or even improved, as would be indicated by the appearance of additional action potentials, particularly low amplitude polyphasic potentials. Thus, this EMG examination, correlated with clinical signs and symptoms, has helped identify which nerves are involved, the anatomic level of the lesion, and the extent of the lesion. Subsequent tests will be useful in monitoring progress and formulating and modifying the treatment program.

CONTRAINDICATIONS AND PRECAUTIONS FOR ELECTROMYOGRAPHIC EVALUATION

All practitioners who administer EMG examinations must be well versed in contraindications and precautions for the procedure. They are obligated to appropriately update their knowledge of these measures by studying reports, tests, and professional publications. Specific contraindications, or conditions, in which great discretion must be used when considering EMG, are bleeding disorders such as hemophilia, patients on anticoagulant medications, and recurrent systemic infections.[86] When performing EMG, sterile techniques must always be strictly adhered to. For Jakob-Creutzfeldt disease and other dementias, acquired immunodeficiency syndrome (AIDS), hepatitis, and any other conditions in which transmission of pathogenic organisms may be hazardous, needle electrodes must never be reused on other patients and are to be disposed of properly.

PLANNING A CLINICAL ELECTRICAL EVALUATION

Before outlining a plan for testing a patient's nerve conduction, electromyographic activity, or other electrophysiologic responses, a detailed physical examination of muscle strength, sensation, coordination, reflexes, and other aspects of neuromusculoskeletal function is selectively performed. In addition, the psychosocial and behavioral status of the patient is assessed, and effective interaction is established with the patient. The findings of these physical and behavioral assessments are then to be studied in light of the patient's clinical signs and symptoms. The clinician then interprets all of this information to formulate a preliminary electrical evaluation plan, which identifies the nerves or muscles to be tested and indicates the sequence of testing.

When planning the electrical evaluation, the first step is to establish the presence of normal or abnormal electrical excitability of nerve or muscle. One of the older, traditional tests such as the reaction of degeneration or a chronaxie test may be a useful screening tool at this point, and the findings may be a helpful guide in making decisions about the need for further electrical evaluation. The neuroanatomic nature of the problem is considered at this preliminary stage of the test, and the test is planned to determine whether an abnormality, if found, is in a local area and restricted to a focal region of a specific peripheral nerve, or whether the pathology extends to a portion of a nerve plexus or possibly to the more general peripheral nervous system.

The clinician may then attempt to determine, through nerve conduction testing, whether the pathology involves the motor or sensory component of the peripheral nerve or both components. As a further analysis of the problem, the examiner may use nerve conduction and electromyographic tests to clarify the presence of demyelinating or axonal changes, or both. Study and interpretation of the results of each aspect of the electrical evaluation will guide the examiner in judging the extent of the pathology, in terms of the completeness or severity of the lesion.

To summarize, the electrical evaluation may provide information to determine the following: (1) the presence of normal or abnormal electrical excitability of the peripheral nervous system and muscle tissue, (2) the neuroanatomic location or limits of the pathology, (3) the involvement of motor or sensory components of the peripheral nerve, (4) the presence of demyelinating or axonal changes, and (5) the extent of the pathologic process. Finally, the clinical report reflects each of these features as may be appropriate for the specific problem being evaluated and includes a summary or impression of the results.

Case Study 2 is presented to illustrate the process of formulating a plan for electrical evaluation, results of the test, and interpretation of the results.

CASE STUDY

2

LMD is a 61-year-old male who has had pain in his right lumbar area, right buttocks, and posterior thigh, and numbness and burning on the bottom of both feet for about 2 months. He reports twisting his back 3 months ago, with sharp pain in the low-back area at the time, which subsided in a week. The current symptoms began later and have become quite severe over the past 3 to 4 weeks. He is generally in good health, except that he has mild diabetes which has been controlled with diet and oral medication for about 2 years. He works as a cook in a restaurant. The patient is referred for electrical evaluation for a possible herniated disc.

Physical Examination. Muscle strength is normal; sensation is intact although numbness and tingling are described at the plantar surfaces of both feet. Reflexes and coordination are normal; straight-leg raising is without discomfort to 35° on right and 65° on left; no other limitations of joint movement are noted. Ambulation is somewhat slow and hesitant and there is a mild antalgic trunk shift to the left. He is alert, attentive, and fully oriented.

ELECTROMYOGRAPHY

Patient ___LMD___ Unit No. _62-78-96_ Referred by _____

Birthdate _5/8/31_ Sex M _X_ F _____

Problem   Pain low back, right buttock and lower extremity; numbness, burning both feet

Date	Muscle	Insertional Activity	Spontaneous Activity	Muscle Action Potentials	Interference Pattern
3/15	rt. gastrocnemius rt. abductor hallucis rt. biceps femoris (long head) rt. lumbar paraspinals	Increased	fibrillation +2 positive sharps +2	Moderately increased polyphasics, normal amplitude and duration	Slightly Reduced
	rt. tibialis anterior rt. peroneus longus lt. gastrocnemius lt. lumbar paraspinals	Normal	None	Normal	Full; normal recruitment

A

FIGURE 4–21. Electromyography and nerve conduction test reports of 3/15 (see Case Study 2, LMD).

Nerve Conduction Test

Patient **LMD**   Unit No. **62-78-96**   Referred by _____

Birthdate **5/8/31**   Sex M **X**   F _____

Problem   Pain low back, right buttock and lower extremity; numbness, burning both feet

Date	Nerve	Latency	Amplitude	Velocity
3/15	rt. peroneal motor ankle-muscle fib. head-ankle F wave	6.2 msec 52 msec	3.5 mV	36 m/sec
	rt. tibial motor ankle-muscle knee-ankle F wave H reflex	7.2 msec 58 msec 34.6 msec	1.5 mV	32 m/sec
	lt. tibial motor ankle-muscle knee-muscle F wave H wave	6.7 msec 56 msec 32 msec	2.0 mV	37 m/sec
	rt. sural	No Response		
	rt. superficial peroneal sensory	No Response		
	lt. sural	No Response		
	lt. superficial peroneal sensory	5.8 msec	4 uV	24 m/sec
	rt. median motor wrist-muscle elbow-wrist	3.6 msec	9.5 mV	48 m/sec
	rt. median sensory index-wrist	3.5 msec	10 uV	40 m/sec

Impression: EMG changes and H reflex conduction are compatible with S-1 nerve root irritation. Nerve conduction findings show slowing in latency and velocity, and reduced amplitude in motor and sensory nerves in both lower extremities, consistent with a demyelinating polyneuropathy. Right median motor and sensory conduction are normal.

Signature   _____

B

FIGURE 4-21. *Continued.*

Planning the Electrical Evaluation. Electromyography is an appropriate test for evaluation of a herniated disc, because irritation or compression of the spinal motor-nerve roots can cause abnormal EMG. Motor and sensory nerve conduction and strength duration and chronaxie are usually normal with radiculopathy unless there is severely advanced denervation of the peripheral nerves, which is rare. The H-reflex conduction response can be delayed in S-1 radiculopathy; theoretically, the F wave can be delayed, but its reliability in evaluation of herniated discs has not been established. Although the patient's complaint of back and thigh pain are compatible with a herniated disc, the symmetrical, bilateral paresthesia suggests a polyneuropathy, for which nerve conduction testing is indicated, particularly sensory conduction. A report of the electrical evaluation of this patient is shown in Figure 4–21. Selection of electrical tests to be performed on this patient was based on analysis of clinical signs and symptoms, along with physical findings and consideration of whether the results of each test could assist in the identification of possible neuropathologies. The test results of this patient provided information on most of the features discussed in the summary on planning a clinical electrical evaluation. Electrical testing is but one part of total patient evaluation. Whether a simple screening test is used, for example, the RD test, or a more complex evaluation procedure is performed, for example, EMG, electrical testing is a critical aspect of total evaluation.

SUMMARY

This chapter reviews the historical application of clinical electrophysiologic evaluation procedures, including those currently in use, and briefly addresses new procedures and investigative studies that have potential for clinical application. Traditional tests widely used in earlier time periods, namely, the reaction of degeneration, strength-duration curve, chronaxie, galvanic twitch-tetanus ratio test, as well as the nerve excitability test, which remains in use, are explained. Furthermore, indications for and the clinical significance of these tests are discussed.

Electrical evaluation procedures common to contemporary clinical practice are described, that is, motor and sensory nerve conduction tests, including F-wave and H-reflex studies, evoked potential tests, and electromyography. Their clinical indications are enumerated, and interpretation of their measurement outcomes is discussed.

One patient case study is used throughout the chapter in order to illustrate application of several tests. Each test performed on the patient is reported, followed by a discussion of the results and implications of the test.

The author proposes an incorporation of data obtained from other patient assessments, such as muscle strength and sensory tests, in the development of a systematic plan for electrophysiologic evaluation. Finally, another case study demonstrates application of the theoretical process of analyzing clinical information in formulating an appropriate plan for electrical testing as part of comprehensive patient evaluation.

REFERENCES

1. Licht, S: History of electrodiagnosis. In Licht, S (ed): Electrodiagnosis and Electromyography, ed 3. Elizabeth Licht, New Haven, 1971, p 1.
2. Duchenne, GB: Treatise on Localised Electrisation, London, 1871.
3. Adrian, ED: The electrical reactions of muscles before and after injury. Brain 39:1, 1916.

4. Fischer, E: Physiology of skeletal muscle. In Licht, S (ed): Electrodiagnosis and Electromyography, ed 3. Elizabeth Licht, New Haven, 1971, p 80.
5. Shriber, WJ: A Manual of Electrotherapy, ed 4. Lea & Febiger, Philadelphia, 1975, p 145.
6. Patterson, RP: Instrumentation for electrotherapy. In Stillwell, GK (ed): Therapeutic Electricity and Ultraviolet Radiation, ed 3. Williams and Wilkins, Baltimore, 1983, p 105.
7. Wynn Parry, CB: Strength-duration curves. In Licht, S (ed): Electrodiagnosis and Electromyography, ed 3. Elizabeth Licht, New Haven, 1971, p 241.
8. Harris, R: Chronaxie. In Licht, S (ed): Electrodiagnosis and Electromyography, ed 3. Elizabeth Licht, New Haven, 1971, p 218.
9. Li, CL and Bak, A: Excitability characteristics of the A- and C-fibres in a peripheral nerve. Exp Neurol 50:67, 1976.
10. Oester, YT and Licht, S: Routine electrodiagnosis. In Licht, S (ed): Electrodiagnosis and Electromyography, ed 3. Elizabeth Licht, New Haven, 1971, p 201.
11. Boulrière, F: Excitability and aging. J Gerontol 3:191, 1948.
12. Rutan, F: Measurement of nerve excitability. Phys Ther 47:1035, 1967.
13. Campbell, EDR, et al.: Value of nerve-excitability measurements in prognosis of facial palsy. Br Med J 2:7, 1962.
14. Laumans, EPJ: Nerve excitability tests in facial paralysis. Arch Otolaryng 81:478, 1965.
15. Gasser, HS and Erlanger, J: A study of the action potential of nerve with cathode ray oscillograph. Am J Physiol 62:496, 1922.
16. Adrian, ED and Bronk, DW: The discharge of impulse in motor nerve fibres. J Physiol 67:119, 1929.
17. Harvey, AM and Masland, RL: A method for the study of neuromuscular transmission in human subjects. Bull Johns Hopkins Hosp 68:81, 1941.
18. Hodes, R, Larrabee, MG, and German, W: The human EMG in response to nerve stimulation and the conduction velocity of motor axons. Arch Neuro Psychiat 60:340, 1948.
19. Dawson, GD and Scott, JW: The recording of nerve action potential through the skin in man. J Neurol Neurosurg Psychiat 12:259, 1949.
20. Dawson, GD: Cerebral responses to electrical stimulation of peripheral nerve in man. J Neurosurg Psychiat 10:137, 1947.
21. Rodriquez, AA and Oester, YT: Fundamentals of electromyography. In Licht, S (ed): Electrodiagnosis and Electromyography, ed 3. Elizabeth Licht, New Haven, 1971, p 297.
22. Gilliatt, RW: History of nerve conduction studies. In Licht, S (ed): Electrodiagnosis and Electromyography, ed 3. Elizabeth Licht, New Haven, 1981, p 412.
23. Kimura, J: Electrodiagnosis in Diseases of Nerve and Muscle: Principles and Practice, ed 2. FA Davis, Philadelphia, 1989, p 581.
24. Kimura, J: Electrodiagnosis in Diseases of Nerve and Muscle: Principles and Practice, ed 2. FA Davis, Philadelphia, 1989, p 55.
25. Kraft, GH: Peripheral neuropathies. In Johnson, EW (ed): Practical Electromyography. Williams & Wilkins, Baltimore, 1980, p 155.
26. Wagman, IH and Lesse, H: Maximum conduction velocity of motor fibers of ulnar nerve in human subjects of various ages and sizes. J Neurophysiol 15:235, 1952.
27. Thomas, JE and Lambert, EH: Ulnar nerve conduction velocity and H-reflex in infants and children. J Appl Physiol 15:1, 1960.
28. Gamstorp, I: Normal conduction velocity of ulnar, median and peroneal nerves in infancy, childhood and adolescence. Acta Paediat Suppl 146:68, 1963.
29. La Fratta, CW and Smith, OH: A study of the relationship of motor nerve conduction velocity in the adult to age, sex, and handedness. Arch Phys Med 45:407, 1964.
30. Cerra, D and Johsnon, EW: Motor nerve conduction velocity in premature infants. Arch Phys Med Rehabil 43:160, 1972.
31. Weber, RJ and Piero, D: Entrapment syndromes. In Johnson, EW (ed): Practical Electromyography. Williams & Wilkins, Baltimore, 1980, p 206.
32. Kimura, J: Electrodiagnosis in Diseases of Nerve and Muscle: Principles and Practice, ed 2. FA Davis, Philadelphia, 1989, p 462.
33. Winckler, G: Le nerf pironier accessoire profond: étude d'anatomie compafee. Arch Anat Histol Embryol 18:181, 1934.
34. Lambert, EH: The accessory deep peroneal nerve: A common variation in innervation of extensor digitorum brevis. Neurology (Minneap) 19:1169, 1969.
35. Young, RR and Shahani, BT: Clinical value and limitations of F-wave determination. Kimura, J: A Comment. Panayiotopoulos, CP: A Reply. Muscle Nerve 1(2):248, 1978.
36. Eccles, JC: The central action of antidromic impulses in motor nerve fibers. Pflugers Arch fur die Gesante Physiologic des Menschen und der Tiere 260:385, 1955.
37. Magladery, JW and McDougal, DB, Jr: Electrophysiological studies of nerve and reflex activity in normal man. Bull John Hopkins Hosp 86:265, 1950.
38. Trontelj, AJ: A study of the F-respones by single fibre electromyography. In Desmedt, JE (ed): New Developments in Electromyography and Clinical Neurophysiology, Vol 3. Karger, Basel, 1973, p 318.

39. Shiller, HH and Stålberg, E: F responses studied with single fibre EMG in normal subjects and spastic patients. J Neurol Neurosurg Psychiatry 41:45, 1978.
40. Cornwall, MW and Nelson, C: Median nerve F-wave conduction in healthy subjects. Phys Ther 64:1679, 1984.
41. Weber, RJ and Piero, DL: F wave evaluation of thoracic outlet syndrome: A multiple regression derived F wave latency predicting technique. Arch Phys Med Rehabil 59:464, 1978.
42. Dorfman, LJ and Bosley, TM: Age related changes in peripheral and centeral nerve conduction in man. Neurology (New York) 29:38, 1979.
43. Nelson, C, et al: Median nerve F wave conduction in healthy subjects over age sixty-five. Electromyogr Clin Neurophysiol 30:219, 1990.
44. Jolly, F: Uber myasthenia gravis pseudoparalytica. Berl Klin Wochenschr 32:1, 1895.
45. Harvey, AM and Masland, RL: The electromyogram in myasthenia gravis. Bull Johns Hopkins Hosp 69:1, 1941.
46. Maclean, IC: Neuromuscular junction. In Johnson, EW (ed): Practical Electromyography. Williams & Wilkins, Baltimore, 1980, p 73.
47. Kimura, J: Electrodiagnosis in Diseases of Nerve and Muscle: Principles and Practice, ed 2. FA Davis, Philadelphia, 1989, p 519.
48. Ozdemir, C and Young, RR: The results to be expected from electrical testing in the diagnosis of myosthenia gravis. Ann NY Acad Sci 274:203, 1976.
49. Eaton, LM and Lambert, EH: Electromyography and electric stimulation of nerves in diseases of motor unit: Observations on myasthenic syndrome associated with malignant tumors. JAMA 163:111, 1957.
50. Desmedt, JE and Borenstein, S: Double-step nerve stimulation test for myasthenic block: Sensitization of postactivation exhaustion by ischemia. Ann Neurol 1:55, 1977.
51. Gilchrist, JM and Sanders, DB: Double-step repetitive stimulation in myasthenia gravis. Muscle Nerve 10:233, 1987.
52. Kimura, J: Electrodiagnosis in Diseases of Nerve and Muscle: Principles and Practice, ed 2. FA Davis, Philadelphia, 1989, p 288.
53. Sanders, DB, Howard, JF, and Johns, TR: Single-fiber electromyography in myasthenia gravis. Neurology 29:68, 1979.
54. Schuchmann, J and Braddom, RL: Sensory conduction. In Johnson, EW (ed): Practical Electromyography. Williams & Wilkins, Baltimore, 1980, p 61.
55. Johnson, EW and Melvin, JL: Sensory conduction studies of median and ulnar nerves. Arch Phys Med Rehabil 48:25, 1967.
56. Gamstorp, I and Shelburne, SA: Peripheral sensory conduction in ulnar and median nerves of normal infants, children and adolescents. Acta Paediatr Scand 54:309, 1965.
57. La Fratta, CW and Canestrani, RE: A comparison of sensory and motor nerve conduction velocities as related to age. Arch Phys Med Rehabil 47:286, 1966.
58. Buchthal, F AND Rosenfalck, A: Evoked action potentials and conduction velocity in human sensory nerves. Brain Res 3:1, 1966.
59. Sethi, RK and Thompson, LL: The Electromyographers Handbook, ed 2. Little, Brown & Co, Boston, 1989.
60. DeLisa, J and Mackenzie, K: Manual of Nerve Conduction Velocity Techniques. Raven Press, New York, 1982.
61. Ma, DM and Liveson, JA: Nerve Conduction Handbook. FA Davis, Philadelphia, 1983.
62. Hoffmann, P: Untersuchungen uber die Eigenreflexe (Schnenreflexe) Menschlicker Muskeln. Springer, Berlin, 1922.
63. Braddom, RL and Johnson, EW: Standardization of H reflex and diagnostic use in S1 radiculopathy. Arch Phys Med Rehabil 55:161, 1974.
64. Sabbahi, MA and Khalil, M: Segmental H-reflex studies in upper and lower limbs of healthy subjects. Arch Phys Med 71:216, 1990.
65. Braddom, RL and Schuchmann, J: Motor conduction. In Johnson, EW (ed): Practical Electromyography. Williams & Wilkins, Baltimore, 1980, p 16.
66. Kriss, A: Setting up an evoked potential (EP) laboratory. In Halliday, AM (ed): Evoked Potentials in Clinical Testing. Churchill Livingstone, London, 1982, p 1.
67. Lehmkuhl, LD: Evoked spinal, brain stem and cerebral potentials. In Wolf, SL (ed): Electrotherapy. Churchill Livingstone, New York, 1981, p 123.
68. Barron, DH and Matthews, BHC: The interpretation of potential changes on the spinal cord. J Physiol 92:276, 1938.
69. Jasper, HH: The ten-twenty system of the international federation. Electroencephalogr Clin Neurophysiol 10:371, 1958.
70. Jones, SJ: Somatosensory evoked potentials: The normal waveform. In Halliday, AM (ed): Evoked Potentials in Clinical Testing. Churchill Livingstone, London, 1982, p 393.
71. Cracco, JB, Cracco, RQ, and Stolone, R: Spinal evoked potential in man: A maturational study. Electroencephalogr Clin Neurophysiol 46:58, 1979.
72. Chatrian, GE: American Electroencephalographic Society: Guidelines for clinical evoked potential studies. J Clin Neurophysiol 1:3, 1984.

73. Halliday, AM: The visual evoked potential in the investigation of disease of the optic nerve. In Halliday, AM (ed): Evoked Potentials in Clinical Testing. Churchill Livingstone, London 1982, p 187.
74. Aepen, G, Doerr, M, and Thoden, U: Huntingdon's disease: Alterations of visual and somatosensory cortical evoked potentials in patients and offspring. In Courjon, J, Mauguiere, F, and Reval, M (eds). Clinical Applications of Evoked Potentials in Neurology. Raven Press, New York, 1982, p 141.
75. Carroll, WM, et al: The incidence and nature of visual pathway involvement in Friedreich's ataxia. Brain 103:413, 1980.
76. Robinson, K and Rudge, P: Centrally generated auditory potentials. In Halliday, AM (ed): Evoked Potentials in Clinical Testing. Churchill Livingstone, London, 1982, p 345.
77. Robinson, K and Rudge, P: Abnormalities of the auditory evoked potentials in patients with multiple sclerosis. Brain 100:19, 1977.
78. Stockard, JJ, Stockard, JE, and Skarbrough, FW: Detection and localization of occult lesions with brainstem auditory responses. Mayo Clin Proc (Rochester) 52:761, 1977.
79. Chiappa, KH, et al: Brainstem auditory evoked responses in 200 patients with multiple sclerosis. Ann Neurol 7:135, 1980.
80. Tsobokawa, T, et al: Assessment of brainstem damage by auditory brainstem response in acute severe head injury. J Neurol Neurosurg Psychiatry 43:1005, 1980.
81. Robinson, K and Rudge, P: The use of auditory potentials in neurology. In Halliday, AM (ed): Evoked Potentials in Clinical Testing. Churchill Livingstone, London, 1982, p 373.
82. Goodgold, J and Eberstein, A: Electrodiagnosis of Neuromuscular Disease, ed 3. Williams & Wilkins, Baltimore, 1983, p 45.
83. Kimura, J: Electrodiagnosis in Diseases of Nerve and Muscle: Principles and Practice, ed 2. FA Davis, Philadelphia, 1989, p 37.
84. Stålberg, E and Trontelj, J: Single Fibre Electromyography. The Miraville Press Limited. Old Woking, Surrey, UK, 1979.
85. Goodgold, J and Eberstein, A: Electrodiagnosis of Neuromuscular Diseases, ed 3. Williams & Wilkins, Baltimore, 1983 p 1.
86. Kimura, J: Electrodiagnosis in Disease of Nerve and Muscle: Principles and Practice, ed 2. FA Davis, Philadelphia, 1989, p 227.
87. Goodgold, J and Eberstein, A: Electrodiagnosis of Neuromuscular Disease, ed 3. Williams & Wilkins, Baltimore, 1983, p 64.
88. Buchthal, F, Guld, C, and Rosenfalck, P: Action potential parameters in normal human muscle and their dependence on physical variables. Acta Physiol Scand 32:200, 1954.
89. Chu-Andrews, J and Johnson, RJ: Electrodiagnosis: An Anatomical and Clinical Approach. JB Lippincott, Philadelphia, 1986, p 230.
90. Buchthal, F and Rosenfalck, P: Action potential parameters in different human muscles. Acta Psychiatr 30:125, 1955.
91. American Association of Electromyography and Electrodiagnosis: Glossary of Terms. Muscle Nerve Supplement, Oct, 1987.
92. Kimura, J: Electrodiagnosis in Diseases of Nerve and Muscle: Principles and Practice, ed 2. FA Davis, Philadelphia, 1989, p 249.
93. Stålberg, E and Antoni, L: Computer-aided EMG analysis. In Desmedt, JE (ed): Progress in Clinical Neurophysiology, Vol 10, Computer-Aided Electromyography. Basel, Karger, 1983, p 186.
94. Stålberg, E, et al: Automatic analysis of the EMG interference pattern. Electroencephalogr Clin Neurophysiol 56:672, 1983.
95. Wiechers, DO and Warmolts, JR: Anterior horn cell diseases. In Johnson, EW (ed): Practical Electromyography. Williams & Wilkins, Baltimore, 1980, p 135.
96. Goodgold, J and Eberstein, A: Electrodiagnosis of Neuromuscular Diseases. ed 3. Williams & Wilkins, Baltimore, 1983, p 207.
97. Weingarden, HP, Mikolich, LM, and Johnson, EW: Radiculopathies. In Johnson, EW (ed): Practical Electromyography. Williams & Wilkins, Baltimore, 1980, p 91.
98. Kimura, J: Electrodiagnosis in Diseases of Nerve and Muscle: Principles and Practice, ed 2. FA Davis, Philadelphia, 1989, p 535.
99. Goodgold, J and Eberstein, A: Electrodiagnosis of Neuromuscular Diseases, ed 3. Williams & Wilkins, Baltimore, 1983, p 98.
100. Goodgold, J and Eberstein, A: Electrodiagnosis of Neuromuscular Diseases, ed 3. Williams & Wilkins, Baltimore, 1983, p 104.
101. Jebsen, RH: Motor conduction velocities in the median and ulnar nerves. Arch Phys Med Rehabil 48:185, 1967.
102. Jebsen, RH: Motor conduction velocities in proximal and distal segments of radial nerve. Arch Phys Med Rehabil 47:597, 1966.
103. Melvin, JL, Harris, DH, and Johnson, EW: Sensory and motor conduction velocities in the ulnar and median nerves. Arch Phys Med Rehabil 47:511, 1966.
104. Di Benedetto, M: Posterior interosseus branch of the radial nerve: Conduction velocities. Arch Phys Med Rehabil 53:266, 1972.

105. Kimura, J: Electrodiagnosis in Diseases of Nerve and Muscle: Principles and Practice, ed 2. FA Davis, Philadelphia, 1989, p 332.
106. Jabre, JF: The superficial peroneal sensory nerve revisited. Arch Neurol 38:666, 1981.
107. Downie, A and Scott, TR: An improved technique for radial nerve conduction studies. J Neurol Neurosurg Psychiatry 30:332, 1967.
108. Izzo, KL, et al: Sensory conduction studies of the branches of the peroneal nerve. Arch Phys Med Rehabil 62:24, 1981.
109. Schuchmann, JA: Sural nerve conduction: A standardized technique. Arch Phys Med Rehabil 58:166, 1977.

SUGGESTED READINGS

Chu-Andrews, J and Johnson, RJ: Electrodiagnosis: An Anatomical and Clinical Approach. JB Lippincott, Philadelphia, 1986.

Goodgold, J and Eberstein, A: Electrodiagnosis of Neuromuscular Diseases ed 3. Williams & Wilkins, Baltimore, 1983.

Johnson, EW: Practical Electromyography. Williams & Wilkins, Baltimore, 1981.

Kimura, J: Electrodiagnosis in Diseases of Nerve Muscle: Principles and Practice, ed 2. FA Davis, Philadelphia, 1989.

Liveson, JA: Peripheral Neurology: Case Studies in Electrodiagnosis, ed 2. FA Davis, Philadelphia, 1991.

CHAPTER 5

Transcutaneous Electrical Nerve Stimulation (TENS) for Management of Pain and Sensory Pathology

Meryl R. Gersh, M.M.Sc., P.T.

The pain experience has been a part of man's existence since the beginning of time. Attempts to modify pain via electricity date back to the era of Hippocrates[1] but the first written record of electrotherapeutic analgesia is attributed to Scribonius Largus in 46 A.D.[2] John Wesley,[3] a religious leader and founder of the Methodist Church, was also a student of electrotherapy and detailed the "cure" of various ailments including sciatica, hysteria, headache, kidney stone, and gout in his treatise, "Desideratum: or Electricity Made Plain and Useful by a Lover of Mankind and of Common Sense," published in 1759. In the early 19th century, Sarlandiere[4] described the use of electrical stimulation of acupuncture points (electroacupuncture) for treatment of rheumatism, gout, neuralgia, migraine headache, alcoholism, and ataxia.

In 1926, electrotherapy was placed in the hands of the general consumer with products such as the Renulife (violet-ray) Generator.* The manufacturers of this product claimed to improve health and cure a wide variety of ailments by "increasing circulation, charging the blood with health-giving oxygen and nutrition . . . and dissolving and carrying away poison and inflammation."[5] However, because of unsubstantiated claims such as these, and a dearth of clinical investigation and publication, electroanalgesia fell into disrepute until the dissemination of the gate-control theory of pain by Melzack and Wall[6] in 1965. This concept of pain modification via the introduction of sensory input gained wide acceptance in the scientific community and fostered the

---

*Renulife Electric Company, Detroit, Michigan.

development of dorsal column stimulation by Norman Shealy[7] for the management of intractable back pain. Shealy began to use a prototype of the modern transcutaneous electrical nerve stimulation (TENS) unit to evaluate patients for dorsal column stimulator implantation and found serendipitously that these patients responded favorably to transcutaneous stimulation by reporting significantly reduced pain during the evaluation process. In the early 1970s, the manufacture of the modern TENS units led to successful pain control in patients with a wide variety of acute and chronic neurologic and musculoskeletal disorders.

More recently, investigations have been performed to evaluate the effect of TENS on osteogenesis, circulatory imbalances, pruritus, and angina pectoris.[8-11] While widely used, the clinical efficacy of TENS has not been clearly established by well-controlled scientific study.

The purposes of this chapter are to summarize the current body of knowledge regarding the neurophysiologic bases for electroanalgesia, and describe various clinical applications of TENS. A schema will be presented to suggest general guidelines for (1) the evaluation of the patient with pain for whom TENS might be indicated, (2) the selection of preferred electrode placement sites and electrical stimulus characteristics, and (3) the assessment of treatment outcomes. These guidelines will be applied to a specific case history. Contraindications and precautions for TENS application will be reviewed, and suggestions for future clinical investigations will be presented.

BIOPHYSICAL PRINCIPLES

The neurophysiologic principles of pain perception and modulation are reviewed in detail in Chapter 2 of this text. The development of TENS has long been associated with the publication of the gate control theory of pain by Melzack and Wall[6] in 1965. These investigators proposed that sensory perception was the result of activation of transmission (T) cells in the dorsal horn of the spinal cord, which in turn resulted from a balance of peripheral input along large (A-alpha and A-beta) and small (A-delta and C) diameter afferent nerve fibers (Fig. 2–4). Activity from both large and small afferent neurons directly activate the T cell. However, noxious input transmitted through small-diameter fibers also inhibits inhibitory interneurons in the dorsal horn, thus decreasing the effect of presynaptic inhibition on the T cell from the interneurons and ultimately resulting in a net increase in perception of painful input.

In contrast, activity traveling along large diameter afferent fibers activates the inhibitory interneurons, thus facilitating presynaptic inhibition of the T cell and ultimately resulting in a "closing of the spinal gate" or a decrease in the perception of sensory activity. In the early 1970s TENS was viewed as a form of comfortable peripheral sensory input that could decrease pain perception by preferentially increasing the large diameter afferent fiber input and facilitating presynaptic inhibition of the T cell, thus decreasing pain perception. For instance, TENS has been demonstrated to be effective in relieving pain associated with postherpetic neuralgia, a disease which results in degeneration of large diameter afferent fibers.[12] Conventional TENS, applied to the painful region, or to a segmentally related region in which the population of large diameter fibers remains intact, effectively controls the pain associated with postherpetic neuralgia purportedly by activating the remaining large diameter afferent fibers that lie in close proximity to the pathologically active small diameter afferent neurons in the neuraxis.[13]

The gate control theory was criticized for failing to account for a variety of painful conditions in which small diameter afferents were preferentially destroyed and for not considering the role of higher centers in conscious pain perception.[14] Melzack and Casey,[15] in 1968, suggested a modification of the gate control theory to account for activation of higher centers. They added the limbic and reticular systems, both of which are known to influence pain perception, emotional phases of affect, and motor responses. Higher centers in the neocortex also monitor painful afferent input by comparing it to past experiences and learned responses. Melzack and Casey further suggested that a "central control trigger" activated by input to these higher centers might influence activity in the dorsal horn via descending systems and contribute to pain modulation as well. Thus, a mechanism for pain control via distraction, meditation, or relaxation was suggested.

As described in Chapter 2, other mechanisms proposed for pain modulation via afferent stimulation include a simple antidromic blocking of afferent impulses from nociceptors[16] as well as reflex activation of sympathetic neurons which results in vasomotor responses and relief of ischemic pain.[9]

One of the more intriguing theories of stimulation-produced analgesia (SPA) involves the production and utilization of endogenous opiates, such as endorphins and enkephalins.[17] In 1978, Basbaum and Fields[18] proposed a negative-feedback loop mechanism to account for analgesia resulting from low rate, high amplitude (acupuncturelike) TENS. They suggested that the noxious input associated with acupuncturelike TENS activated ascending pathways leading to awareness of pain. Along these pathways, certain axons that synapsed within medullary reticular formation nuclei were identified. Output from these nuclei was transmitted to the periaqueductal gray (PAG) region of the midbrain and to the thalamus. These regions possess high concentrations of endogenous opiates and opiate receptors and, when activated, facilitate cells in the nuclei raphe magnus (NRM) and reticularis gigantocellularis (RCG). Output from these nuclei in turn descends to the spinal cord and makes enkephalinergic synapses, which inhibit spinal release of substance P, a substance implicated as a neurotransmitter among axons conveying noxious information. Thus, the application of acupuncturelike TENS may activate a negative feedback loop that ultimately blocks further transmission of noxious information.

Administration of naloxone, an opiate antagonist, will reverse endorphin-mediated analgesia or return an elevated pain threshold to pretreatment values.[19] Direct stimulation of the PAG region results in diffuse, profound analgesia, which is reversed by naloxone, according to several investigators.[20,21] In addition, Sjolund, Terenius, and Eriksson[22] measured increased levels of endorphins in the cerebrospinal fluid following electroacupuncture.

The presence of an endorphin-mediated analgesic mechanism activated by acupuncturelike TENS has been confirmed or implied by many researchers.[22-25] Facchinetti and colleagues[26] reported increased levels of plasma beta-endorphin following 30 minutes of stimulation with conventional TENS. Hughes and associates[27] demonstrated an increase in plasma beta-endorphin with both high rate/low amplitude and low rate/high amplitude TENS applied for 30 minutes.

In contrast, O'Brien and associates[28] applied high rate, low rate, or placebo TENS to acupuncture points Li4 (Hoku point) and Li10, in 42 subjects, for a period of 2 hours and failed to reveal any significant changes in pain perception or plasma beta-endorphin levels under any of the experimental conditions. Hansson and colleagues[29] also failed to confirm activation of an endorphin-mediated analgesic mechanism associated with low- or high-rate TENS in patients with acute orofacial pain. Consideration of the differences between clinical pain and experimentally induced pain may offer an explanation of these conflicting results. The clinical pain experience involves pathology as well as sensory, motor, affective, and cultural components and results in a complex set of physiologic and behavioral responses. Fear, anxiety, depression, and a sense of loss of control are often associated with the presence of clinical pain. In contrast, pain that is experimentally induced by electrical, thermal, or other sensory stimuli, produces a more discretely defined sensory experience. The subject knows that the pain is self-limiting, is not associated with pathology, and that its duration and intensity are under his or her control. Fear, anxiety, and the loss of control are not components of the experimental pain experience. Since some investigators[24-28] evaluated the role of endorphin-mediated analgesia on experimentally induced pain, while others[29] evaluated this mechanism in patients with clinical pain, it is not surprising to find conflicting reports of TENS' influence on endorphin-mediated analgesia. In addition, patients with clinical pain may demonstrate impaired ability to produce or utilize endorphins, when compared to healthy individuals. The role that endorphins play in either high- or low-rate induced electroanalgesia requires additional definition and confirmation. Care must also be taken not to apply the results of investigations on healthy subjects to patients with clinical pain.

The mechanisms described above provide plausible explanations for the ways in which TENS can modulate pain perception. As methods of histochemical and electrophysiologic data acquisition become more sophisticated, additional neurophysiologic mechanisms, as well as confirmation or refutation of present ones, will add to our understanding of TENS-induced analgesia.

CLINICAL APPLICATIONS OF TENS

Acute Pain Conditions

POSTOPERATIVE INCISIONAL PAIN

One of the most successful applications of TENS continues to be control of postoperative incisional pain. This acute pain is well-localized, well-defined, and generally self-limiting in its time course and severity. Patients often are provided with a preoperative exposure to TENS for the setting of appropriate stimulus parameters. Sterile disposable electrodes are applied parallel to the incision during surgery, and electrical stimulation commences in the recovery room immediately following wound closure and dressing. TENS is usually provided for 48 to 72 hours following surgery, with the patients regulating the stimulus amplitude and thus exercising control over their pain experience.

A variety of objective measures suggesting the analgesic effect of TENS are easily applied to this patient population. These measures include pain-medication request and intake records, early ambulation or mobility, respiratory spirometry, compliance with physical therapy, respiratory therapy, nursing interventions, length of intensive care unit (ICU) or hospital stay, and incidence of postoperative ileus or atelectasis, in addition to the patient's subjective pain report. These easily obtained objective data provide the clinician with an excellent opportunity to assess the efficacy of TENS in the management of postoperative incisional pain.

Investigators[30-45] have evaluated the analgesic effects of TENS in patients who had undergone cholecystectomies or other abdominal surgery, thoracotomies, laminectomies, and other types of orthopedic surgery. The methods of application of TENS and measures used to evaluate treatment outcomes are summarized in Tables 5–1 and 5–2. Studies which include detailed descriptions of electrode placements, stimulus parameters and schedules, and a variety of objective outcome measures offer the most complete picture of TENS efficacy and are most easily replicated. In addition, the results of these studies are strengthened because TENS is compared to placebo, "sham" TENS, control, or "no treatment" groups.[30,33,45]

Several investigators[34,37,45] examined the effect of postoperative TENS applied for brief periods of time, rather than on a continuous 24-hour basis. In these investigations the effects of TENS analgesia were evaluated by the patient's ability to perform a brief but usually uncomfortable task, such as respiratory spirometry or shoulder flexion, rather than by medication intake or functional activities. Patients who received actual TENS, rather than a placebo treatment did perform these brief tasks better than their control-group counterparts. However, this short-term application of TENS may have limited value for the general postoperative patient population for whom analgesia of longer duration is desirable.

Attention should be paid to the patient's own sensory requirements regarding selection of stimulation parameters and administration of analgesic medication when postoperative pain studies are undertaken. Warfield, Stein, and Frank[36] evaluated the effect of TENS on pain report, narcotic use, and duration of ICU stay in patients who had undergone thoracotomy for lung resection. Twenty-four patients received preoperative education regarding TENS. Twelve patients received TENS postoperatively, applied through electrodes placed parallel to the incision, while 12 patients received sham TENS in a similar fashion. TENS was administered continuously for the first 48 hours postoperatively. Pulse duration, rate, and amplitude were identically set for all patients receiving actual TENS. Patients receiving TENS reported lower pain levels on a 0 to 10 visual analog scale than patients receiving sham TENS. The difference between groups was most dramatic during the first 24 postoperative hours. Patients receiving actual TENS also had shorter stays in the ICU and tolerated chest physical therapy more comfortably. No significant differences were noted among groups in the areas of postoperative complications, nausea, or narcotic use. However, of critical importance is the observation that narcotics were administered according to a schedule determined by the nursing staff, rather than on request by the patient. In addition, the predetermined setting of identical stimulus parameters for all patients may not have permitted patients the full advantage of TENS set to each individual's own needs and tolerance. The preset stimulus levels may have been uncomfortable for some patients and inadequate to produce analgesia for others. Consideration of each patient's response to, and tolerance of, electrical stimulation is critically important to the successful application of TENS for pain control.

In addition, drug-intake history may be a confounding factor in evaluating the effect of TENS on postoperative pain. Solomon, Viernstein, and Long[39] evaluated the effect of TENS on patients following laminectomy. The authors noted that TENS was most effective for managing pain in the "drug-naive" patients; that is, patients who had not used narcotic medication for more than 2 weeks in the 6 months prior to surgery. Clearly, this finding implies that the lack of effectiveness of TENS in patients with chronic pain may be due to the history of significant prescription drug intake often associated with these patients.

TABLE 5–1 Transcutaneous Electrical Nerve Stimulation Application Methods for Postoperative Pain

Primary Author	Diagnosis	Electrode Placement	Pulse Duration (μs)	Pulse Rate (Hz)	Amplitude (mA)	Frequency Duration of Treatments
Ali[30]	Cholecystectomy	Paraincisional	128–200	50	Comfort	Continuous × 48 hours
Sodipo[32]	Abdominal surgery	Paraincisional				
Taylor[33]	Abdominal	Paraincisional	80	40	Comfort	60 minutes every 4 hours
Stratton[34]	Thoracotomy	Greatest pain			Submotor	10 minutes
Warfield[36]	Thoracotomy	Paraincisional				Continuous × 48 hours
Liu[37]	Thoracotomy	Paraincisional	100	1.5–150	Subsensory, 0–10	20 minutes
Schuster[38]	Laminectomy	Paraincisional	40	80	0–90 V	Continuous × 18–24 hours
Smith[43]	Arthrotomy of knee	Paraincisional	50–250	3–150	Comfort	Continuous for length of hospital stay

TABLE 5–2 Evaluation Methods for Transcutaneous Electrical Nerve Stimulation Treatment for Postoperative Pain

Primary Author	Diagnosis	Subjective Pain Rating	Medication Intake	Physical Evaluations	Other
Ali[30]	Cholecystectomy	–	+	Pulmonary functions	Complications
Sodipo[32]	Upper abdominal surgery	–	+	Pulmonary functions	Ileus
Taylor[33]	Upper abdominal surgery	+	+	Ambulation	
Stratton[34]	Thoracotomy	–	–	Pulmonary functions	
Warfield[36]	Thoracotomy	+	+	Tolerance of chest rehabilitation	Complications; ICU stay
Liu[37]	Thoracotomy	+	–	Independence in functional activities	
Schuster[38]	Laminectomy	–	+		Complications
Smith[43]	Arthrotomy of knee	–	+	Ambulation; straight-leg raise	Length of hospital stay

– indicates evaluation not used.
+ indicates evaluation used.

The avoidance of side effects associated with narcotic medication, including drowsiness, ileus, respiratory depression, and gastrointestinal upset, is a desirable benefit of postoperative electroanalgesia via TENS and is emphasized in a study by Pike[42] of patients who used TENS continuously for 8 to 17 hours following surgery for total hip replacement. Twenty patients who used TENS required significantly fewer doses of pethidine than 20 patients who did not use TENS. Analgesic medication was available upon request to all patients. As anticipated, patients who used TENS had a much lower incidence of nausea, vomiting, and drowsiness than patients in the control group.

Several components of postoperative TENS application that have been found to maximize the likelihood of a successful treatment are presented in Table 5 – 1. Patients should be carefully evaluated preoperatively, and any history of narcotic use should be noted. They should be introduced to the TENS treatment protocol preoperatively whenever possible, in order to determine optimal electrode placement sites and stimulus parameters, and to allay the patient's fear or apprehension associated with electrical stimulation. Finally, ongoing staff education and training, and development of protocols are critical to the successful implementation of a postoperative pain management program incorporating TENS.[46]

One of the most successful applications of electroanalgesia has been the management of postoperative incisional pain. This type of pain is acute, predictable, well-localized, and often of limited duration. Preferred application procedures and objective, functional parameters for evaluation of treatment outcomes have been clearly defined and replicated. Patient and cost benefits may include reduced narcotic intake and resultant central nervous system (CNS) depression, early mobility, fewer incidences of postoperative pulmonary complications, and, in some cases, reduced length of ICU or hospital stay. Electroanalgesia should be considered as a potentially effective supplement or alternative to traditional postoperative analgesic interventions.

ORTHOPEDIC PAIN

Dougherty[47] discussed TENS as an alternative to drugs for the management of acute and chronic pain. He reported the results of treating a wide variety of orthopedic and neurologically based pain with conventional TENS applied over trigger points or peripheral nerves supplying the painful areas. While most patients exhibited good pain relief as measured by decreases in reported pain level, increased mobility, and improved function, Dougherty presented neither specific application techniques nor criteria for measuring treatment outcomes and did not include a control or placebo group in his study. In the past, many investigations of the efficacy of TENS were merely reports of uncontrolled data collection as presented in Dougherty's paper. A critical review of objective evaluations of TENS treatments is presented here.

Levy and colleagues[48] examined the effect of conventional TENS on intra-articular temperature, pressure, and synovial inflammation in rabbits' knee joints that had been rendered acutely arthritic by an injection of urate crystals. There was a decrease in the volume of synovial fluid and leukocyte count in the treated joints, while the untreated joints demonstrated massive leukocyte infiltration, neutrophilic exudate, capillary congestion, and other signs of acute inflammation. While the limitations of applying information from animal models to clinical situations is appreciated, Levy's report suggests that application of conventional TENS may reduce or limit the acute-inflammatory response, thereby reducing the pain often associated with this condition.

Kaada's study[49] provides an example of the application of low rate, high amplitude

TENS on an acupuncture point. In 1984 Kaada reported the results of treating peritendinitis calcarea of the rotator cuff muscles with TENS. Patients had previously been treated with roentgen irradiation, injections of local anesthetic and hydrocortisone, which had resulted in no relief of symptoms. All patients reported pain and demonstrated limited shoulder range of motion upon initial evaluation. Radiographic evidence of calcium deposits was collected prior to and at regular intervals following initiation of TENS treatment. Significant relief of pain and improved function at the 3-week evaluation was demonstrated by 10 of 11 patients. This improvement was maintained in all but one patient throughout the duration of follow-up evaluation. Calcium deposits persisted in the patients with asymptomatic shoulders but were eliminated or greatly reduced in 7 of the 11 symptomatic shoulders. While the presence of calcium deposits may not be correlated with the severity of symptoms, the results of this study indicate that TENS may accelerate the resorption of calcium and appears to accelerate the natural course of healing as indicated by the reduction in symptoms and restoration of movement and function.

Paris and colleagues[50] also applied low rate, high amplitude stimulation to acupuncture points on the ear and involved lower extremity of patients with acute ankle sprains. They found that those patients who received TENS in addition to standard physical therapy management of cold, elevation, compression, and non-weight-bearing gait, demonstrated earlier resolution of pain and edema as well as an earlier return of normal ankle range of motion and pain-free weight bearing, than those patients receiving only standard physical therapy treatments. The neurophysiologic basis for the clinical efficacy of acupuncture point stimulation remains to be clarified.

PAIN OF GYNECOLOGIC ORIGIN

The analgesic benefits of TENS during labor and delivery have long been recognized in Europe and are presently being evaluated in the United States.[51] As early as 1977, Augustinsson and colleagues[52] evaluated the effectiveness of TENS for relief of pelvic and back pain associated with the first and second stages of labor. During the first stage of labor, the pain was most successfully controlled by application of TENS paraspinally at the T_{10} and T_{11} nerve root levels. Pain associated with the second stage of labor and delivery required a stimulus amplitude strong enough to elicit muscle fasciculations, applied paraspinally at the S_2-S_4 levels. Although 98 of 147 patients who received TENS during labor also requested pudendal or epidural blocks for adequate pain control, patient acceptance of TENS as an adjunctive treatment for pain control was high. No side effects of stimulation were noted among mothers or babies, and the authors concluded that TENS should be considered as an alternative method of pain control during labor and delivery, particularly if administration of anesthetic medication is contraindicated.

The work of other investigators[53-61] confirms the efficacy of TENS as an alternative or adjunct method of pain relief during labor. Advantages of TENS over conventional analgesic methods used during labor include the administration of a safe, noninvasive, readily reversible analgesia that does not effect the vital functions of the mother or child during or immediately following delivery. It has also been reported that TENS facilitated the mother's ability to concentrate on breathing and relaxation techniques, and provided another opportunity for involvement of the labor coach in the birthing process.[54] The major disadvantage of using TENS during labor and delivery is the occasional interference with fetal monitoring secondary to the electrical signal generated by the TENS device. This inconvenience may be addressed by temporarily lowering the TENS amplitude or turning the device off while fetal monitoring is done. Bundsen and Ericson[62] developed a special filter to suppress the stimulus artifact from the TENS unit, so that accurate, continuous monitoring of the fetal electrocardiogram could take place with the TENS unit remaining active.

Riley[63] and Polden[64] reported that TENS was effective in managing postoperative incisional pain following caesarean section. Mothers requested less pain medication and were more alert, awake, and better able to actively participate in the care and bonding with their babies than mothers receiving narcotic medication for control of incisional pain. Deep breathing, coughing, and early ambulation were also facilitated. In addition, no medication was passed to the newborns through breast milk, so that breast feeding and associated bonding could commence sooner than with mothers receiving narcotic medications.

An additional application of TENS during pregnancy was described by Fisher and Hanna[65] for the management of meralgia paresthetica. TENS was used to control the pain associated with irritation of the lateral femoral cutaneous nerve in three women during the second trimester of pregnancy. TENS was described as "a highly successful, non-invasive, non-neurolytic technique which does not carry fetal risk" and should be considered as a viable alternative to pain medication for women who are pregnant and for whom ingestion of certain medications carry significant risk.

Use of TENS as an alternative to medication in the management of dysmenorrhea has recently been evaluated by several investigative teams. Dawood and Ramos[66] compared the analgesic effects of conventional TENS, placebo TENS, and ibuprofen (400 mg) for relief of menstrual pain in 32 women. TENS was applied through three electrodes placed in an inverted triangle on the abdomen at the level of the umbilicus. Conventional TENS more significantly relieved self-rated menstrual discomfort, diarrhea, clot formation, and fatigue compared to placebo TENS or ibuprofen, and was well accepted by 82 percent of the subjects as a viable alternative to medication for the management of dysmenorrhea.

Lundeberg, Bondesson, and Lundstrom[67] compared the effect of conventional, low-rate (acupuncturelike) TENS, and placebo TENS in 21 women with dysmenorrhea and reported that the most significant pain reduction occurred with conventional TENS. Indeed, patients reported less adequate pain control with the acupuncturelike TENS, than with placebo stimulation.

While acupuncturelike TENS was found to be effective in the management of dysmenorrhea by Neighbors and colleagues,[68] Mannheimer and Whalen[69] found that 72.2 percent of subjects using conventional TENS reported a statistically significant reduction in menstrual pain, compared with only 51.8 percent using low-rate acupuncturelike TENS and 26.1 percent using placebo TENS. Mean duration of pain relief was 4.2 hours for the conventional group and 2.5 hours for the low-rate group. The acupuncturelike TENS was less well tolerated that the conventional TENS because ongoing rhythmic muscle contractions in the legs associated with this form of TENS interfered with ambulation and other activities.

TENS offers a viable alternative to medication for substantial relief of dysmenorrhea. Most studies suggested that, while low-rate TENS was more effective than placebo stimulation in decreasing pain, conventional TENS provided more effective relief of temporary discomfort than low-rate TENS. Additional investigation of optimal stimulation settings and electrode placements are indicated, as is the clarification of neurophysiologic modes of action associated with various application techniques. In addition, the cost effectiveness of units used for this application should be considered by consumers, clinicians, and manufacturers alike.

In summary, TENS offers a safe, noninvasive method of analgesia for women during labor and delivery. However, some women report that the electrical stimulation interferes with their ability to concentrate on the breathing methods also used to manage parturition pain. Potential interference with fetal monitoring devices must also be considered. TENS offers an alternative to medication for the management of postoperative pain following caesarean section, allowing the mother to nurse her infant soon after delivery without transmitting narcotics to the child through her breast milk. In addition infant-mother bonding may be facilitated if the mother is not under the sedative influences of narcotic medication. Finally, while data supporting the use of electroanalgesia for dysmenorrhea are not conclusive, trends suggest that TENS may be as effective as oral medication and may offer the woman who is intolerant of these medications a viable alternative for managing dysmenorrhea. A careful cost-benefit analysis is clearly indicated prior to deciding upon the optimal method of analgesia.

OROFACIAL PAIN

The evaluation of TENS analgesia in patients with acute orofacial pain also provides an excellent environment for comparing the effects of various types of TENS on acute, well-controlled discomfort of uniform etiology.[70,71] In 1983 Hansson and Ekblom[70] reported the results of using TENS for relief of acute dental pain in 62 patients. Patients experiencing pain for a duration of 1 to 4 days were randomly assigned to groups receiving sham TENS, high rate TENS (100 Hz), or low rate TENS (2 Hz). Patients had taken no pain medication for 6 hours prior to the TENS treatment. All TENS was applied through surface electrodes to the face in the region that pain was localized. Amplitude was set at two to three times the sensory threshold for the high rate stimulation and three to five times sensory threshold to evoke a muscle contraction for the low rate stimulation and was administered for 15 to 30 minutes. Pain estimates were reported by the patients using a simple descriptive scale and visual analog scale (VAS) prior to treatment, during treatment, and 30 minutes following treatment.

Maximum pain relief of more than 50 percent after 15 to 30 minutes of stimulation was reported by 9 of 22 patients receiving high rate TENS and 11 of 20 patients receiving low rate TENS. Pain relief of more than 50 percent was also reported by 8 of 20 patients receiving sham TENS. Superior pain relief from TENS rather than from the aspirin was reported by 12 of 23 patients who had taken aspirin prior to attending the clinic. Duration of pain relief was not evaluated after 30 minutes following stimulation, and no significant differences were observed in the analgesic effect of high versus low rate TENS.

Ekblom and Hansson[72] continued the investigation of TENS analgesia for acute dental pain by applying the modes of stimulation described in the preceding study to the Hoku acupuncture point, between the first and second metacarpals, to 30 of 50 patients experiencing acute dental pain. Two additional treatment groups, of 10 subjects each, received either actual or placebo vibratory stimulation of the Hoku point at 100 Hz, and 500 to 800 μm of pressure. Patients again reported their pain prior to, during, and following treatment, using the simple descriptive scale and the VAS. Thirty percent of patients receiving actual TENS or vibration reported a diminution of pain after 25 to 30 minutes of treatment, compared with 20 percent of patients receiving placebo treatments. In both cases, pain relief outlasted the treatment time. When the results of this study are compared with the previous study, it appears that a greater number of patients experienced pain reduction when intrasegmental stimulation was applied directly to the area in which the pain was localized, rather than when the Hoku point was stimulated. Further clinical investigation is indicated to discover the optimal electrode placements and stimulus parameters for electroanalgesia in patients with dental pain.

Chronic Pain Conditions

Early studies of the analgesic effects of TENS for relief of chronic pain were comprised largely of patients with widely divergent diagnoses and symptom complexes. Investigators attempted to define similarities in pain control for patients with vastly different pain histories and pathologies. Little care was taken to evaluate specific etiologies of pain related to specific neurologic, orthopedic, or circulatory deficiencies, and then determine appropriate application techniques to achieve electroanalgesia by modifying the neurologic, orthopedic, or circulatory environment. While well intended, these early studies provided gross generalizations regarding the effectiveness of TENS-produced analgesia, with little understanding of the importance of several factors critical to the successful application of TENS. Careful patient screening and evaluation, systematic application, documentation, and evaluation of the specific electrical parameters used to produce electroanalgesia, fastidious objective evaluation of treatment outcomes, and ultimately, the determination of the optimal relationships among pain etiology, perception, and control through electrical stimulation are critical to the efficacious application of TENS for patients suffering from chronic pain. A historical perspective of the development and refinement of clinical research in TENS may be obtained by consulting the chronological bibliography on TENS compiled by Michael Nolan.[73]

Attempts have been made to determine optimal electrode placement and stimulus settings for the management of pain of specific origins. Wolf, Gersh, and Rao[74] evaluated the effect of TENS in 114 patients reporting chronic pain secondary to peripheral neuropathy, peripheral nerve injury, radiculopathy, or musculoskeletal trauma. Electrodes were systematically placed at the site of pain or along the nerve trunk or related nerve roots subserving the painful region. Conventional TENS was applied at frequencies of 50 to 100 Hz; pulse durations and amplitudes were set to evoke profound, comfortable paresthesia without associated muscle contraction. Treatments were provided to both inpatients and outpatients for 30 to 45 minutes. Treatment outcomes were evaluated by patient report of pain before and after treatment using VAS and several components of the McGill Pain Questionnaire (MPQ).[75] Patients with peripheral neuropathy (most of those being patients with postherpetic neuralgia) responded favorably to TENS, experiencing the greatest degree and duration of pain reduction. Patients with chronic pain secondary to radiculopathy responded least favorably. No relationship was discerned between specific electrode placements, stimulus parameters, etiology of pain, and treatment outcome. Patients with fewer prior-treatment interventions, including surgery and history of narcotic use, responded more favorably to TENS and experienced more complete and longer lasting analgesia. Follow-up evaluation on 25 patients who experienced initial pain control and who then rented TENS units for use at home indicated that the analgesic effects of TENS decreased as time progressed. These diminished benefits may have been due to decreased patient compliance, increased patient responsibility, and the removal of the physical therapist from the treatment regime when independent application of TENS by the patient became a requirement. Early intervention with TENS and the presence of a health care professional during treatment may have contributed to the overall efficacy of TENS for pain relief in patients with chronic pain.

LOW-BACK PAIN

A wealth of information is available regarding TENS for control of low-back pain (LBP). Long-term use of TENS permitted some patients to decrease their pain medication intake and others to return to work or resume normal activity levels.[76,77]

Several investigators have compared the analgesic effects of TENS to those of other analgesic interventions. Melzack, Vetere, and Finch[78] compared the effects of TENS to massage in 41 patients with chronic LBP. Twenty patients received low rate, high amplitude TENS through electrodes applied to the lumbar paraspinal muscles and lateral thigh two times per week for 30 minutes per treatment. Each patient received a total of 10 treatments. Twenty-one patients received 10 treatments of massage through suction cups applied over the lumber paraspinal muscles, in order to reduce variation in the therapist's administration of massage. Treatment was discontinued or changed if the patient reported that massage did not help, requested a change of treatment, or reported an increase in pain.

Treatment outcomes, measured by patient report of pain using portions of the MPQ and a VAS, as well as evaluation of lumbosacral range of motion (ROM) and straight-leg raising, indicated that TENS was significantly more effective in decreasing pain and allowing increased mobility than massage applied through suction. The results may have been skewed toward the TENS treatment, if patients, not used to the unconventional treatment of massage as it was applied here, reported discomfort and requested a change of treatment. The outcomes may not be compared to results of treatment with manual massage.

Lundeberg[79] compared the effects of high and low rate TENS, high and low rate vibration, and placebo vibration in 60 patients with axial or extremity myofascial or musculoskeletal pain. Eighty percent of the patients reported significant relief of pain with some form of peripheral stimulation or vibration. No significant differences in effectiveness were determined between the 100 Hz or 200 Hz vibration and the high- or low-rate TENS. Ongoing comparison of electrical stimulation to other analgesic interventions will provide a more complete understanding of pain etiology and enable us to more consistently offer treatments affording specific patients effective pain relief.

Several investigators have studied the effects of electrically induced analgesia in patients with chronic pain of apparent nonorganic origin. Lehmann, Russell, and Spratt[80] compared the effects of conventional TENS, low rate electroacupuncture, and placebo TENS in 54 patients participating in an inpatient pain rehabilitation program. These patients reported chronic LBP with a preponderance of nonorganic findings related to their pain complaints. While electroacupuncture was most effective in producing analgesia, measured by patient report on a VAS, none of the treatments resulted in improved function, increased participation in activities of daily living (ADL) or increased compliance with recommended exercise programs. In addition, patients with chronic pain and nonorganic findings who tend to exaggerate pain or exhibit extensive pain behavior incompatible with physical findings, can contaminate clinical research results. Every effort should be made to identify and control for the nonorganic chronic pain patient when evaluating the efficacy of analgesic interventions.

Fried, Johnson, and McCracken[81] reviewed questionnaires completed by 563 patients who had experienced chronic LBP and dysfunction, and had been receiving financial compensation for injuries sustained on the job. These patients had used TENS in a long-term home rehabilitation program. Forty-four percent reported that, after 6 months of treatment, they were free from disability and had returned to work. An additional 36.2 percent were capable of participating in a modified work schedule or environment. Benefits associated with the TENS included decreased need for pain medication, improved sleep patterns, and decreased pain. The investigators concluded that a substantial number of patients with chronic pain who also received workman's compensation could benefit from TENS. Clearly, additional well-controlled evaluations of this patient group are warranted, especially considering the cost of long-term health care for these patients.

ARTHRITIS

Several investigators[82-86] have reported the analgesic effects of TENS in patients with arthritic pain. In 1981, Taylor, Hallett, and Flaherty[82] studied 10 patients with nonoperative osteoarthritis of the knees. In a double-blind crossover design, five patients were treated with conventional TENS set at a comfortable sensory level, while the remaining patients received a placebo unit designed to produce sound but no stimulation. Electrodes were placed about the knee. Patients treated themselves at home for 30 to 60 minutes as needed and were instructed to use the unit as often as necessary. After 2 weeks the patients returned to the hospital for evaluation, received the other type of unit, and returned home for another 2 weeks of treatment. After another evaluation, patients were told that they could use the unit that offered them the best results at home for one more month.

Treatment outcomes were evaluated on the basis of subjective pain report, distance of ambulation, and pain-medication intake. The actual TENS was significantly more effective than the placebo TENS in producing satisfactory analgesia, as indicated by subjective pain report and medication ingestion, and was therefore the unit of choice for continuation of treatment at home. Optimal analgesia was reported while the stimulation was on, and pain relief lasted a maximum of several hours following cessation of treatment. Patients who chose to continue treatment at home for an additional month reported decreased analgesic effectiveness over time. These results are consistent with those reported by other investigators[74] and indicate that TENS is an acceptable analgesic alternative for patients with osteoarthritis who are not surgical candidates.

Smith, Lewith, and Machin[83] and Lewis, Lewis, and Sturrock[84] reported conflicting results in two separate studies of patients with osteoarthritic knee pain. Smith, Lewith, and Machin reported that significantly more patients receiving conventional TENS (66.7 percent) demonstrated pain relief based upon pain report, activity logs, and medication intake than those receiving a placebo treatment (26.7 percent). In contrast, Lewis, Lewis, and Sturrock were unable to determine differences between the TENS and placebo. Perhaps those patients receiving TENS first were conditioned to believe that the placebo treatment would be as effective. The concept of placebo response is discussed in detail later in this chapter.

Mannheimer, Lund, and Carlsson[85] have extensively studied the effects of various modes of TENS on patients with pain and dysfunction secondary to rheumatoid arthritis (RA). TENS was applied to the dorsal and volar surfaces of the wrist in 19 patients with RA. The stimulus amplitude was set to provoke an intense paresthesia in the fingers during one trial, and a weak, local vibratory sensation in a second trial. A third application of TENS was delivered paraspinally to the T_3 nerve root, with the amplitude adjusted to evoke a mild, vibratory sensation.

Treatment outcomes were assessed by subjective pain report as well as by objective measures of strength of the wrist through limb loading. Limb loading consisted of having the patient grip and hold a handle loaded with a weight. The weight was chosen so that the patient could not hold it for more than 30 seconds without experiencing onset or increased pain in the wrist. Eighteen of nineteen patients demonstrated increased load time, and subjective pain relief in response to the intense stimulation, compared to 14 of 19 patients responding similarly to the milder stimulation. Only one patient reported pain relief, not associated with increased load time, in response to the paraspinal stimulation. All four patients who were re-evaluated at 6 and 24 hours following treatment continued to demonstrate increased limb-load capability and pain relief at 6 hours, and three of the four continued to demonstrate these benefits at 24 hours following treatment. The results of this study emphasize the functional gains that may be realized with TENS. Caution should be exercised to protect the affected joints, however, especially in the presence of significant pain reduction.

In 1979, Mannheimer and Carlsson[86] continued their research with patients with RA. TENS was applied to the wrist in the manner described above. Patients received conventional TENS, low rate TENS, or burst TENS for 10 minutes each, applied in random order. Amplitude was set to evoke tolerable paresthesia in the fingers. Treatment outcomes were again measured by subjective pain report and limb-load time. Optimal results in terms of intensity and duration of analgesia and limb-load tolerance were reported in relation to the conventional TENS application. The poorer results associated with low rate TENS may be related to the total current delivered to the patient in each of the stimulation trials. Differences may also be related to the activity of different autogenous analgesic mechanisms facilitated at various frequencies of stimulation.

OSTEOGENESIS

One additional orthopedic application of TENS, that of facilitating osteogenesis in patients with nonunited fractures, is discussed by Kahn.[8] He provided radiographic evidence of improved callous formation in three patients with nonunited fractures of more than 6-months duration. Electrodes were placed on either side of the fracture site and stimulus parameters were set to provide a long "on" time (lowest rate and widest pulse duration available). Amplitude was adjusted to the sensory threshold. Stimulation was provided at home for 30 to 60 minutes, three to four times a day. Improved callous formation was observed after 1 month of treatment in one patient and after 10 weeks of treatment in the other two patients. The osteogenesis observed in these cases was a serendipitous finding, since the original intent of treatment was pain control. Further studies of TENS for osteogenesis have not been reported, but are clearly indicated. Additional discussion of electrical stimulation for osteogenesis is provided in Chapter 10.

PAIN OF NEUROLOGIC ORIGIN

Patients with a variety of neuropathic pain syndromes have been successfully treated with TENS. Patients with pain secondary to postherpetic neuralgia,[87] amputation,[88–89] peripheral neuropathy,[90] Guillain-Barré syndrome,[91] Sudeck's atrophy,[92] and trigeminal neuralgia[93] have achieved varying degrees of analgesia with TENS applied to the areas of pain or related acupuncture points. Parameters have been set according to conventional TENS guidelines, as well as in the low-rate ranges.

The neurologic syndromes listed above have in common the characteristic of sensory deprivation. Whether secondary to peripheral nerve injury or systemic peripheral neuropathy, input from large diameter afferent fibers appears to have been diminished. Conventional TENS, through the spinal gate mechanism or through activation of higher pain inhibitory centers, may augment the individual's capacity to modify pain perception by providing increased large diameter afferent input along intact nerve fibers, thus restoring a balance of sensory activity in the nervous system.[94] Based on this premise, any treatment or activity that increases large diameter afferent activity (massage, movement, vibration, or heat) would serve to activate suprasegmental inhibition and promote analgesia. Ongoing investigation into the mechanisms of pain perception and modification related to specific etiologies are warranted if health professionals are to optimally use all treatments currently available in appropriate combinations to maximize successful treatment outcomes.

A devastating pain condition in which a limb is often rendered useless by intractable pain and associated trophic changes is reflex sympathetic dystrophy syndrome (RSDS). While not always the case, RSDS frequently occurs following partial or complete nerve injury and includes trauma, associated pain, and immobilization (either imposed or volitional). A hallmark of RSDS is the obvious disruption of a normal balance of sympathetic nervous system activity in the area of the injury, possibly triggered by either abnormal central feedback mechanisms or pathologic synapses (ephapses) that form between primary afferent nerve fibers and sympathetic afferent fibers in close proximity with one another.[94,95]

The first phase of RSDS is often characterized by the occurrence of painful trauma, followed by either external or self-imposed immobilization. Patients with early signs of RSDS tend to experience significant pain and desire to shield the limb from all external stimuli. They immobilize the limb because it is painful to move it. This immobilization appears to generate secondary symptoms of RSDS which include edema and inflammation. The second phase of RSDS, during which the limb is exceedingly painful, hyperesthetic, and during which patients protect the limb from all stimuli and function, is marked by hyperactivity of the sympathetic efferents, resulting in local vasoconstriction, cyanosis, lowered skin temperature, hyperhydrosis, disruption of hair and nail growth, and associated skin, muscle, and bony atrophy.[96] Indeed, near-normal characteristics of function of the limb have been restored by the blocking of sympathetic efferent activity either by a temporary sympathetic ganglion block or sympathectomy.[97] However, in some cases, anesthetic blocks only temporarily relieve the symptoms of RSDS, and surgical disruption of the sympathetic pathways can result in other complications.

The application of TENS may be associated with alterations in sympathetic tone.[9,98,99] Owens, Atkinson, and Lees[99] noted only slight increases in digit temperature when TENS was applied to healthy subjects. Wong and Jette[98] reported increases in sympathetic nervous system activity, represented by significant decreases in skin temperature in the ipsilateral digits when high rate (85 Hz), low rate (2 Hz), and burst (two bursts per second with seven pulses per burst and a carrier frequency of 85 Hz) were applied separately to four acupuncture points in the upper extremities of 12 healthy subjects. No temperature changes were observed with placebo stimulation. In contrast, Kaada[9] reported significant increases in skin temperature in six patients with circulatory impairment secondary to Raynaud's syndrome or diabetes mellitus when low-rate TENS was applied to the Hoku point. Wong and Jette[98] explained the discrepancy in their results compared with those reported by Kaada as follows: "It is possible that sympathetic vasoconstrictive nerve fibers may have been directly stimulated by the TENS, or that blood was shunted from the skin to muscles contracting secondary to the low frequency stimulation." An alternative explanation is the difference in the capacity of the normal versus abnormal sympathetic nervous system to respond to external stimulation.

Reports of successful management of RSDS with TENS, particularly in children, suggest that a normal balance of sympathetic nervous system activity may be restored with the application of TENS, and pain and other symptoms are relieved.[100–104] Leo[104] reported the complete resolution of a lower extremity RSDS in a 10-year-old child using low-rate, high-amplitude acupuncturelike TENS applied to upper-extremity acupuncture points and associated auriculotherapy points on the ear for two treatments. No special considerations regarding application of TENS in children are reported other than careful patient education and observance of the child's tolerance to the electrical stimulation.

Kaada[9] described the use of acupuncturelike TENS on the Hoku point (Li4) to modulate abnormal sympathetic activity. Mannheimer and Lampe[105] reported successful treatment of RSDS using conventional TENS for a patient who had sustained a Colles fracture. They applied TENS to acupuncture points throughout the affected arm, as well as to segmentally related paraspinal areas. The reader is referred to Mannheimer and Lampe's discussion in *Clinical Transcutaneous Electrical Nerve Stimulation* for a more complete discussion of treatment alternatives.[105]

Additional Clinical Applications

CIRCULATORY FACILITATION

In 1979, Owens, Atkinson, and Lees[99] reported slight increases in ipsilateral finger temperature in healthy subjects following application of conventional TENS to the ulnar groove. Kaada[9] reported in 1982 on the possible interactions between TENS and sympathetic nervous-system activity when he evaluated the effect of TENS on pain and peripheral circulation in patients with Raynaud's syndrome or diabetic peripheral neuropathy. Kaada studied the effect of acupuncturelike TENS on pain and skin temperature in the hands and feet of four patients with Raynaud's syndrome affecting their hands and feet, and two patients with severe peripheral neuropathy secondary to diabetes mellitus affecting both feet. He applied acupuncturelike TENS to the Hoku point of one hand at 2 to 5 Hz, 0.2 ms pulse duration, and an amplitude that evoked nonpainful muscle contractions (2 to 4 times the sensory threshold). The second electrode was placed on the ulnar border of the same hand. Patients received TENS for 30 to 45 minutes once daily during their hospital stay. Subjective pain measures were evaluated on a five-point scale, every 15 minutes for 2 hours prior to, during, and for 24 hours following treatment. Skin temperature of the fingers and toes were recorded simultaneously. Skin temperatures as low as 22 to 24°C were raised to 31 to 34°C 15 to 30 minutes after treatment began. The temperature elevation lasted 4 to 6 hours after treatment ended.

Smaller temperature elevations were noted when an electrical stimulus at 180 Hz was applied. In normally warm extremities, skin temperature rose 0.5 to 2.0°C. The core temperature remained unchanged. Changes associated with the rise in skin temperature included presence of rubor where cyanosis had been observed and significant decreases in pain. Kaada also reported that unilateral stimulation of the Hoku point induced temperature and pain changes in all involved extremities. In one patient, manual needle acupuncture of the same Hoku point induced similar changes.

Kaada then administered 0.8 to 1.6 mg of naloxone and observed no reversal of the circulatory or analgesic effects resulting from the TENS. This observation indicated the need to look for an explanation other than an endorphin-mediated mechanism to explain the beneficial effects associated with the low rate TENS. Kaada reported that the patients who had previously undergone sympathectomies experienced more dramatic temperature changes and pain reduction than those with intact sympathetic nervous systems. In addition, three female patients with no history of migraine headache, two of whom had undergone sympathectomies, reported onset of migraine-type headaches associated with the TENS-induced vasodilation, possibly due to unchecked vasodilation in the cranial vessels. The headaches were successfully aborted with oral analgesics. These responses imply an interaction between the sympathetic nervous system and TENS. Patients with intact sympathetic nervous systems experienced a lesser degree of vasodilation and temperature increase, possibly because of the vasoconstrictive influence of sympathetic tone. The failure of naloxone to reverse the effects of TENS refutes an endorphin-mediated system, and the systemic vasodilation that was observed suggests a mechanism that is not limited to segmental spinal regulation. Furthermore, while a mechanism subserving the restoration of peripheral circulation was not suggested by the investigator, it may be hypothesized that, in patients with a preponderance of sympathetic output, electrical stimulation may somehow normalize this autonomic influence.

Kaada also reported that one patient with Raynaud's syndrome and one patient with diabetes, both of whom suffered foot pain prior to treatment, were able to maintain normal skin temperature and freedom from pain by using the TENS for 30 to 45 minutes every 2 or 3 days in the prescribed manner. Patients with hand pain were less successful with home treatment, especially during times of upper extremity activity or when exposed to outdoor cold.

ANGINA PECTORIS

More recently, Mannheimer and associates[11] investigated the application of TENS for relief of pain associated with angina pectoris (AP). They first established the safety of applying TENS to the cardiac region by applying electrical stimulation directly to the cardiac muscle during open-heart surgery. They reported that no arrhythmias were induced at current densities less than 50 mA/m². They then delivered electrical stimulation on the painful external chest wall of 10 male patients with medically stabilized AP. TENS was applied at a rate of 70 Hz, pulse duration of 0.2 ms, and an amplitude less than that which evoked pain (15 to 50 mA). Bike-ergometry testing, performed before and after TENS treatment, indicated improved work capacity, decreased S-T segment depression on electrocardiogram, and decreased recovery time in all 10 patients following treatment. Long-term follow-up of 23 similar patients also indicated a decrease in the frequency of anginal attacks and a decreased ingestion of nitroglycerine.

In a related study, Mannheimer and colleagues[106] reported similar control of anginal pain and myocardial ischemia in patients who experienced experimentally induced angina through a temporary pacemaker. While the placebo effect was not ruled out by the design of these studies, the authors suggest that the reduction of anginal symptoms may have been related to the modification of sympathetic activity influencing the cardiac system.

HEADACHE

While the efficacy of TENS for management of headache pain has been inconsistent, consideration of this application is appropriate when evaluating the influence of TENS on peripheral circulation. Solomon and Guglielmo[107] studied the effect of TENS applied transcranially using the Pain Suppressor* in 62 patients with migraine or tension headache. This unit differs from most TENS units by supplying a higher rate (12,000 to 20,000 Hz), lower amplitude (0 to 4 mA), and shorter pulse duration (0.030 ms) stimulus. Electrodes were placed either bilaterally on the head at the site of pain or the occiput, or at the Hoku point on the right hand, if headache pain was generalized. The level of stimulation was set at either sensory threshold, subsensory threshold, or zero (placebo). Patients were treated for 15 minutes. A decrease of pain of at least 20 percent was reported by 55 percent of the patients treated with sensory threshold stimulation as measured by subjective pain report on a scale of 0 to 10. This success was compared to similar results in 28 percent of the patients receiving subsensory stimulation and 28 percent of those patients receiving the placebo. Pain relief was not related to headache type or location.

Several factors may have contributed to the results of this study. The stimulus amplitude provided by the Pain Suppressor unit may not be adequate to modify pain perception through any mechanism. The only measure of pain relief was a subjective pain report. The inclusion of objective measures of headache pain might have provided evidence of treatment efficacy. These measures may include peripheral circulation (skin temperature) in the case of migraine headache and muscle activity (electromyography) in the case of tension headache. There is evidence that stimulation of the Hoku point may actually exacerbate migraine headache.[9] Additional, well-controlled investigations of headache-pain modulation through conventional and acupuncturelike TENS are warranted.

MICROCURRENT FOR PAIN CONTROL

Recently, interest has developed in the application of minute amounts of electrical current (10 to 600 μA) for the management of a wide variety of acute and chronic pain conditions. While the benefits of microamperage for facilitation of wound healing have been carefully evaluated and documented in peer-reviewed journals,[108,109] reports claiming major advantages of microcurrent over conventional forms of TENS and other treatment interventions have remained largely the domain of manufacturers' testimonials, public-interest articles, sports magazine features, and nonreviewed journals.

Microamperage electrical nerve stimulation (MENS) is applied to regions of pain or injury with the intention of restoring a biological electrical balance to facilitate tissue healing and subsequent pain control.[110] As previously mentioned, the efficacy of MENS for wound healing has been established, although the theoretical bioelectric mechanism

---

*Pain Suppression Labs, Clifton, NJ.

by which wound healing is facilitated has not been well substantiated. The relationship between pain secondary to neurologic, orthopedic, or soft-tissue injury and disruption of normal bioelectric potentials has not been clearly established, and, presently, there are no well-designed, carefully controlled studies in the professional literature to support claims than MENS is a safe, efficacious modality for pain control. Careful, critical evaluation and documentation of this type of TENS for the specific goal of pain management is therefore the obligation of every health professional who incorporates MENS into his or her treatment regimen.

CONSIDERATIONS FOR APPLICATION

Electrode Systems

A wide variety of electrodes are available to meet patients' special needs (Fig. 5–1A and 5–1B). The most frequently used electrodes are made of a carbon-silicone material, available in various shapes and sizes, which require a conductive gel or paste to improve conductivity. They are held in place with paper tape or patches. Carbon-silicone electrodes gradually lose conductivity and should be replaced every 6 months, or earlier if the surface appears worn, dull, or discolored.

Self-adhesive electrodes made of karaya gum or synthetic polymers conform to irregular skin surfaces well, adhere without the need for tape, do not require additional gel for improved conductivity, may be worn continuously for several days, and offer an alternative to the patient who experiences skin irritation associated with gel or tape.

Sterile conductive tape strips are often applied adjacent to a surgical site, after wound closure, in the operating room. This application permits the postoperative activation of TENS in the recovery room immediately following surgery. Sterile electrodes may then be replaced as needed during wound-dressing changes.

Several lead-wire systems are manufactured to connect electrodes to TENS devices. Consideration should be given to the length of the leads, so patients are free to move without tangling them, and to the durability of the wires and pin connectors. Some lead wires are bifurcated and allow the connection of several electrodes to the device through one main cable. While this arrangement facilitates treatment of several painful sites simultaneously, the current density available at each electrode for a set amplitude is reduced by a factor equaling the number of electrodes connected to one lead-wire terminal. Thus a greater current amplitude may be required for treatment, and battery life is shortened.

Determination of Electrode Placement

Preferred stimulation sites for treatment of specific types of pain have not been clearly determined. Electrodes have been placed at the site of pain, adjacent to the spinal column at the spinal nerve roots segmentally related to the involved dermatome, scleratome, or myotome, along the course of the peripheral nerve(s) subserving the painful region, upon related motor points, trigger points, or acupuncture points, and on seemingly unrelated extrasegmental sites that may contribute to excitation of suprasegmental and cortical pain inhibitory centers.[105] Mannheimer and Lampe[105] provided a comprehensive review of the anatomic and physiologic interrelationships among these

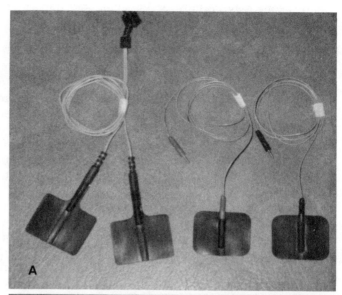

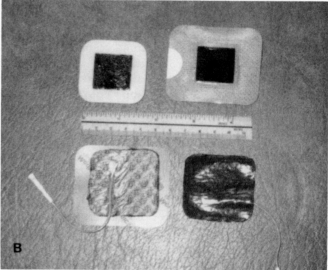

FIGURE 5–1. Types of TENS electrodes. (*A*) Electrodes pictured are made of the carbon-silicone combination and require that a conductive gel be applied prior to use. Lead wires are attached. (*B*) Those pictured have a self-adhesive conductive-polymer surface and do not require an additional conductive medium.

apparently discrete sites proposed for electrical stimulation. While a detailed discussion is beyond the scope of this chapter, a brief summary of the relationship among motor points, trigger points, and acupuncture points is necessary for the reader to understand the effective stimulation of these sites for pain control and symptom resolution.

The motor point is an anatomically discrete area at which the peripheral motor nerve pierces the surface of the muscle. The neurovascular hilus of the muscle at which nerve fibers and blood vessels pierce the surface of the muscle to provide afferent and efferent nerve supplies to muscle fibers, spindles, Golgi tendon organs, circulatory components, and free-nerve endings is located in this region. The greatest density of sensory end organs is also located here, resulting in a region in which both sensory and motor axons may be most easily stimulated transcutaneously. Clinically this location exhibits high electrical conductance (low skin impedance). Additionally, motor points in muscles segmentally related to an area of pathology show increased tenderness to palpation, as do hyperesthetic points located paraspinally, even in the absence of nerve-root irritation.

Trigger points are hypersensitive areas of skin overlying muscles or connective tissue, characterized by tenderness and hardness, hyperesthesia, and resultant referred pain when palpated. Various theories have been presented on the etiology of trigger points, including fibrosis of muscle tissue, disruption of the sarcoplasmic reticulum, resulting in chronic localized muscle fiber activity, presence of irritable muscle spindles, and pressure on the dura mater, giving rise to extrasegmental referred pain.[111-116] Consequently, there is little agreement on whether trigger points are anatomically distinct entities.

While a detailed review of acupuncture is impossible within the scope of this chapter, of the thousands of acupuncture points known to exist, the 50 to 100 that are used clinically correlate anatomically with the location of superficial nerve branches and sensory end organs.[105] Many meridians follow the courses of peripheral nerves. Some acupuncture points correlate anatomically with sites commonly used for motor and sensory nerve conduction studies, and others with sites commonly used for conventional nerve blocks. The clinical efficacy of TENS applied to acupuncture points for pain control for lumbosacral pathology and for restoration of sympathetic nervous system equilibrium has been well established in clinical investigations.[117-119]

Clinical commonalities among motor, trigger, and acupuncture points include tenderness to palpation when segmentally related pathology is present, decreased resistance to electricity, production of referred pain on palpation, and in some cases, shared anatomic locations. When stimulating a trigger point, a motor point or acupuncture point is also likely to be stimulated. Mannheimer and Lampe referred to these anatomically discreet locations as "specific points."[105]

Selection of Preferred Stimulation Sites (PSS)

Once the nature, location, and structural source of pain has been discerned, the spinal cord segments and peripheral nerves innervating that structure should be identified. Preferred stimulation sites (PSS) along the innervating structures may be located using motor point, trigger point, or acupuncture point charts or tables, or by palpation and knowledge of anatomy. These charts are referenced by Mannheimer and Lampe.[105] Specific points may also be located by palpation of tender or rigid areas, or by electrical determination of sites of low electrical resistance using an ohmmeter, a device which determines electrical impedance. The ohmmeter is a feature of point locator devices that assist in mapping out optimal stimulation sites prior to applying TENS. The clinician can also "search" for regions of high conductivity by holding one electrode of a TENS circuit, giving the patient the second electrode, turning on the electrical current, and placing the clinician's index finger of the hand holding the electrode on the skin overlying the course of the peripheral nerve innervating the painful region. As the finger moves along the skin, the patient will report sites at which the electrical stimulus is perceived most acutely. These are points of low skin resistance and are most susceptible to electrical stimulation.[120] The selection of PSS specifically related to the type of stimulation mode used will be discussed in the section describing electrical stimulation modes.

The configuration (orientation) of electrode placement sites varies with the particular treatment application. If effective pain control is not accomplished with the first electrode-placement selection, alternative placements should be attempted. Electrodes may be placed (1) unilaterally; (2) bilaterally; (3) proximal and/or distal to a painful region, ensuring perception of electrically induced paresthesias throughout the entire distribution of referred pain; (4) in a "V" configuration (as described previously for management of dysmenorrhea); (5) in a crisscross configuration (interferential), so that current pathways from each channel ideally intersect at the painful site, as in the case of joint pain; (6) on segmentally related myotomes, either close to or remote from the painful region; (7) on a contralateral homologous segmentally related site, when hyperesthesia prevents ipsilateral stimulation of the painful site; or (8) at a remote, unrelated specific point, where stronger stimulation is used presumably to activate suprasegmental inhibitory centers. Transcranial stimulation for headache pain is recommended by Pain Suppression Labs,* but its use is not often documented in the literature, as it is listed as contraindicated in the manuals of some equipment manufacturers. Additional considerations for electrode selection and placement will be discussed as appropriate to subsequent sections.

Modes of Stimulation

Originally, the objective of TENS was to promote analgesia through stimulation of Class I afferent fibers, those densely myelinated, fast-conducting sensory fibers whose activity facilitates segmental inhibition at the level of the spinal gate.[6] In recent years, TENS has been applied to myotomes and motor points that are segmentally related to the area of pain in an attempt to achieve analgesia through suprasegmental inhibition that may be endorphin-mediated. The *adequate stimulus*, that electrical stimulus of sufficient amplitude, pulse duration, and rise time, is different for various sensory and motor fibers. The characteristics of the adequate stimulus for each of these fibers are reviewed in Chapters 1 and 2.

WAVEFORM

A variety of waveforms are available with different TENS devices. The specific characteristics of stimulating waveforms are discussed in detail in Chapter 3. Most TENS units generate a constant current, asymmetric, biphasic waveform with a net zero DC component. Untoward polar effects secondary to alkalosis or acidosis under the electrodes, and iontophoretic reactions are essentially avoided, particularly when each of the electrodes of a single channel are of equal surface area. However, because of the asymmetric shape of the two phases of the wave, one phase (associated with one electrode) may indeed be more "active" than the other and capable of exerting a greater excitatory effect because of a greater vertical deviation from the baseline. More even effects under the electrodes may be achieved by changing electrode connections, selecting more (or less) easily excited electrode placement sites, or changing the size of one electrode relative to the other.

To date no one waveform has been determined to be more effective than another in producing electroanalgesia. However, occasionally an individual patient will respond

---

*Clifton, NJ.

TABLE 5–3 Stimulus Specifications of Commercial TENS Units*

Manufacturer	DC/AC	Pulse Duration (μs)	Pulse Rate (Hz)	Amplitude (mA)	Waveform	Modulations
Pain suppressor	?	?	12,000–20,000	0–4	?	None
Basix	?	0–400	2–152	0–60	?	Amplitude width, rate burst
Stimtech Stimburst	AC	50–250	3–150	0–50	Asymmetric-biphasic	Burst only
Dynex III	AC	40–250	2–110	0–60	Modified-biphasic	Burst, width
N-Tron TTS 2600	AC	40–200	2–10; 20–1000	0–60	Asymmetric-biphasic	Burst, rate, width
Medtronic Eclipse	AC	30–250	2–125	0–60	Asymmetric-biphasic rectangular	Burst, rate, width, and combinations
MRL Neuroprobe III	DC	?	1–128	0–1.0	Square-wave	None
Napcor Micropulse	?	?	0.6, 10, 20, 40, 300	0.020, 0.200, or 0.600	?	None
Richmar HV-VI (high-voltage pulsed current)	DC	45	2–120	0–500 volts 0–60 mA	Twin-peak monophasic pulse	None

*Manufacturers' addresses appear in the Appendix on page 191.

more favorably to one waveform than another. It is therefore advantageous to have access to more than one waveform (i.e., more than one TENS device) in clinical practice.

STIMULUS PARAMETERS

The stimulus parameters of several TENS units are summarized in Table 5–3. Any electrical stimulator capable of producing a pulsed (interrupted) waveform, with pulse frequencies of 1 to 150 Hz, pulse durations of 0.040 to 0.300 ms, and intensities of 0 to 60 mA, may be used for TENS treatments. Additionally, TENS treatments may be administered with high-voltage, pulsed, stimulators, microcurrent devices, and other low-voltage devices, providing parameters are appropriately selected. A balanced biphasic waveform (described in Chapter 3) is preferred to avoid skin irritation secondary to electrochemical reactions. A prototype of a TENS unit is described in Figure 5–2. TENS may be applied using various combinations of stimulus parameters, described in the following sections and summarized in Table 5–4.

HIGH RATE CONVENTIONAL TENS

The most frequently used mode of stimulation for electroanalgesia is high rate conventional TENS. The target of this stimulus is the large diameter afferent fiber, which is implicated in activating segmental inhibition at the spinal gate in the substantia gelatinosa (refer to Chapter 2 for a more detailed discussion of the gate control theory of pain). Electrodes are usually applied at or near the site of pain, or on segmentally related dermatomes. Suggested pulse rates are 75 to 100 Hz, pulse durations are of less than 0.200 ms, and pulse amplitude is set to produce a comfortable paresthesia in the area of pain or underlying the electrodes. The amplitude required to evoke such paresthesia may be two or three times the sensory threshold. Mannheimer and Lampe suggested an

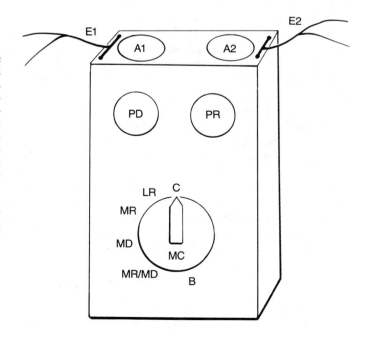

FIGURE 5–2. A prototype of a TENS device. E1 and E2 are bifurcated electrode leads for channels 1 and 2 respectively. A1 and A2 are the amplitude controls for channels 1 and 2 respectively. PD is the control for pulse duration (width). PR is the control for pulse rate (frequency). MC is the control for modulation selection; C– conventional mode; LR–low ratee (e.g., modifies PR control to a range of 2 to 10 pps rather than 20 to 100 pps); MR–modulates rate; MD–modulates pulse duration; MR/MD–modulates pulse duration and rate; B–selects a burst mode.

TABLE 5–4 Modes of TENS Stimulation

Mode	Amplitude Range to Produce	Pulse-Rate Range (pps)	Pulse-Duration Range (ms)	Indications
High rate conventional TENS	Comfortable paresthesia	75–100	<0.200	Acute or chronic pain; temporary relief
Low rate acupuncturelike TENS (LRAT)	Motor threshold	1–4	0.200–0.300	Acute or chronic pain; circulatory facilitation; longer-duration analgesia
Brief, intense TENS	Muscle fasciculations or tetany	150	>0.300	Brief, profound analgesia during uncomfortable procedures

initial setting of 80 Hz, 0.040 to 0.060 ms, and adequate amplitude to produce paresthesia.[105] Following 5 to 10 minutes of treatment, they suggested that pulse duration be increased in an attempt to broaden or deepen the perceived sensation, and thus recruit additional sensory-nerve fibers. Increasing the pulse rate will increase the firing frequency of the large diameter afferent fibers that have already been recruited, and thus increase input to the segmental inhibitory centers in the substantia gelatinosa. In contrast, increasing the pulse amplitude will recruit additional afferent and efferent nerve fibers, possibly resulting in undesirable noxious sensations or muscle contraction.

Analgesia resulting from conventional stimulation has a short induction time and does not usually provide long-lasting pain control beyond the stimulation session. The effectiveness and duration of relief has been related to the length of application time and intensity of perceived paresthesia in the painful area. Therefore, conventional TENS may be applied for prolonged periods of time. If motor activity is avoided, direct excitation of suprasegmental inhibitory centers by conventional TENS, applied to areas remote to the site of pain, is unlikely. Analgesia resulting from the application of conventional TENS is *not* reversed by naloxone, negating the likelihood of an endorphin-mediated analgesic mechanism to account for the beneficial effects.

The accommodation of sensory-nerve fibers to conventional TENS is frequently observed. To reduce this accommodation, characteristics of the stimulus can be changed at regular intervals and may be done manually by the clinician or patient, but is more conveniently done by setting a modulation mode on the TENS device, if such a mode is offered. In a modulation mode, the pulse rate, duration, and/or amplitude will vary automatically between the level set at the outset of treatment and some level below that at regular intervals. The resultant change in current density or rate reduces the likelihood of accommodation of sensory fibers. Since modulation features vary with individual devices, clinicians are referred to the operating manual of the specific device that they apply to understand best the use of that device.

LOW RATE ACUPUNCTURELIKE TENS

Low rate acupuncturelike TENS (LRAT) results in the stimulation of both sensory and motor nerves in the area of pain or in a segmentally related myotome. The activation of suprasegmental inhibition through an endorphin-mediated mechanism has been implicated in electroanalgesia using LRAT, because this analgesia is naloxone reversible.[19] Electrodes may be applied to the skin overlying a motor nerve, or a motor point, in the area of pain, or in a segmentally related myotome. Electrodes do not have to be placed on a specific acupuncture point since this mode of TENS derives its name from the low rate used, a rate shared with application techniques of electrical or manual acupuncture, rather than from common sites of stimulation. The pulse rate is set at 1 to 4 Hz, pulse duration at 0.200 to 0.300 ms, because the chronaxie of motor nerves is longer than that of sensory nerves, and amplitude is set to produce visible, but comfortable muscle twitches (usually three to five times the sensory threshold). There is a latency between the initiation of stimulation and the onset of analgesia, usually a delay of 30 to 45 minutes, further suggesting an induction time for neurohumorally mediated suprasegmental inhibition of pain. Analgesia usually outlasts the time of stimulation by several hours to several days.[9,85] Treatment time is usually 45 minutes or less, depending on the fatigability of the muscles being stimulated. The duration of analgesia is directly related to the tolerance of strong muscle contractions for 30 to 45 minutes.[121]

A point locator (Fig. 5-3), is a device that permits pinpoint stimulation of PSS at either low or high rates. Because of the small surface area of the stimulating probe, the current density is very high, allowing stimulation to be applied for shorter periods of time (increments of 15 or 30 seconds), yet still resulting in prolonged analgesia.

A related mode of stimulation is that of pulse trains or bursts. In this case, a burst of pulses is generated at a low rate (one to four bursts per second). Each burst, however, contains a higher-frequency carrier wave that may vary from 5 to 7 Hz, to 100 Hz. The peripheral nervous system recognizes each burst as a "pulse" and thus responds to this burst stimulation as it would to low rate pulsed stimulation. However, motor activity occurs at a lower amplitude when a low rate burst (pulse train) mode is used, as compared to an individual low rate pulsed mode, because a greater pulse charge is generated by the burst waveform. Therefore, patients may tolerate muscle contractions at lower current intensities for longer periods of time, or more comfortably, with less

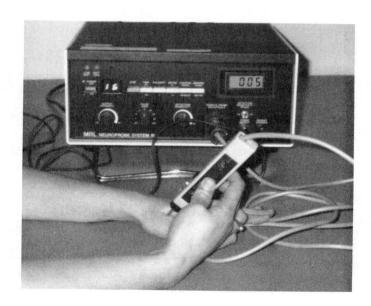

FIGURE 5-3. A point locator permits identification of preferred stimulation sites by electrically detecting regions of low skin impedance. Stimulation of the Hoku acupuncture point is shown.

recruitment of C-fiber activity. In addition, a carrier frequency of 100 Hz, packaged in 2 bursts per second, provides the stimulus capabilities of both conventional and LRAT.

The clinical efficacy of LRAT has been established in patients with Raynaud's syndrome, diabetic peripheral neuropathy,[9] rheumatoid arthritis,[85] trigeminal neuralgia,[93] and other chronic pain conditions. Eriksson and colleagues[93] found that patients with chronic facial pain who had not responded favorably to conventional TENS did experience analgesia when LRAT was applied to segmentally related myotomes. LRAT provides a viable alternative to conventional TENS in the management of a variety of acute- and chronic-pain conditions.

BRIEF INTENSE TENS

A mode of stimulation used to induce short-term electroanalgesia during uncomfortable procedures such as wound debridement is that of brief intense TENS. Electrodes are usually placed surrounding or proximal to the site of potential pain, pulse rate is set to the maximum available (usually about 150 Hz), and amplitude is surged to induce strong, intermittent muscle fasciculations. Stimulation may be applied for as long as 15 minutes before muscle fatigue dictates a rest period. After a few minutes, the stimulation may be resumed.

The resultant analgesia permits performance of brief but uncomfortable procedures, including wound debridement, dental work, joint mobilization, or friction massage.[86,122-123] Particularly in the case of joint mobilization, the clinician must weigh the consequences of removing pain as a protective mechanism and exercise extreme caution during the procedure.

Patient Evaluation

Critical evaluation of the patient with pain is prerequisite to the successful application of TENS. During the initial interview the clinician should discern the chief complaint or medical diagnosis, the relevant medical and surgical history, previous and current treatments that have been employed, and current and recent medication intake data. In addition, the clinician should take a careful family, social, and vocational history to learn the patient's perception of the effects that the pain and dysfunction have on these important areas.

A careful, consistent evaluation of the patient's perception of the intensity, quality, and distribution of the pain, as well as the variation of pain level relative to posture, activity, medication intake, or time of day is important to be able to assess treatment outcomes. Several methods of subjective pain evaluation are commonly used in the clinical setting. The first is a simple descriptive scale (SDS). Two examples of such a device, illustrated in Figure 5–4, use a four- or five-point scale based upon the patient's selection of a word that best describes pain at present or pain associated with specific activities. The value of this scale is limited by its lack of sensitivity in detecting small changes in pain states.[124]

The numerical rating scale (NRS), shown in Figure 5–5, is a verbal or written determination of a pain level on a scale from 1 to 10, in which 1 represents no pain and 10, excruciating pain. The NRS provides better discrimination of small changes in pain intensity than does the SDS.

The visual analog scale is a 10-cm line, oriented vertically or horizontally, with one end indicating "no pain," and the other end representing "pain as bad as it can be." The

1 = nil   4 = severe

2 = mild   5 = excruciating

3 = moderate

☐ none   ☐ slight   ☐ moderate   ☐ severe   ☐ very severe

FIGURE 5–4. Examples of simple descriptive scales.

patient is asked to mark a place on the line that indicates his or her present pain rating (Figure 5–6).

Downie and colleagues[124] evaluated the degree of agreement among these scales in patients with rheumatic diseases and found a high correlation between the three scales. The scales are simple to understand and do not demand a high degree of literacy or sophistication from the patient, as other pain measurement tools do, such as the semantic differentiation scales described below. The NRS, SDS, or VAS may be used before, during, and following treatment to evaluate changes in the patient's perception of pain relative to treatment, or the scales may be completed throughout the course of a day to assess changes in pain intensity relative to activity or time of day.

Semantic differentiation scales are comprised of word lists and categories representing the sensory, affective, and evaluative components of the pain experience. Words are

| 1 | 2 | 3 | 4 | 5 | 6 | 7 | 8 | 9 | 10 |

| 10 |
| 9 |
| 8 |
| 7 |
| 6 |
| 5 |
| 4 |
| 3 |
| 2 |
| 1 |

FIGURE 5–5. Examples of numerical rating scales.

No Pain 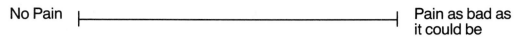 Pain as bad as
it could be

FIGURE 5–6. The visual analog scale.

categorized by whether they describe temporal, spatial, pressure, or thermal character-istics of pain (sensory), fear, anxiety, and tension qualities of the pain experience (affective) or the overall cognitive experience of pain (evaluative). Words within each category are rank ordered in terms of intensity. The word lists were developed and ranked by physicians, students, and patients.[125]

One of the most commonly used word lists was developed by Melzack and Torge-son[125] for the McGill Pain Questionnaire (Figure 5–7).[75] Patients are asked to select a word from any of 20 categories that best describes their pain experience. Not all categories need be selected by any one patient. Several numerical indices regarding the scope, quality, and intensity of the pain experience can be calculated from this inven-tory. A number of words chosen (NWC) score (0 to 20) is calculated by simply adding up the number of words selected by the patient. A pain-rating index (PRI) can be calculated by adding the rank sums of the assigned intensity values for each of the three categories of words selected, or for all categories together.

Semantic differential scales are more difficult and time consuming to complete, and demand a sophisticated literacy level, a sufficient attention span, and a normal cognitive state by the patient. They are therefore less convenient to use in the clinical environment but have value when a more detailed analysis of patients' perceptions of their pain is needed, as in a pain clinic or clinical research setting.

The patients' rating of their pain relative to changing postures, activities of daily living, work, recreational and social activities, and time of day is important in identify-ing factors which aggravate or relieve pain and may contribute to identification of functional or structural sources of pain that can then be treated. Patients can complete daily activity/pain logs and medication intake records prior to beginning treatment, and maintain these logs during a course of treatment, and after treatment has been com-pleted. Improvement in patients' activity performance is at least as important as im-provement in their subjective pain rating, particularly in documenting efficacy of treat-ment for reimbursement.[126] Such logs can also reveal causes of exacerbations of pain, or signs of malingering, in the face of otherwise efficacious treatment.

The patient should complete a diagram describing the spatial distribution of his or her pain (Fig. 5–8). Different colored pencils or signs may be used to distinguish superficial from deep pain, sharp from dull, light from intense, and so forth. This diagram assists in determining the structural sources of pain and forms the basis upon which initial electrode placements may be selected and documented.[105] Patients may complete new diagrams at regular intervals to indicate changes in distribution, quality, intensity, and source of pain.

The MPQ is a widely used pain inventory that combines several short pain-inten-sity rating scales with a semantic differential scale, a spatial distribution diagram, and open-ended interview questions.[75] A short form of this inventory, recently published, facilitates its use in the clinic.[127]

In addition to using the detailed subjective pain evaluation tools described above, the clinician should perform a physical examination, including assessment of strength, mobility, sensation, posture, spinal function, soft-tissue quality, neurologic integrity, gait, and endurance. Intact cutaneous sensation often facilitates the achievement of

What does your pain feel like?

Some of the words below describe your *present* pain. Indicate which words describe it best. Leave out any word group that is not suitable. Use only a single word in each appropriate group—the one that applies *best.*

1		2		3		4	
1	Flickering	1	Jumping	1	Pricking	1	Sharp
2	Quivering	2	Flashing	2	Boring	2	Cutting
3	Pulsing	3	Shooting	3	Drilling	3	Lacerating
4	Throbbing			4	Stabbing		
5	Beating			5	Lancinating		
6	Pounding						

5		6		7		8	
1	Pinching	1	Tugging	1	Hot	1	Tingling
2	Pressing	2	Pulling	2	Burning	2	Itchy
3	Gnawing	3	Wrenching	3	Scalding	3	Smarting
4	Cramping			4	Searing	4	Stinging
5	Crushing						

9		10		11		12	
1	Dull	1	Tender	1	Tiring	1	Sickening
2	Sore	2	Taut	2	Exhausting	2	Suffocating
3	Hurting	3	Rasping				
4	Aching	4	Splitting				
5	Heavy						

13		14		15		16	
1	Fearful	1	Punishing	1	Wretched	1	Annoying
2	Frightful	2	Gruelling	2	Blinding	2	Troublesome
3	Terrifying	3	Cruel			3	Miserable
		4	Vicious			4	Intense
		5	Killing			5	Unbearable

17		18		19		20	
1	Spreading	1	Tight	1	Cool	1	Nagging
2	Radiating	2	Numb	2	Cold	2	Nauseating
3	Penetrating	3	Drawing	3	Freezing	3	Agonizing
4	Piercing	4	Squeezing			4	Dreadful
		5	Tearing			5	Torturing

FIGURE 5–7. Semantic differential word list from the McGill Pain Questionnaire. (From Melzack,[75] p 277, with permission.)

electroanalgesia. The distribution of the intact-cutaneous sensation should preferably be in the painful region or a segmentally related dermatome. When this is not the case, remote sites may be stimulated.

Application of TENS

Once TENS has been selected as a treatment, electrode placement sites and a mode of stimulation are chosen. The treatment is then initiated. The skin should be cleansed, rinsed, and dried to diminish skin-electrode impedance. It may be necessary to shave

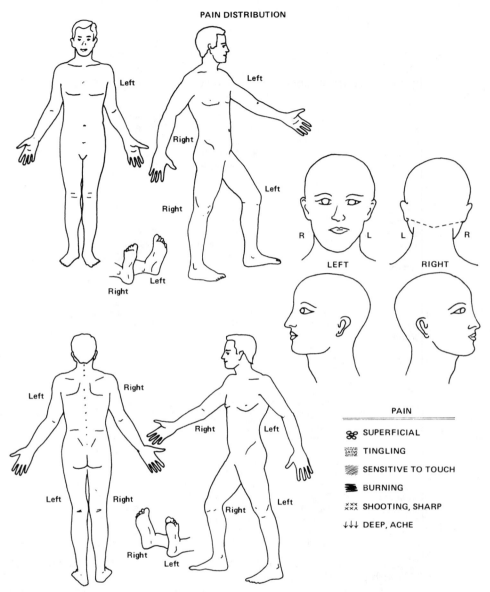

FIGURE 5–8. Example of diagrams used to indicate the spatial distribution of a patient's pain. (From Mannheimer and Lampe,[105] p 192, with permission.)

hair from some areas before applying electrodes. Electrodes are affixed to the selected sites. Stimulus parameters are set by the clinician or the patient, with the clinician's instruction, and the patient is encouraged to increase the stimulus amplitude to a comfortable level (conventional TENS) or to a motor threshold (LRAT). By controlling the stimulus amplitude, patients assume active roles in their treatment. They also are secure in the knowledge that they are in control of the intensity of the sensation that the TENS evokes, and thus, any apprehension regarding *electrical stimulation* specifically may be allayed. Patients should describe the sensation perceived under the electrodes as tingling or buzzing (conventional TENS) rather than burning or pricking, which may indicate an undesirable high skin resistance to current flow. These noxious sensations may be alleviated by conscientious skin preparation, even distribution of conductive gel along the total surface area of the electrode, or relocation of the electrodes to an alternative site of low skin impedance. After 5 to 10 minutes of treatment, patients should report a tingling, buzzing, tapping, or vibratory sensation deep to the electrodes, and throughout the area between the electrodes. If the stimulated area is the painful area, or if a segmentally related area is being stimulated, patients should begin to report a decrease in pain within 30 minutes of initiation of treatment. The clinician should note and record the latency of onset of analgesia (effective time of onset).[105] If analgesia does not occur, electrode placement and stimulus settings should be re-evaluated and alternative treatment procedures should be attempted at that time or at the next scheduled appointment.

Mannheimer and Lampe[105] provided the following guidelines for duration of TENS treatment based upon their clinical experiences. TENS may be continued for up to 1 hour following onset of analgesia, but should then be turned off so that the patient may evaluate the duration of analgesia that persists once stimulation has ceased. There will frequently be a carryover period of analgesia equal to the duration of stimulation. The patient may begin stimulation again once the pain returns. The "rest period" from stimulation is essential to (1) minimize the patient's dependency on stimulation, (2) assess the analgesic value of the stimulation, (3) prolong battery life, (4) minimize skin irritation, and (5) allow the patient to attempt some function or activity without stimulation to better assess carryover analgesia during activity.

TENS may be applied daily by the patient as needed for effective pain control, as long as the patient understands the concept of noncontinuous stimulation and the importance of increasing activity and function commensurate with pain relief. For patients suffering from acute pain that is anticipated to be of short duration, such as postoperative incisional pain, continuous 24-hour stimulation for several days may be indicated. Once the acute pain is relieved, most patients will voluntarily discontinue the TENS treatment. For patients with pain of longer duration or chronicity, discontinuous stimulation may be applied as long as it is effective.

When selecting a TENS system for application by the patient, several factors must be considered. The unit chosen should be durable, the control dials clearly labeled and easy to manipulate, the unit simple to understand and use, and the batteries easy to change or recharge. For some patients, the size, weight, and cosmesis of the unit is important. The selected electrode system should be easy to apply and should minimize skin irritation. Electrode leads should be long enough to permit freedom of movement without pulling loose from the electrodes or unit, and short enough to be concealed in clothing without tangling.

Recommendations for Home Programs

For a home program of TENS analgesia to be appropriate, the patients must be willing to assume responsibility for their treatment and capable of doing so. They should be able to follow directions to carry out an efficacious home program as outlined by the clinician. Many patients will need assistance with electrodes, especially with those placed paraspinally, so the availability of an assistant at home may be necessary in a home program. A complete set of instructions to the patient will include information on the operation of the unit, battery charging and/or changing, care of the unit and supplies, an outline of preferred and alternative electrode placements and stimulation parameters, a suggested schedule of treatment times and "rest periods," warnings regarding misuse of the unit (a complete list of precautions is described later), information on the avoidance and treatment of skin irritation, and the address and phone number of a local distributor to contact for additional supplies (tapes and gel) and troubleshooting. The clinician's name and phone number should also be provided on the written instructions.

Most third-party providers will reimburse a percentage of a 30- or 60-day rental fee for a TENS unit. This trial period is essential because a number of patients will no longer need or decide not to use the TENS after a brief experience with a home program. Studies have concluded that the apparent efficacy of TENS seems to diminish over time in a home program, particularly among patients for whom the intervention of a health care professional was an integral part of the treatment.[74] Third-party providers will often pay up to 80 percent of the purchase price of a unit if certain criteria are met: (1) the pain is intractable, (2) the pain is anticipated to persist for a long time, and (3) the TENS was effective in relieving pain during a 30-day trial period. The 1-month rental fee is most often applicable toward the purchase price of the unit.[105]

Regular follow-up evaluations of a patient participating in a home program is essential to the continued success of the program, the patient's safety and well-being, and the evaluation of the efficacy of TENS for long-term analgesia. Patients participating in home programs should be re-evaluated by the clinician at 2 weeks, 1 month, 3 months, 6 months, and then every 6 months thereafter for the duration of the home program. During these visits clinicians can assess the outcomes of the home treatment. They can troubleshoot any problems with the treatment protocol or device, evaluate and correct malfunctions that may have occurred since the last visit, recommend alternative application procedures if appropriate, and adjust exercise or activity recommendations as indicated. The patient's daily treatment time, schedule, changes in physical activity, vocational or social behavior, lifestyle, medication intake, and intervening medical problems should be solicited and recorded either by patient interview or questionnaire. Conscientious follow-up on a scheduled basis will increase the likelihood of effective analgesia with TENS in a home (patient-regulated) program.

Even under optimal conditions, some patients will not accept the responsibility of managing a home program. Patients should be carefully screened to assess their willingness and capability of complying with a home program using TENS. Some TENS devices offer the clinician the ability to monitor how long or how often the TENS was used at home.* Some patients will be more inclined to comply with a therapeutic regimen if they know that their compliance is being monitored. Another option available to motivate the noncompliant patient is to make further physical therapy treatment contingent upon compliance with a home program. In any case, patients who are unwilling or unable to assume an active role in their rehabilitation process are not candidates for the TENS home program.

---

*Neurotech, Inc., 85 Flagship Drive, Suite A, North Andover, MA 01845.

CONTRAINDICATIONS AND PRECAUTIONS

Two contraindications to the use of TENS have been clearly stated by the Federal Food and Drug Administration.[128] TENS should not be used for a patient with a synchronous (demand) cardiac pacemaker. TENS should not be applied over the carotid sinus because stimulation of the vasovagal reflex could result in a life-threatening hypotensive response or cardiac arrest.

It was proposed by Eriksson, Schuller, and Sjolund[129] in 1978 that TENS operating at a conventional rate could interfere with the operation of synchronous cardiac pacemakers. More recently, conventional TENS applications were evaluated by several investigators.[130,131] Electrodes were placed on sites remote to the cardiac region as well as directly over the left-lateral chest wall. No interference with *continuous* pacing was experienced with application of TENS in either study. While TENS electrodes should generally not be placed in the cardiac region on patients with cardiac pathology, TENS may be applied if needed on an individual case basis, provided that vigilant, continuous cardiac monitoring is employed and emergency medical assistance is readily available. However, FDA regulations still preclude TENS use in patients with *demand* cardiac pacemakers.

Several practice precautions are enumerated by the Food and Drug Administration:[128] (1) Application of TENS to the abdominal or lumbar area during pregnancy may produce adverse effects, although none have been documented to date. The FDA warns against all electromedical modality use in pregnant women. However, successful use of TENS for management of labor pain or meralgia paresthetica have been described. (2) TENS should not be applied over the eyes. (3) TENS should not be applied internally because it may damage mucosal linings. (4) TENS should not be applied transcranially or in the upper cervical region in patients with histories of cerebrovascular accidents, transient ischemic attacks, or seizures, unless brain function is carefully monitored during stimulation. (5) Responsibility for treatment or adjustment of stimulation parameters should not be given to patients with cognitive impairment. Special care should be taken to secure lead wires, electrodes, and potentiometers when treating disoriented or cognitively impaired patients, or young children.

Adverse Responses to TENS

Although rare, reports of adverse skin responses are occasionally noted. Skin irritation may be caused by an electrical reaction, an electrochemical response, an allergic response to electrodes, gel, or tape, or a mechanical irritation caused by shearing forces between adhesive substances and the skin.[105,132-133] The source of irritation must be identified and TENS application modified accordingly before abandoning TENS as a viable treatment.

Electrically induced thermal burns can occur if current density is too high beneath or between electrodes. The smaller the electrode contact area, the higher the current density. An electrode contact surface of at least 4 cm² is required for safe stimulation with the intensities commonly used for TENS.[134] Similarly, the interelectrode distance must be at least equal to the diameter of the electrodes to avoid excessive current density between electrodes.[105]

Micropunctate electrothermal burns occur when current is unevenly distributed in areas under the electrodes. This uneven spread of current is due to poor skin-electrode contact secondary to uneven gelling of the electrode or uneven body contour in the stimulated area. Conductive gel should be evenly distributed along the entire electrode surface which should conform to the body contour. In addition, in areas where open wounds are present, skin impedance is lower than at the surrounding intact area, and current would be concentrated at the wound site. Therefore electrodes should not be applied over regions where open wounds are present.

Because most TENS units are constant-current devices with zero net DC charge, the incidence of electrochemical burns is rare. However, if an electrochemical burn is suspected, the TENS device should be evaluated for a potential DC component. If one is found, another device should be selected for treatment.

Allergic reactions to electrodes, gel, or tape are the most common form of adverse skin response. The component of treatment eliciting the allergic response may be identified by placing the electrode, gel, and tape on three different body sites remote to the area of treatment and observing the skin response. If a carbon-silicone electrode is the offending component, a karaya or conductive polymer electrode may be substituted.[132] If a gel containing propylene glycol is responsible for the adverse response, a different conductive gel or conductive polymer electrode not requiring gel may be used.[133] If the adhesive tape produces an allergic reaction, a different tape may be substituted, electrodes may be held in place with elastic straps or bandages, or a self-adhering electrode may be selected.

Occasionally adhesive tape produces skin irritation because of shearing forces that occur between the tape and the skin. Care should be taken when applying and removing tape to minimize these forces. Mannheimer and Lampe[105] suggested that tape should be affixed from the center outward, rather than from one end to the other. Tape should be carefully removed in the direction that the hair lies in the region. Consideration should be given to body movements occurring in the area of tape application. A series of short tapes, applied with space between each tape, will permit more freedom of movement than one long strip of tape. In addition, tension exerted by lead wires pulling on the electrode and tape may be minimized by forming a "tension loop" of excess lead-wire length, 6 to 10 inches from the electrode, and taping the lead wire down just below the loop, allowing greater freedom of movement without shearing forces. Awareness of the contraindications and precautions associated with TENS, and a thoughtful approach to the problems associated with TENS applications will enhance the successful use of TENS for a greater number of patients.

FACTORS AFFECTING RESPONSE TO TREATMENT

Placebo Response

The term *placebo* is derived from the Latin verb *placere*, to please. In clinical terms, a placebo is defined as a procedure resembling an actual treatment but known to be ineffective for the patient's condition.[94] The patient's favorable response to a placebo may be accounted for by the factors of hope and expectation inherent in the treatment process.[135] Placebos are used as controls in clinical trials to determine the efficacy of a therapeutic intervention. They may also be used to facilitate a patient's beliefs that he or she is "feeling better, or healing" when an active treatment may not be known, available, or in the patient's best interest.

For a placebo to be effective, patients must believe that they are receiving actual treatment. A placebo is simply substituted for a procedure with some intrinsic remedial value. However, because the perception of sensory stimulation is thought to be an integral part of efficacious TENS treatments, a convincing placebo TENS treatment is difficult to administer. Thornsteinsson and coworkers[136] evaluated the placebo effect of TENS in a double-blind study. Patients were told that they might or might not feel a tingling paresthesia associated with the TENS treatment, and were directed to attend to changes in pain level rather than the presence or absence of a cutaneous sensation. Analgesia in response to placebo TENS occurred in 32 percent of the trials, compared with a 48-percent analgesic response to actual electrical stimulation. A placebo effect in the range of 25 to 35 percent is similar to the effect noted in double-blind studies of analgesic medications.

Langley and associates[137] used a double-blind noncrossover design to compare the analgesic effects of conventional TENS, acupuncturelike TENS, and placebo TENS in 33 patients with hand pain and dysfunction secondary to chronic rheumatoid arthritis. Each group of patients was directed to observe the TENS waveform on an oscilloscope. In the case of the placebo TENS, while the patients did not receive actual stimulation, a random pattern of pulse waves was generated on the oscilloscope screen. Comparison of treatment groups revealed nonsignificant differences among groups in outcome measures of resting pain, grip pain, or joint tenderness. In fact, 54 to 63 percent of the patients in each group reported pain relief or greater than 50 percent compared with pretreatment pain ratings. The authors suggested that the focus of attention (on an oscilloscope or on a sensory stimulus) can provide a significant change in pain perception. Since a constant visual focal point was provided for all three treatment groups, similar analgesic results were observed. Special care must be taken when evaluating the placebo factor of TENS to provide a believable sham treatment, either as a control, or in addition to a control (no treatment) group.

Several factors influence the placebo response. Some patients will respond to placebo interventions in certain situations and not others. Increases in pain intensity or related anxiety have been shown to increase the likelihood of a favorable response, perhaps by increasing the motivation to respond favorably.[138-140] Expectation of analgesia, based upon a patient's past experience with a related treatment, or upon enthusiastic suggestion of success by the health professional administering the treatment, will enhance the placebo response.

Other factors that enhance the placebo response include associated side effects such as nausea, dizziness, or sedation, and a high-powered, technologically advanced professional environment. Finally, testimonials of treatment efficacy from valued health professionals, family, friends, or celebrities also add credence to the treatment simulated by the placebo.

Several mechanisms of action for the analgesic response to placebo have been proposed. Chen[141] described the importance of cognitive factors, including a belief system and expectation of analgesia, in facilitating a favorable placebo response. The role of endorphin-mediated pain modulation in the analgesic effect of placebo has been supported by some investigators and refuted by others.[142,143]

Certainly there is an element of placebo response to any treatment administered by caring, concerned health professionals who communicate enthusiastic belief in the efficacy of their treatment. The placebo response is a component of efficacious patient management. The placebo component may be used ethically and effectively as long as it is understood and administered in the best interests of the patient.

Other Factors

Reynolds and associates[144] examined the predictive value of pain questionnaires in selecting patients who would most likely respond favorably to TENS treatments. The results of their study indicate that older, retired individuals with pain of less than 1-year duration, who had undergone limited or no surgery, and who did not use narcotic analgesic medications were most likely to benefit from TENS. Site of injury, sensory deficit, and identifiable financial secondary gains did not affect treatment outcomes.

A study by Johansson and colleagues[145] revealed that pain of neurogenic origin was more successfully treated than pain of psychogenic or somatogenic origin. In a related study, Richardson and associates[146] determined that patients with psychogenic pain obtained greater relief from a placebo injection of saline than from TENS, which actually exacerbated pain in some patients.

Mannheimer and Lampe[105] suggest several methods for improving the analgesic effectiveness of TENS treatment. They advocate a vigilant and ongoing evaluation of stimulation sites, stimulus parameters, and patient response, with attendant adjustment of stimulation sites and settings as needed. They suggest that stimulation in the painful region, at a trigger, motor, or acupuncture point is more effective than stimulation at a remote site, and encourage a gradual increase in stimulus amplitude, until a strong stimulation is well tolerated by the patients. Weaning patients from analgesic medication, particularly from narcotic or addictive medications prior to the initiation of TENS treatment, also enhances positive treatment outcomes. Finally, patient education and vigilant follow-up of a patient's progress, once a home treatment program is initiated, are essential to achieving optimal electroanalgesia with TENS. Mannheimer and Lampe[105] provide a detailed description of these considerations in their text.

CASE STUDY

Illustration of the integration of TENS into a multidimensional rehabilitation program for the specific purpose of alleviating pain and facilitating normal function follows—after the source of pain has been accurately identified.

A 34-year-old woman sustained injury to the left knee when she tripped while walking down a gravel driveway. She initially reported pain and stiffness, and demonstrated slight edema on the patellar ligament. Pain was exacerbated during weight bearing and when the patient climbed stairs, as well as during active knee flexion. Pain increased over the next few days and the patient sought medical treatment.

Radiological evaluation revealed no significant bony injury or soft-tissue discontinuity. The injury was diagnosed to be a strain of the patellar tendon and the patient was placed in a long leg-knee extension brace for 3 weeks, while allowed to bear full weight during ambulation. During this time, the patient reported being unable to bear weight on the limb without significant pain, which was localized at the lateral knee joint line. She was re-evaluated by an orthopedic surgeon who confirmed the diagnosis and encouraged the patient to ambulate without the knee brace, and to begin strengthening and range of motion exercises to restore normal knee function.

Seven weeks after the initial injury the patient was referred to a physical therapist for supervised strengthening of the quadriceps and hamstring muscles,

TABLE 5–5 Evaluation Measures of Case History Patient

Evaluation	At Initiation of Physical Therapy Treatment	At Discharge
Active knee range of motion (°)	0–115	0–128
Isometric strength on Orthoron* (ft·lb)		
Hamstrings	Left: 55	106
	Right: 115	—
Quadriceps	Left: 25	129
	Right: 141	—

*Cybex Division of Lumex, Ronkonkoma, NY, 11779.

and restoration of normal knee mobility. She demonstrated an antalgic gait, with decreased stance time on the left, and she complained of pain in the infrapatellar region and along the lateral joint line. An extension lag of 10 to 15° was observed during active straight-leg raising. Soft-tissue evaluation for ligamentous discontinuity was negative. Skin tone, color, and temperature were equivalent to the uninvolved extremity. A manual muscle test of the knee musculature revealed ⅗ (fair) strength of both the hamstring and quadriceps muscle groups. Mobility measures and isometric evaluation results on the Orthotron* are listed in Table 5–5. The circumference in the area of the vastus medialis muscle was 2 cm less on the involved lower extremity when compared with the uninvolved extremity, indicating that significant disuse atrophy had occurred.

The patient participated in a physical therapy program consisting of isometric and isokinetic exercises for the hamstrings and quadriceps muscles, passive mobilization of the knee joint, and management of pain and joint stiffness with ultrasound, ice massage, or whirlpool. She ambulated with crutches, bearing only partial weight on her affected leg, because she did not trust the knee's ability to take her full weight. Pain continued to be the major obstacle to regaining normal biomechanical function.

Ten weeks following the injury, the patient underwent exploratory arthroscopic surgery to conclusively rule out any bony or soft-tissue derangement in the knee. No such injury was identified, and the patient resumed her physical therapy program 10 days following surgery. At this time, another physical therapist was asked to evaluate the pain component of this patient's dysfunction. Trophic changes, including decreased skin temperature, cyanosis, shininess, increased sweating, and decreased hair growth, as well as slight edema, were observed around the affected knee joint, when compared to the unaffected knee. In light of the patient's history of longstanding painful dysfunction and immobilization, a secondary complication of RSDS was suspected.

Treatment with conventional TENS was initiated to attempt normalization of sympathetic nervous system activity as well as electroanalgesia. Electrodes from one channel were placed paraspinally on the skin overlying the third lumbar nerve root level, and those from a second channel were placed on the skin overlying the peroneal nerve (at the popliteal fossa, and posterior to the lateral malleolus) (Fig. 5–9) to stimulate peripheral nerves subserving the painful area. Pulse rate was set

*Cybex Division of Lumex, Ronkonkoma, NY, 11779.

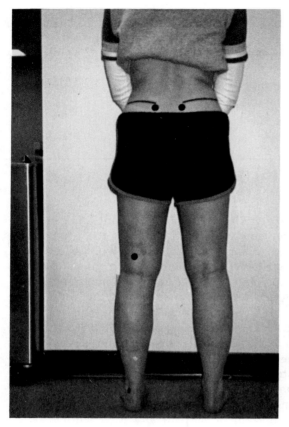

FIGURE 5–9. Electrode-placement sites are identified paraspinally on the skin overlying L_3, origin of the femoral nerve, and on the skin overlying the peroneal nerve at the popliteal fossa and posterior to the lateral malleolus for management of a reflex-sympathetic dystrophy syndrome following a knee injury.

at 100 pps, pulse duration at 0.060 ms, and amplitude was set by the patient to evoke a strong paresthesia in the area of pain, without concommitant muscle contraction. The patient underwent stimulation for 4 or 5 hours daily, at first under the supervision of a physical therapist and then in a home program.

Beneficial treatment outcomes were observed during and immediately following the first treatment. Improvements in skin quality, color, and temperature were observed. The patient reported immediate pain relief during weight bearing, active knee motion, and resisted knee extension. Adequate pain control with the TENS permitted the patient to participate fully in her rehabilitation program, and she regained virtually full function of her injured knee within 4 weeks following initiation of TENS treatment (Table 5–5). When she was able to ambulate bearing full weight on each extremity, she was discharged from physical therapy. Over the next 6 months the patient reported occasional discomfort and slight edema in the knee when she overused it, but she easily controlled these symptoms with ice and elevation of the limb as needed. Symptoms of RSDS did not return.

This case illustrates that accurate identification of the source(s) of pain is critical to the successful treatment of pain with TENS or any other analgesic agent. In the early management of this patient, the source of pain was assumed to be the same as the source of dysfunction, that is, an ill-defined soft tissue injury. If indeed, the soft tissue injury was the only source of pain, the patient should have responded well to the initial treatments of rest and temporary immobilization, followed by modalities and exercise. Once the actual source of pain (RSDS) was identified, the syndrome was easily managed with conventional TENS, applied in the manner recommended by Mannheimer and Lampe.[105] If the patient had not responded favorably to conventional TENS, application of acupuncturelike TENS, modulated, or burst TENS could have been attempted, with electrodes placed on acupuncture points that more rapidly impact circulatory insufficiency or the sympathetic nervous system.[9]

A LOOK TOWARD THE FUTURE

The future of electroanalgesia as an effective treatment alternative depends upon the cooperative efforts of clinicians, manufacturers, and researchers to establish treatment efficacy and adhere to high-quality standards of practice. Concerns regarding the lack of scientific substantiation of TENS applications and the use of electroanalgesic devices by untrained individuals, as well as potential solutions to these problems are presented by Nolan.[147] These and other implications for future integration of TENS into progressive rehabilitation approaches are presented in the following sections.

The Clinician

Clinicians are obligated to become educated consumers of both TENS equipment and information. Clinicians must maintain up-to-date knowledge of current equipment features as well as current basic and clinical research regarding pain mechanisms and treatment efficacy. All too often clinicians rely on industry representatives as their primary source of information regarding TENS. They may receive biased, even inaccurate information regarding the specific features of one device compared to another. Clinicians are responsible for acquiring a sound knowledge base from which they can ask informed questions of industry representatives, and they must critically evaluate TENS devices for efficacy, quality, and value, and in turn, provide optimal cost-effective care for patients.

In addition, clinicians are obligated to evaluate carefully and document treatment outcomes by objective as well as subjective measures, relative to the specific treatment procedures used, in order to optimize patient care. If treatment applications and outcomes are carefully evaluated and systematically documented, the clinician will be better able to effectively modify treatment as indicated. Additionally, the clinician will be able to provide the objective data regarding treatment efficacy requested by health insurance providers. Finally, and perhaps most important, carefully documented data can contribute to establishment of a centralized pool of information regarding treatment alternatives and their efficacy. This pool would facilitate dissemination of information that is required for effective use of electroanalgesia in the future.

The Industry

The TENS industry has guided this modality's development and growth by providing a wide variety of stimulus options available in aesthetically pleasing devices. Over the past 10 years, as the number of companies manufacturing devices grew at a remarkable rate, so did the competition and the need to "build a better (or at least a different) mousetrap." Manufacturers have provided consumers with a vast number of stimulus-parameter combinations, including modulations of pulse rate and width, and low, high, and burst frequencies. Unfortunately, there is no scientific evidence suggesting that one pulse rate, pulse duration, amplitude, or a combination of these waveform characteristics is more clinically effective than another in managing most kinds of pain. The TENS industry would contribute significantly to the future development of this modality by supporting research efforts directed at establishing treatment efficacy within specific diagnostic categories or relative to specific stimulus parameters.

Standardized biomedical terminology describing waveform characteristics must be adopted by the TENS industry as well as clinicians and researchers. Presently, each manufacturer seeks to couch his "special waveform features" in different terms encouraging clinicians to become familiar with and use only one or two types of devices, even if a third device would offer a better treatment alternative for a patient. This wide variety of terms used perpetuates the "mystical" quality often associated with electroanalgesia and hampers information exchange and scientific growth. A group of clinicians, educators, researchers, and engineers with a special interest in electrophysiology have clearly defined electrotherapeutic terminology. These standards have been compiled by the Section on Clinical Electrophysiology of the American Physical Therapy Association.*[148] The universal adoption of this terminology by clinicians, researchers, engineers, and manufacturers will facilitate the informed and appropriate use of a variety of TENS devices by clinicians as well as encourage the sharing of information among these groups.

The TENS industry has responded to the expressed needs of clinicians and patients regarding specific device features and electrode systems that minimize adverse skin responses and maximize ease of application. Manufacturers now have the obligation to assist in the objective evaluation of device features in order to retain necessary options, discard others, and contain the high costs associated with durable medical equipment in the future.

The Researcher

The critical need for scientifically acquired data regarding treatment efficacy and optimal stimulation parameters is readily apparent. The effectiveness of electroanalgesia has been best established in the area of postoperative incisional pain. Additional investigations of electroanalgesia related to pain of orthopedic or neurogenic origin, restoration of normal sympathetic function, enhancement of circulation, and basic pain modulation mechanisms must continue to be implemented. Comparison of TENS to placebo or other analgesic procedures in terms of efficacy as well as cost effectiveness is indicated. The application of TENS as a treatment of choice rather than last resort and the integration of TENS into a contingency management program for the patient with chronic pain provide fertile areas for future investigation.[149] This essential research demands a commitment of interest, time, and funding on the part of clinicians, manufacturers, health care consumers, and the government. The strength of this commitment will define the future of TENS.

The combination of efforts described above can guarantee a bright future for

---

*Available from the Publications Department of the American Physical Therapy Association.

electroanalgesia in terms of effectiveness, decreased treatment time and financial cost, and quality patient care. These efforts can elevate the use of TENS to an art based upon scientifically substantiated fact rather than upon assumption, hearsay, supernatural forces, and time-honored empiricism. The ultimate beneficiary is the patient who will be assured of optimal care, including quality equipment, knowledgeable and caring health professionals, and cost-effective as well as symptom-effective management of his or her pain and dysfunction.

SUMMARY

The optimal use of TENS for effective electroanalgesia is established by an understanding of the neurophysiologic mechanisms involved in pain modulation, an appreciation for the variety of stimulation capabilities presently available, and a systematic approach to patient evaluation, treatment application, and modification determined by assessment of treatment outcomes. In this chapter the neurophysiologic principles upon which TENS is based are reviewed, a comprehensive, critical review of clinical applications to date is presented, and a schema by which TENS may be effectively applied and evaluated is developed. Finally, suggestions for cooperation among clinicians, manufacturers, and researchers to facilitate the future growth of this modality are presented.

APPENDIX: Manufacturers' Addresses for Table 5–3

This information is taken from the operations manual of each unit:

Basix, Empi, Inc.
1275 Grey Fox Road
St. Paul, MN 55112

Dynex, Medtronic Nortech Division
10237 Flanders Court
San Diego, CA 92121

MRL Neuroprobe Physio Technology, Inc.
1925 W. 6th Avenue
Topeka, KS 66606

Napcor, Inc.
9541 B. Business Center Drive
Rancho Cucamonga, CA 91730

N-TRON, Division of Henley
International Inc.
104 Industrial Blvd.
Sugar Land, TX 77478

Pain Suppression Labs, Inc.
P.O. Box 441
Elmwood Park, NJ 07404-0441

Richmar Corporation
Route 2, Box 879
Inola, OK 74036

Stimtech, Codman, and Shurtleff, Inc.
Randolph, MA 02368.

REFERENCES

1. Kellaway, P: The William Osler Medal essay: The part played by electric fish in the early history of bioelectricity and electrotherapy. Bull Hist Med 20:112, 1946.
2. Schonoch, W: Die Rezept Sammlung des Scribonius. Jena (1912–1913). Bakken Museum of Electricity in Life, Minneapolis, MN.
3. Wesley, J: The Desideratum: Or Electricity Made Plain and Useful. W Flexney, London 1760.
4. Sarlandiere, JB: Memoires sur l'ectro-puncture. Delaunay, Paris, 1825.

5. Eberhart, NM: Physician's Directions for Renulife Treatments. Renulife Electric Company, Detroit, MI, 1926.
6. Melzack, R and Wall, PD: Pain mechanisms: A new theory. Science 150:971, 1965.
7. Shealy, CN, Mortimer, JT, and Reswich, JB: Electrical inhibition of pain by stimulation of the dorsal column: Preliminary clinical reports. Anesth Analg 45:489, 1967.
8. Kahn, J: Transcutaneous electrical nerve stimulation for non-united fractures. Phys Ther 62:840, 1982.
9. Kaada, B: Vasodilation induced by transcutaneous nerve stimulation in peripheral ischemia (Raynaud's phenomenon and diabetic polyneuropathy). Eur Heart J 3:303, 1982.
10. Ekblom, A, Fjellner, B, and Hansson, P: The influence of mechanical vibratory stimulation and transcutaneous electrical nerve stimulation on experimental pruritus induced by histamine. Acta Physiol Scand 122:361, 1984.
11. Mannheimer, C, et al: Transcutaneous electrical nerve stimulation in angina pectoris. Int J of Cardiol 7:91, 1985.
12. Nathan, PW and Wall, PD: Treatment of post-herpetic neuralgia by prolonged electrical stimulation. Br Med J 3:645, 1974.
13. Gersh, MR and Wolf, SL: Applications of transcutaneous electrical nerve stimulation in the management of patients with pain: State-of-the-art update. Phys Ther 65:314, 1985.
14. Nathan, PW and Rudge, P: Testing the gate control theory of pain in man. J Neurol Neurosurg Psychiatry 37:1366, 1974.
15. Melzack, R and Casey, KL: Sensory, motivational, and central control determinants of pain. In Kenshalo, DR (ed): The Skin Senses. Charles C Thomas, Springfield, IL, 1968.
16. Lee, KH, Chung, JM, and Willis, WD: Inhibition of primate spinothalamic tract cells by transcutaneous electrical nerve stimulation. J Neurosurg 62:276, 1985.
17. Kaada, B, et al: Failure to influence the VIP level in the cerebrospinal fluid by transcutaneous nerve stimulation in humans. Gen Pharmacol 15:563, 1984.
18. Basbaum, AI and Fields, HL: Endogenous pain control mechanisms: Review and hypothesis. Ann Neurol 4:451, 1978.
19. Mayer, DJ, Price, DD, and Rafii, A: Antagonism of acupuncture analgesia in man by the narcotic antagonic naloxone. Brain Res 121:368, 1977.
20. Hosobuchi, Y, Adams, J, and Linchitz, R: Pain relief by electrical stimulation of the central gray matter in humans and its reversal by naloxone. Science 197:183, 1977.
21. Lewis, VA and Gebhart, GF: Evaluation of the periacqueductal central gray (PAG) as a morphine specific locus of action and examination of morphine induced and SPA coincident at PAG loci. Brain Res 124:283, 1977.
22. Sjolund, BH, Terenius, L, and Eriksson, MBE: Increased CSF levels of endorphins after electroacupuncture. Acta Physiol Scand 100:382, 1977.
23. Eriksson, MBE, Sjolund, BH, and Nielzen, S: Long term results of peripheral conditioning stimulation as an analgesic measure in chronic pain. Pain 6:335, 1979.
24. Sjolund, BH and Eriksson, MBE: The influence of naloxone on analgesia produced by peripheral conditioning stimulation. Brain Res 173:295, 1979.
25. Salar, G, et al: Effect of transcutaneous electrotherapy on CSF beta-endorphin content in patients without pain problems. Pain 10:169, 1981.
26. Facchinetti, F, et al: Concommitant increase in nociceptive flexion reflex threshold and plasma opioids following transcutaneous nerve stimulation. Pain 19:295, 1984.
27. Hughes GS, Jr, et al: Response of plasma beta endorphins to transcutaneous electrical nerve stimulation in healthy subjects. Phsy Ther 64:1062, 1984.
28. O'Brien, W, et al: Effect of transcutaneous electrical nerve stimulation on human blood beta endorphin levels. Phys Ther 64:1367, 1984.
29. Hansson, P, et al: Influence of naloxone on relief of acute oro-facial pain by transcutaneous electrical nerve stimulation or vibration. Pain 24:323, 1986.
30. Ali, J, Uaffe, CS, and Serrette, C: The effect of transcutaneous electrical nerve stimulation on postoperative pain and pulmonary function. Surgery 89:507, 1981.
31. Rosenberg, M, Curtis, L, and Bourke, DL: Transcutaneous electrical nerve stimulation for the relief of postoperative pain. Pain 5:129, 1978.
32. Sodipo, JOA, Adedeji, SA, and Olumide, O: Postoperative pain relief by transcutaneous electrical nerve stimulation. Am J Chin Med 8:190, 1980.
33. Taylor, AG, et al: How effective is transcutaneous electrical nerve stimulation for acute pain? Am J Nurs 83:1171, 1983.
34. Stratton, SA and Smith, MM: Postoperative thoracotomy: Effect of TENS on forced vital capacity. Phys Ther 60:45, 1980.
35. Navarthanam, RG, et al: Evaluation of the transcutaneous electrical nerve stimulator for postoperative analgesia following cardiac surgery. Anesth and Intensive Care 12:345, 1984.
36. Warfield, CA, Stein, JM, and Frank, HA: The effect of transcutaneous electrical nerve stimulation on pain after thoracotomy. Ann Thorac Surg 39:462, 1985.
37. Liu, YC, Liao, WS, and Lien, IN: Effect of transcutaneous electrical nerve stimulation for post-thoracotomic pain. J Formosan Med Assoc 84:801, 1985.

38. Schuster, GD and Infante, MC: Pain relief after low back surgery: The efficacy of transcutaneous electrical nerve stimulation. Pain 8:299, 1980.
39. Solomon, RA, Viernstein, MC, and Long, DM: Reduction of postoperative pain and narcotic use by transcutaneous electrical nerve stimulation. Surgery 87:142, 1980.
40. Richardson, RR and Siqueira, EB: Transcutaneous electrical neurostimulation in post-laminectomy pain. Spine 5:361, 1980.
41. Issenman, J, et al: Transcutaneous electrical nerve stimulation for pain control after spinal fusion with Harrington rods. Phys Ther 65:1517, 1985.
42. Pike, PMH: Transcutaneous electrical stimulation: Its use in the management of postoperative pain. Anesthesia 33:165, 1978.
43. Smith, MJ, Hutchins, RC, and Hehenberger, D: Transcutaneous neural stimulation use in postoperative knee rehabilitation. Am J Sports Med 11:75, 1983.
44. Harvie, KW: A major advance in the control of postoperative knee pain. Orthopedics 2:129, 1979.
45. Alm, WA, Gold, ML, and Weil, LS: Evaluation of transcutaneous electrical nerve stimulation in podiatric surgery. J of Am Podiatr Med Assoc 69:537, 1979.
46. Smith, CM and LaFlamme, CA: Managing a TENS program in the operating room. AORN J 32:411, 1980.
47. Dougherty, RJ: TENS: An alternative to drugs in the treatment of acute and chronic pain. Presented at the 34th Annual Scientific Assembly, Am. Acad. of Family Physicians, San Francisco, CA, Oct 4, 1982.
48. Levy, A, et al: Transcutaneous electrical nerve stimulation in experimental acute arthritis. Arch Phys Med Rehab 68:75, 1987.
49. Kaada, B: Treatment of peritendinitis calcarea of the shoulder by transcutaneous nerve stimulation. Acupunct Electrother Res Int J 9:115, 1984.
50. Paris, DL, Baynes, F, and Gucker, B: Effects of the Neuroprobe in the treatment of second degree ankle inversion sprains. Phys Ther 63:35, 1983.
51. Erkola, R, Pikkola, P, and Kanto, J: Transcutaneous nerve stimulation for pain relief during labor: A controlled study. Ann Chire Gynaecol 69:273, 1980.
52. Augustinsson, LE, et al: Pain relief during delivery by transcutaneous electrical nerve stimulation. Pain 4:59, 1977.
53. Keenan, DL, Simonsen, L, and McCrann, DJ: Transcutaneous electrical nerve stimulation for pain control during labor and delivery. Phys Ther 5:1363, 1985.
54. Grim, LC and Morey, SH: Transcutaneous electrical nerve stimulation for relief of parturition pain. Phys Ther 65:337, 1985.
55. Bundsen, P, et al: Pain relief in labor by transcutaneous electrical nerve stimulation: Testing a modified stimulation technique and evaluation of the neurological and biochemical condition of the newborn infant. Acta Obstet Gynecol Scand 61:129, 1982.
56. Harrison, RF, et al: Pain relief in labor using transcutaneous electrical nerve stimulation: A TENS/TENS placebo controlled study in two parity groups. Br J Obstet Gynaecol 93:739, 1986.
57. Harrison, RF, et al: A comparative study of TENS, entonox, pethidine + promethazine and lumboar epidural block for pain relief in labor. Acta Obstet Gynecol Scand 66:9, 1987.
58. Tawfik, MO and Badraoui, MHH: The value of transcutaneous nerve stimulation during labor in Egyptian mothers. Pain (Suppl 1):S146, 1981.
59. Stewart, P: Transcutaneous electrical nerve stimulation as a method of analgesia in labor. Anesthesia 34:361, 1979.
60. Heywood, A, Frank, M, and McAteer, E: Efficacy and safety of TENS in labor (Abstract). Third European Congress of Obstetric Anesthesia and Analgesia. Dublin, Ireland, June 24, 1986.
61. Robson, JE: Transcutaneous nerve stimulation for pain relief in labor. Anesthesia 34:357, 1979.
62. Bundsen, P and Ericson, K: Pain relief in labor by transcutaneous electrical nerve stimulation: Safety aspects. Acta Obstet Gynecol Scand 61:1, 1982.
63. Riley, JE: The impact of TENS on the post-caesarean patient. J Obstet Gynecol Neonatal Nurs 11:325, 1982.
64. Polden, M: Transcutaneous nerve stimulation and post-caesarean section. Physiotherapy 71:350, 1985.
65. Fisher, AP and Hanna, M: Transcutaneous electrical nerve stimulation in meralgia paresthetica of pregnancy. Br J Obstet Gynaecol 94:603, 1987.
66. Dawood, MY and Ramos, J: Transcutaneous electrical nerve stimulation for treatment of primary dysmenorrhea: A randomized, cross-over comparison with placebo TENS and ibuprofen. Am College of Obstetricians and Gynecologists, Las Vegas, NV, April 27, 1987.
67. Lundeberg, T, Bondesson, L, and Lundstrom, V: Relief of primary dysmenorrhea by transcutaneous electrical nerve stimulation. Acta Obstet Gynecol Scand 64:491, 1985.
68. Neighbors, LE, et al: TENS for pain relief in primary dysmenorrhea. Clin J Pain 3:17, 1987.
69. Mannheimer, JS and Whalen, EC: The efficacy of TENS in dysmenorrhea. Clin J Pain 1:75, 1985.
70. Hansson, P and Ekblom, A: TENS as compared to placebo TENS for relief of acute oro-facial pain. Pain 15:157, 1983.
71. Murphy, GJ: Electrical physical therapy in treating temporomandibular joint patients. J of Craniomandibular Practice 1:67, 1983.

72. Ekblom, A and Hansson, P: Extrasegmental transcutaneous electrical nerve stimulation and mechanical vibratory stimulation as compared to placebo for the relief of acute oro-facial pain. Pain 23:223, 1985.

73. Nolan, MF: A chronological indexing of the clinical and basic science literature concerning transcutaneous electrical nerve stimulation (1967–1987). American Physical Therapy Association Section on Clinical Electrophysiology, Washington, DC, 1987.

74. Wolf, SL, Gersh, MR, and Rao, VR: Examination of electrode placement and stimulating parameters in treating chronic pain with conventional transcutaneous electrical nerve stimulation. Pain 11:37, 1981.

75. Melzack, R: The McGill Pain Questionnaire: Major properties and scoring methods. Pain 1:277, 1975.

76. Santiesteban, AJ: The role of physical agents in the treatment of spine pain. Clin Orthop 179:24, 1983.

77. Brill, MM and Whiffin, JR: Application of twenty-four hour burst TENS in a back school. Phys Ther 65:1355, 1985.

78. Melzack, R, Vetere, P, and Finch, L: Transcutaneous electrical nerve stimulation for low back pain: A comparison of TENS and massage for pain and range of motion. Phys Ther 63:489, 1983.

79. Lundeberg, T: The pain suppressive effect of vibratory stimulation and transcutaneous electrical nerve stimulation compared to aspirin. Brain Res 294:210, 1984.

80. Lehmann, TR, Russell, DW, and Spratt, KF: The impact of patients with non-organic physical findings on a controlled trial of TENS and electroacupuncture. Spine 8:625, 1983.

81. Fried, T, Johnson, R, and McCracken, W: Transcutaneous electrical nerve stimulation: Its role in the control of chronic pain. Arch Phys Med Rehabil 65:228, 1984.

82. Taylor, P, Hallett, M, and Flaherty, L: Treatment of osteoarthritis of the knee with transcutaneous electrical nerve stimulation. Pain 11:233, 1981.

83. Smith, CR, Lewith, GT, and Machin, D: Transcutaneous nerve stimulation and osteoarthritic pain. Physiotherapy 69:266, 1983.

84. Lewis, D, Lewis B, and Sturrock, RD: Transcutaneous electrical nerve stimulation in osteoarthritis: A therapeutic alternative. Ann Rheum Dis 43:47, 1984.

85. Mannheimer, C, Lund, S and Carlsson, CA: The effect of transcutaneous electrical nerve stimulation on joint pain in patients with rheumatoid arthritis. Scand J Rheumatol 7:13, 1978.

86. Mannheimer, C and Carlsson, CA: The analgesic effect of transcutaneous electrical nerve stimulation in patients with rheumatoid arthritis: A comparative study of different pulse patterns. Pain 6:329, 1979.

87. Meyerson, BA: Electrostimulation procedures, effects, presumed rationale and possible mechanisms. Adv Pain Res Ther 5:495, 1983.

88. Winnem, MF and Amundsen T: Treatment of phantom limb pain with transcutaneous electrical nerve stimulation. Pain 12:299, 1982.

89. Carabelli, RD and Kellerman, WC: Phantom limb pain: Relief by application of TENS to contralateral extremity. Arch Phys Med Rehabil 66:466, 1985.

90. Gersh, MR, Wolf, SL, and Rao, VR: Evaluation of transcutaneous electrical nerve stimulation for pain relief in peripheral neuropathy. Phys Ther 60:48, 1980.

91. McCarthy, JA and Zigenfus, RW: Transcutaneous electrical nerve stimulation: An adjunct in the pain management of Guillain-Barré syndrome. Phys Ther 58:23, 1978.

92. Bedenheim, R and Bennett, JH: Reversal of a Sudek's atrophy by the adjunctive use of transcutaneous electrical nerve stimulation. Phys Ther 63:1287, 1983.

93. Eriksson, MBE, Sjolund, BH, and Sundberg, G: Pain relief from peripheral conditioning stimulation in patients with chronic facial pain. J Neurosurg 61:149, 1984.

94. Fields, HL: Pain. McGraw Hill, New York, 1987, pp 316, 150, 309.

95. Tahmoush, AJ, Malley, J and Jennings, JR: Skin conductance, temperature, and blood flow in causalgia. Neurology 33:1483, 1983.

96. Kleinert, HE, Norberg, H, and McDonough, JJ: Surgical sympathectomy: Upper and lower extremity. In Omer, GE et al (eds): Management of Peripheral Nerve Problems. WB Saunders, Philadelphia, 1980, p 285.

97. Livingstone, WK: Pain Mechanisms. Macmillan, New York, 1943, p 91.

98. Wong, RA and Jette, DU: Changes in sympathetic tone associated with different forms of transcutaneous electrical nerve stimulation in healthy subjects. Phys Ther 64:478, 1984.

99. Owens, S, Atkinson, ER, and Lees, DE: Thermographic evidence of reduced sympathetic tone with transcutaneous nerve stimulation. Anesthesiology 50:62, 1979.

100. Headley, B: Historical perspective of causalgia: Management of sympathetically maintained pain. Phys Ther 67:1370, 1987.

101. Frampton, VM: Pain control with the aid of transcutaneous nerve stimulation. Physiotherapy 66:77, 1982.

102. Richlin, D, et al: Reflex sympathetic dystrophy: Successful treatment by transcutaneous nerve stimulation. J Pediatr 93:84, 1978.

103. Stilz, RJ, Carron, H, and Sanders, DB: Case history number 96: Reflex sympathetic dystrophy in a six year old. Successful treatment by transcutaneous nerve stimulation. Anesth Analg 56:438, 1977.

104. Leo, KC: Use of electrical stimulation at acupuncture points for the treatment of reflex sympathetic dystrophy in a child. Phys Ther 63:957, 1983.

105. Mannheimer, JS and Lampe, GN: Clinical Transcutaneous Electrical Nerve Stimulation, FA Davis, Philadelphia, 1984, pp 192, 210, 230, 234, 268, 273, 301, 406, 530, Chapters 4, 8, and 12.

106. Mannheimer, C, et al: The effects of transcutaneous electrical nerve stimulation in patients with severe angina pectoris. Circulation 71:308, 1985.
107. Solomon, S and Guglielmo, K: Treatment of headache by transcutaneous electrical stimulation. Headache 25:12, 1985.
108. Carley, PJ and Wainapel SF: Electrotherapy for acceleration of wound healing: Low intensity direct current. Arch Phys Med Rehabil 66:443, 1985.
109. Barron, JJ, Jacobson, WE, and Tidd, G: Treatment of decubitus ulcer: A new approach. Minn Med 68:103, 1985.
110. Becker, RO and Selden, G: The Body Electric. Morrow, New York, 1985.
111. Simons, DG: Special review: Muscle pain syndromes, Part II. Am J Phys Med 55:15, 1976.
112. Travell, J: Pain mechanisms in connective tissue. In Ragan, C (ed): Connective Tissues: Transactions of the Second Conference. Josiah Macy, Jr, Foundation, New York, 1952, p 86.
113. Mennell, JM: The therapeutic use of cold. JAOA 74:1146, 1975.
114. Zohn, DA and Mennell, JM: Musculoskeletal Pain. Little, Brown & Co, Boston, 1976, p 190.
115. Cyriax, J: Textbook of Orthopedic Medicine, Vol. 1, ed 6. Williams & Wilkins, Baltimore, 1975, p 32.
116. Gunn, CC and Milbrandt, WE: Utilizing trigger points. The Osteopathic Physician 44:29, 1977.
117. Gunn, CC and Milbrandt, WE: Review of 100 patients with "low back sprain" treated by surface electrode stimulation of acupuncture points. Am J of Acupunct 3:224, 1975.
118. Fox, EJ and Melzack, R: Transcutaneous electrical nerve stimulation and acupuncture: Comparison of treatment for low back pain. Pain 2:141, 1975.
119. Laitinen, J: Acupuncture and transcutaneous electrical nerve stimulation in the treatment of chronic sacrolumbalgia and ischalgia. Am J Chin Med 4:169, 1976.
120. Berlant, SR: Method of determining optimal stimulation sites for transcutaneous electrical nerve stimulation. Phys Ther 64:924, 1984.
121. Sjolund, BH: Peripheral nerve stimulation suppression of C-fiber evoked reflex in rats, Part I, Parameters of continuous stimulation. J Neurosurg 6:612, 1985.
122. Andersson, DA and Holmgren, E: Analgesic effects of peripheral conditioning stimulation III: Effect of high frequency stimulation; segmental mechanisms interacting with pain. Acupunct Electrother Res 3:23, 1978.
123. Strassburg, HM, Krainick, JV, and Thoden, V: Influence of transcutaneous nerve stimulation on acute pain. J Neurol 217:1, 1977.
124. Downie, W, et al: Studies with pain rating scales. Ann Rheum Dis 37:378, 1978.
125. Melzack, R and Torgeson, WS: On the language of pain. Anesthesiology 34:50, 1971.
126. Nolan, MF: Documenting patient care with transcutaneous electrical nerve stimulation: Suggestions for reducing reimbursement denials. Clinical Management in Physical Therapy 8:16, 1988.
127. Melzack, R: The short form McGill Pain Questionnaire. Pain 30:191, 1987.
128. Food and Drug Administration Guidelines for Electromedical Devices, 1975.
129. Eriksson, MA, Schuller, H, and Sjolund, BH: Letter: Hazard from transcutaneous nerve stimulation in patients with pacemakers. Lancet 1:1319, 1978.
130. Rasmussen, MJ, et al: Can TENS be safely used in patients with permanent cardiac pacemakers? Mayo Clin Proc 63:443, 1988.
131. Shade, SK: Use of transcutaneous electrical nerve stimulation for a patient with a cardiac pacemaker. Phys Ther 65:206, 1985.
132. Bolton, L: TENS electrode irritation. J Am Acad Dermatology 8:134, 1983.
133. Zugarman, C: Dermatitis from transcutaneous electrical nerve stimulation. J Am Acad Dermatol 6:936, 1982.
134. FDA Drug Bulletin, July–August, 1975.
135. Evans, FJ: The placebo response in pain reduction. Adv Neurol 4:289, 1974.
136. Thornsteinsson G, et al: The placebo effect of transcutaneous electrical stimulation. Pain 5:31, 1978.
137. Langley, GB, et al: The analgesic effects of transcutaneous electrical nerve stimulation and placebo in chronic pain patients. Rheumatol Int 4:119, 1984.
138. Levine, JD, et al: Role of pain in placebo analgesia. Proc Nat Acad Sci USA 76:3528, 1979.
139. Evans, FJ: Expectancy, therapeutic instructions, and the placebo response. In White, L, et al (eds) Placebo: Theory, Research, and Mechanisms. Guilford Press, New York, 1985.
140. Shapiro, AK: Factors contributing to the placebo effect. Am J Psychother 18:73, 1964.
141. Chen, ACN: Behavioral and brain evoked potentials evaluation of placebo effects: Contrast of cognitive mechanisms and endorphin mechanisms. Program Abstracts: Second General Meeting of the American Pain Society, 1980, p 12.
142. Levine, JD, Gordon, NC, and Fields, HL: Evidence that the analgesic effect of placebo is mediated by endorphins. Pain Abstracts, Vol 1, Second World Congress on Pain, International Association for the Study of Pain, Seattle, 1978, p 18.
143. Mihic, D and Binkert, E: Is placebo analgesia mediated by endorphin? Pain Abstracts, Vol 1, Second World Congress on Pain, International Association for the Study of Pain, Seattle, 1978, p 19.
144. Reynolds, AC, et al: Chronic pain therapy with transcutaneous electrical nerve stimulation: Predictive value of questionnaires. Arch Phys Med Rehabil 64:311, 1983.
145. Johansson, F, et al: Predictors for the outcome of treatment with high frequency transcutaneous electrical nerve stimulation in patients with chronic pain. Pain 9:55, 1980.

146. Richardson, RR, et al: Transcutaneous electrical neurostimulation in functional pain. Spine 6:185, 1981.
147. Nolan, MF: Selected problems in the use of transcutaneous electrical nerve stimulation for pain control. An appraisal with proposed solutions: A Special Communication. Phys Ther 68:1694, 1988.
148. Terminology for Electrophysiology and Electrotherapeutics, American Physical Therapy Association, Section on Clinical Electrophysiology, 1991.
149. Fordyce, W: Treating chronic pain by contingency management. Adv Neurol 4:583, 1974.

SUGGESTED READINGS

Echternach, JL (ed): Pain. In Clinics in Physical Therapy. Churchill Livingstone, New York, 1987.

Fields, HL: Pain. McGraw Hill, New York, 1987.

Mannheimer, J and Lampe, G: Clinical Transcutaneous Electrical Nerve Stimulation. FA Davis, Philadelphia, 1984.

Nolan, MF: A Chronological Indexing of the Clinical and Basic Science Literature Concerning TENS, 1967–1987. Published by the American Physical Therapy Association Section on Clinical Electrophysiology, 1987.

CHAPTER 6

Electrotherapeutic Alternatives for the Treatment of Pain

Luther C. Kloth, M.S., P.T.

Through the centuries, electricity from various natural sources has been applied to the body for treatment of numerous symptoms and afflictions. The ability to generate and control electricity led to the development of numerous electrical devices that delivered current in various forms to the body. Published during the early 19th century were a multitude of anecdotal case reports that described beneficial treatment outcomes or cures by transcutaneously applied electricity of painful maladies.[1,2]

One of the first battery-powered devices with surface electrodes marketed for pain control appeared in 1919. This device, called the Electreat, provided fixed-pulse frequency and duration with a variable amplitude adjustment.[3] In 1950, Bernard[4] of France and Nemec[5] of Austria published reports on diadynamic and interference currents, respectively. Both of these currents are applied transcutaneously and have been used by physical therapists around the world since the 1950s for treatment of acute and chronic pain. Another type of current also applied noninvasively, and in widespread use for management of pain, has been available in the United States since the late 1950s. This current, driven into the tissue under high voltage, delivers a paired monophasic, pulsed waveform. The first devices of this type appeared in the marketplace around the time that Melzack and Wall published their gate control theory of pain modulation in 1965.[6] Shortly thereafter, Shealy, Mortimer, and Reswick[7] began surgical implantation of electrodes directly on the dorsal columns of the spinal cord in an attempt to modulate noxious-impulse transmission in patients with chronic intractable pain. In the early 1970s when Long[8,9] and Shealy[10,11] used transcutaneous electrical nerve stimulation (TENS) to determine which patients would respond most favorably to dorsal column stimulation, they found that, in many patients, TENS was almost as effective in decreasing pain perception as direct dorsal column stimulation. Subsequent to this finding, a number of private medical electronic companies and various research granting agencies provided financial support to study electrical stimulation with surface electrode delivery systems for the treatment of individuals with acute and chronic pain. These studies paved the way for development and incorporation of electronic components into miniaturized, portable TENS devices and the rediscovery by physicians that electrical stimulation applied transcutaneously was a viable alternative to analgesic medication for pain amelioration.

The latter half of the 19th century became known as the "golden age of medical electricity," and, during that period, many physicians in the United States used electrotherapy in their practices.[12] However, during much of the 20th century, the medical use of electricity fell into disrepute with most physicians because of clinical advances in biochemistry and pharmacology. During this lull in the use of therapeutic electricity by physicians, physical therapists continued to use diadynamic, interference, and high voltage pulsed currents applied transcutaneously for inducing electroanalgesia.

Other types of current such as sinusoidal alternating current (AC) in various modulated and nonmodulated forms, monophasic and biphasic pulsed waveforms, and continuous and interrupted direct current applied through a probe electrode to acupuncture points have also been used for pain control. Most of the electrical current types and stimulation delivery systems used for management of pain have utilized noninvasive techniques. The acronym TENS as used in this chapter pertains to the *generic* use of all electrical stimulus waveforms delivered transcutaneously to produce electroanalgesia. With this information in mind the purposes of this chapter are to:

1. Discuss biophysical and electrophysiologic principles related to the use of alternative currents (e.g., nontraditional currents) in treating pain, including interference current, currents for the transcutaneous stimulation of acupuncture points, impulse current, diadynamic current, alternating current, and high voltage pulsed current.
2. Discuss the alternative stimulus variables with respect to efficacy of producing electroanalgesia.
3. Present clinical decision-making paradigms that illustrate the importance of current and device selection, stimulus variables, electrode placement, and treatment schedule.
4. Identify precautions and contraindications to be considered before any kind of TENS device is administered for treating pain.

BIOPHYSICAL AND ELECTROPHYSIOLOGIC PRINCIPLES

Low and High Voltage Devices

All of the electrotherapeutic devices used to modulate pain by noninvasive methods may be classified as either low or high voltage TENS devices. Most commercially available electrical stimulators are low voltage devices capable of generating pulses of relatively longer duration (250 μs [1.0 μs = 10^{-6} s] to 1 s or longer) and therefore, require lower voltages (up to 150 V) to drive total current of up to 80 mA (1.0 mA = 10^{-3} A) into the tissue.[13-15] In contrast, high voltage devices generate pulses of much shorter duration (5 to 100 μs) which require voltages in excess of 150 volts, but not more than 500 volts to drive total current, up to approximately 2.0 mA, into the tissue.[13-15]

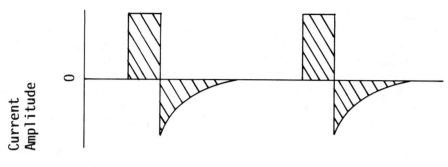

Time

FIGURE 6–1. Pulse charge (charge per pulse) is the sum of charges of the component phases. Each pulse consists of two phases represented by the shaded areas. Phase charge (charge per phase) is the charge within each phase (integrated sum of current amplitude × time; area under the curve measured in microcoulombs). (From Snyder-Mackler, L and Robinson, A: Clinical Electrophysiology: Electrotherapy and Electrophysiologic Testing, p 13. © 1989, the Williams & Wilkins Co., Baltimore.)

With the exception of microamperage stimulators, which deliver less than 1.0 mA of current, low voltage TENS devices deliver a greater quantity of electricity (charge) to the tissue with each pulse than high voltage TENS devices. For example, the charge delivered to tissues within a few minutes by continuous or interrupted direct current from a low voltage device may approach 10,000 μC (1.0 μC = 10^{-6} C) which is equivalent to 10 mA of total current.[15] In contrast, high voltage devices may deliver only 12 to 15 μC at a total current of 2 mA during the same period of time.

The amount of charge delivered to the tissues by each pulse from any TENS device is represented by the area under the curve of the pulse waveform.[13] (Fig. 6–1) This quantity is very important because it influences the type of nerve fiber that will be excited and the type of response that will be produced, that is, non-noxious-sensory, motor, or noxious-sensory response. It is important to know that the quantities of total and net charge in microcoulombs delivered to the tissue by monophasic pulses are equal and always greater than zero.[13,15] The net charge delivered to the tissue from unbalanced *asymmetrical* biphasic pulses is also greater than zero. Only biphasic *symmetrical* and balanced asymmetrical biphasic pulses deliver a net charge of zero to the tissue because ionic flow produced by a phase charge in one direction equals ionic flow produced by the other phase charge in the opposite direction. This concept is discussed in detail in Chapter 3.

When the quantity of residual positive or negative charge builds up in the tissue, there is increased likelihood of producing undesirable electrochemical irritation of the skin. These deleterious changes may be manifested by erythema and blistering or burning of the skin. Tissue changes such as these are most apt to occur with currents that contaminate the tissue with excess residual charge, characteristic of long-duration monophasic pulses, unbalanced asymmetric biphasic pulses, and continuous direct current (see Chapter 3). Accumulation of negative charges in the tissue raises the pH, causing an increase in alkaline concentration, while residual positive charges lower the pH, causing an increase in acid concentration. These undesirable polar effects from alkaline and acid pH changes are most likely to occur with direct current at the cathode (−) and anode (+), respectively. Thus, the presence of skin irritation may indicate a DC-component residual charge in the tissues. Pulses with zero net charge or minimal net DC component such as symmetrical AC, biphasic symmetrical, and balanced biphasic asymmetrical waveforms do not cause significant skin irritation. Additionally, monophasic pulsed current from high voltage devices does not permit accumulation of deleterious residual charge because of its very brief pulse duration and low pulse charge.

Total (average) current is the absolute quantity of current delivered to the tissue per second[14] and is dependent on the variables of pulse amplitude, pulse rate (frequency), and pulse and phase duration. Increasing one or more of these variables will increase the charge that excites different peripheral nerve fibers. Small diameter A-delta and C fibers require more charge for depolarization while large diameter A-alpha and beta fibers need less charge.[16-18] The implication is that by selecting the appropriate combination of stimulus variables (amplitude and duration), the amount of charge delivered will be sufficient to excite either large diameter axons that mediate afferent non-noxious input related to touch, proprioception, and kinesthesia, or primarily small diameter axons that convey nociceptive information.[19] Alon[15] advocates that maximum phase charge should reach between 20 and 40 μC to assure perceptually discriminatory excitation of non-noxious sensory, motor, and pain fibers. [The United States Food and Drug Administration recommends that the pulse charge of any device sold as a TENS stimulator for treatment of pain not exceed 25 μC if the electrodes are applied transthoracically.[20]] Most traditional TENS devices allow the user to vary the amount of charge by adjustment of all stimulus variables, but most of the alternative forms of TENS (high voltage pulsed current, interference current, diadynamic current, alternating current, and currents used to stimulate acupuncture points) allow adjustment of only amplitude and frequency. This correctly implies that alternative current forms deliver pulses with fixed durations. In general, the individual pulse durations available from these devices range between 50 μs and 10 ms. Alon[15] has indicated that a short duration (less than 100 μs) monophasic or biphasic waveform, applied transcutaneously with a progressive increase in amplitude, increases one's ability to sequentially discriminate between non-noxious, motor, and noxious stimulation. However, eliciting these responses in this sequence assumes that the three nerve-fiber types associated with these responses are all located about the same distance from the stimulating electrode. Obviously, this assumption is invalid because the explanation for the sequential recruitment of nerve fibers found at various tissue depths depends on the quantity of charge delivered in a waveform that is primarily dependent on the combination of phase/pulse amplitude and duration. A short phase/pulse duration of 100 μs or less with sufficient amplitude will preferentially excite non-noxious sensory fibers before exciting motor and nociceptor fibers. However, all three fiber types in a mixed peripheral nerve are usually excited simultaneously with phase/pulse durations of 300 μs or longer.

Many traditional TENS devices allow the phase/pulse amplitude, duration, and sometimes the rate/frequency to be varied over time (modulated). Although the intent of these modulations is to reduce nerve fiber accommodation, present clinical reports fail to support this assumption,[21,22] and enhanced clinical efficacy has not been demonstrated.

As mentioned earlier, the quantity of charge delivered to the tissue influences the type of nerve fiber that will be excited and the response (sensory, motor, or pain) that will be elicited. The quantity of charge (μC) that reaches the nerve fiber from transcutaneous stimulation cannot be known; however, it is influenced by factors such as electrode size and number, distance between electrodes, distance from electrodes to nerve fibers, electrode and tissue impedance, and electrode placement site.[23] Less charge is required when smaller and/or fewer electrodes are used, when the interelectrode distance is small, and when electrodes are placed over areas of low impedance, often corresponding to areas with high density innervation, such as over acupuncture points, motor points, and superficial nerves.[24-26]

During the past two decades reports of clinical studies have appeared in the literature in which various electrical stimulation devices were used to study the efficacy of TENS in relieving pain, strengthening muscle,[27-29] or improving blood flow.[30,31] Unfortunately most of the supportive studies dealing with noninvasive electroanalgesia have used traditional TENS devices, which leads the uninformed reader to believe that data provided from these studies support only the use of traditional TENS equipment for efficacious pain suppression. On the contrary, if the stimulus variables reported in these traditional TENS studies can be reproduced by any other low or high voltage electrical stimulation device (e.g., interference current or high voltage pulsed current devices), these alternative devices can similarly deliver the adequate stimulus necessary to achieve electroanalgesia. It is notable that Alon, Allin, and Inbar[17] reported producing adequate stimulation with a prototype stimulator capable of providing phase and pulse variables in both low and high voltage ranges. They concluded that the physiologic responses remain similar as stimulus variables arbitrarily change from low to high voltage at 150 V.

Modes of Stimulation

Before identifying and describing stimulus characteristics of alternative low and high voltage electrical stimulators used clinically for electroanalgesia, it is necessary to review the stimulus variables associated with electroanalgesia delivered by traditional TENS devices. Subsequently, stimulus variables available from alternative devices are reviewed and may be compared with the traditional TENS currents. As clinical decision-making models related to electroanalgesia are presented later in this chapter, the reader will appreciate why different electrical stimulation devices can be interchanged for treating various pain syndromes.

For a TENS treatment to most efficaciously ameliorate pain, it is essential that electrical impulses with sufficient amplitude, duration, and frequency be applied to the target tissues so that electrical, (tingling) paresthesia and rhythmical muscle-contraction responses are produced simultaneously or independently.[26] Assuming the stimulus has sufficient amplitude and duration, both responses are produced when the pulse frequency exceeds 20 pps (pulses per second) for pulsed current or 20 Hz for alternating current.

Mannheimer[23,24] and Mannheimer and Lampe[25] have described four stimulation modes for producing electroanalgesia with traditional TENS devices: the conventional mode used most often to treat acute, superficial pain associated with inflammation; the acupuncturelike stimulation mode, for chronic inflammatory or neurogenic pain; the burst mode which may be considered a frequency-modulated conventional or acupuncturelike TENS mode; and the brief, intense mode, a high-amplitude, somewhat uncomfortable level of stimulation used when brief periods of analgesia are required to permit otherwise painful treatments to be done. The stimulation settings and clinical applications of each of these modes are presented in detail in Chapter 5 and serve as a basis for comparison of the alternative electrical currents described in this chapter.

LOW VOLTAGE CURRENT ALTERNATIVES TO TRADITIONAL TENS

Interference Current

When sine waves of constant amplitude but slightly different frequencies from two independent low voltage AC circuits are superimposed on the same time axis (Fig. 6–2), a higher amplitude wave is produced secondary to summation of current (millamperage) values at specific points in time (A and C) when the sine waves from each circuit are exactly in phase. At another point on the same time axis (B), an upward phase of circuit 1 cancels a downward phase of circuit 2 resulting in a summated-wave amplitude of zero. This summation and cancellation of current values produces the amplitude-modulated beats that are characteristic of interference current (IFC)[32,33] and may be thought of as bursts. The term *beat* is not a commercial name. Rather it is a physical phenomenon in which amplitude modulation occurs by summation of two intersecting sine waves that are either exactly in phase or are one, two, three, or more wavelength(s) out of phase with the other wave. The source of the converging sine waves may be from

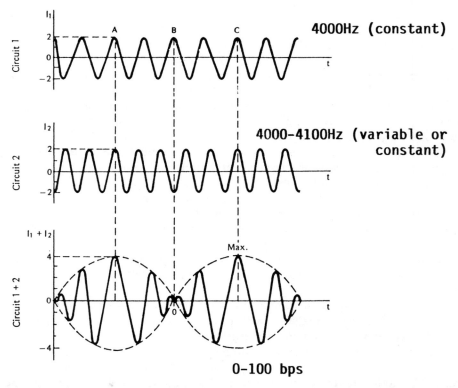

FIGURE 6–2. Amplitude-modulated beats of IFC produced by summation and cancellation of superimposed phases from two independent AC circuits. A difference of 100 Hz between the two circuits gives a beat frequency of 100 bps. (Adapted from Kloth, L: Interference Current. In Nelson, R and Currier, D (eds): Clinical Electrotherapy. Appleton & Lange, Norwalk, CT, 1987, p 186.)

light, electricity, or sound. For example, the piano tuner listens to beats between sounds of two vibrating objects (i.e., a piano string and a tuning fork) to establish agreement of frequency.[34]

The beat frequency is equal to the number of times each second the current amplitude increases to its maximum value and then decreases to its minimum value, or simply the difference between the frequencies in circuits 1 and 2. In Figure 6-2, a constant-beat frequency of 100 bps (beats per second) would accurately represent a difference of 100 Hz between carrier frequencies of 4000 Hz in circuit 1 and 4100 Hz in circuit 2. However, any beat frequency within the range of 0 to 100 bps may be produced by selecting a frequency in circuit 2 that lies within the range of 4000 to 4100 Hz. Conversely, if one wishes to modulate the number of beats per second, this may be accomplished by allowing the frequency in circuit 2 to cyclically vary through all or part of the range of 4000 to 4100 Hz. For example, varying the frequency in circuit 2 between 4090 to 4100 to 4090 Hz would actually deliver a modulated beat frequency which varies between 90 to 100 to 90 bps. Various programmed beat-frequency amplitude modulations can be selected on most IFC devices. Thus, like most traditional TENS devices, which allow modulation of pulse rate, amplitude, and/or pulse duration to decrease neural accommodation, most IFC devices also allow modulation of these variables. For example, with an IFC device generating a carrier frequency of 4000 Hz, the duration of each cycle within a beat remains constant if the beat frequency remains constant. However, if the beat frequency is varied over time, the cycle duration within the beats will also vary. It can be seen in Table 6-1 that for a constant beat frequency of 100 bps, each beat will have a duration of 10 ms and will contain 40 cycles or pulses, each of which has a duration of 250 μs. If, however, the beat frequency is varied from 100 to 10 bps then the beat duration, as well as the number of cycles per beat and the duration of the cycles within each beat, will also vary. In this case the individual cycle duration will change from 250 to 25 μs. Thus, it is the individual cycles of alternating current that may be amplitude, frequency, or duration modulated in IFC. Beat amplitude and frequency modulations were described earlier and beat-duration modulation as shown in Table 6-1 is inversely related to beat frequency.

It may also be observed from Table 6-1 that beat durations are considerably longer than the pulse-duration ranges discussed earlier for traditional TENS devices. At a 4 kHz carrier frequency each of the 100 bps lasts 10 ms and represents a single multiphasic, amplitude-modulated burst (beat) containing 40 cycles, each with a duration of 250

TABLE 6-1 Beat and Cycle Durations as a Function of Beat Frequency Assuming a Carrier Frequency of 4 kHz

Beat Frequency (bps)	Beat Duration (ms)	Cycles per Beat (Hz)	Cycle Duration (μs)
100	10.0	40	250.0
80	12.5	50	200.0
50	20.0	80	125.0
25	40.0	160	62.5
10	100.0	400	25.0
5	200.0	800	12.5
2	500.0	2000	5.0
1	1000.0	4000	2.5

μs (Fig. 6–2). Each beat produces neuroexcitatory responses similar to single monophasic and biphasic pulses of traditional TENS devices. The major difference between IFC beats and traditional TENS pulses is that the former are capable of delivering much higher maximum total current to the tissues (70 to 100 mA) compared to traditional TENS devices (10 to 50 mA). This means that the total charge delivered to the tissue by an IFC beat will usually be greater than the charge delivered by a single pulse from a traditional TENS device. Thus, with amplitude set at the highest comfortably tolerated level and a beat frequency of 1 to 5 bps when IFC is delivered through small electrodes, sufficient charge is provided to satisfy the electroanalgesia requirements of rhythmic muscle contractions characteristic of the acupuncturelike mode of traditional TENS. Recall that this stimulus choice for pain relief calls for stimulating proprioceptive and kinesthetic receptors by eliciting rhythmic contractions from large, deep muscles without producing a tingling electrical paresthesia. IFC applied according to this paradigm would be most applicable for treatment of deep, aching, chronic pain.

If a beat frequency of 2 bps is selected, each beat would contain 2000 cycles (Table 6–1), and if the IFC stimulus amplitude is adjusted to produce a comfortable tingling electrical paresthesia (associated with the 2000 cycles per beat) without a muscle contraction, then primarily A-alpha and beta afferent fibers are recruited. This paradigm corresponds with the low amplitude TENS burst mode which is really a modulated form of the conventional TENS mode in which the sensation perceived is electrical paresthesia with a rhythmic sensory pulsing at 2 bps. Thus, IFC applied in this manner would be appropriate for treating acute, superficial, or chronic, deep, aching pain. By increasing the IFC stimulus amplitude to a level that produces strong, comfortable muscle contractions at a rate of 2 bps, plus a strong degree of electrical paresthesia, a paradigm corresponding to the high amplitude burst mode is produced which combines characteristics of both conventional and acupuncturelike TENS. This combination of stimulus characteristics produces sufficient charge to effectively treat pain syndromes of a chronic, deep, aching nature.

Some advocates of IFC for the treatment of musculoskeletal pain that originates in deep tissues explain erroneously that IFC preferentially penetrates more deeply than other forms of TENS, based on the rationale that skin impedance decreases in response to higher frequencies of alternating current. While it is true that skin impedance declines and conduction of current improves with increasing AC frequency, the decline in skin impedance results from the decreased pulse charge generated at higher frequencies of AC, and *not* from an increase in frequency alone. In this regard IFC is not unique in its ability to penetrate the tissues, since tissue impedance can be reduced by any TENS device that allows selection of very-short-duration pulses or phases (less than 100 μs).[15]

Finally, IFC may be applied in such a manner that beat characteristics produce stimulus responses that correspond to those elicited by brief, intense TENS. Setting the beat frequency between 100 and 120 bps produces beat durations between 10 and 8 ms, respectively. By setting the amplitude to the maximum tolerable output, a strong continuous tingling paresthesia combined with mild to moderate muscle fasciculations or tetany will be produced. By simultaneously exciting motor and sensory nerve fibers, analgesia may be induced within 15 minutes. However, one should be cautioned that muscle ischemia may occur if tetanic contractions are maintained for that period of time. As suggested earlier, the rapid onset of analgesia induced by this combination of stimulus variables may be used to permit surgical debridement, painful mobilization/passive elongation, or other uncomfortable procedures to be performed. An additional benefit of IFC is its derivation from biphasic symmetrical sine waves which do not contaminate the tissues with undesirable residual charge; therefore, skin irritation from electrochemical reactions is negligible.

Although theories have been developed to explain how IFC modulates pain,[35] unfortunately, there is a paucity of clinical studies to confirm the efficacy of IFC for suppressing pain. Burghart[36] observed relief of pain associated with osteoarthritis in 39 patients without accelerated cell-sedimentation rate, who had not benefited from other therapies. In her book, *Treatment with Interferential Current*, Nicolova-Troeva[37] described various clinical applications of IFC, usually in combination with other therapies but without control or placebo treated groups. Her most convincing reports on pain relief describe the use of IFC at 100 bps for inducing sympathetic ganglion block in treating pain and symptoms associated with thromboangitis obliterans and Raynaud's disease. However, the validity of her study specifically related to IFC results is questionable, because patients with both diagnoses received preliminary treatments with vasodilating drugs, novacaine block, or hydrotherapy.

The placebo effect of IFC has been studied under controlled clinical conditions in patients with symptoms of recurrent jaw pain. Taylor and associates[38] assigned 20 patients with recurrent jaw pain and reduced jaw opening to one of two groups: an IFC treatment group and an IFC placebo group. Subjects in the treatment group received three 20-minute treatments to the involved temporomandibular joint (TMJ) and masticatory muscles with predetermined IFC stimulation characteristics. The placebo group received the exact IFC procedure as the treatment group except subjects were told that they would receive a subthreshold current sensation. Although jaw pain for both the treatment and placebo groups decreased over the three treatment sessions, the differences between the two groups were not statistically significant. Also, no statistically significant increase in jaw opening occurred between the two groups of subjects over the three treatment sessions. Thus, a short-term treatment period with IFC had no greater therapeutic effectiveness on jaw pain or range of motion than a placebo procedure. Additional clinical studies are needed to determine whether other treatment protocols using various combinations of IFC stimulation frequency, intensity, and duration may be more effective for treatment of pain syndromes.

Transcutaneous Electrical Stimulation of Acupuncture Points

When pulsed or direct currents from low voltage devices, including traditional TENS, are applied transcutaneously to acupuncture, trigger, or motor points through a small-diameter (less than 5 mm) metal probe electrode, the current density and the transcutaneous resistance are very high. Terms such as hyperstimulation, acupoint stimulation, and auriculotherapy (which pertains to stimulation of acupuncture points on the ear) only imply that a special electrode delivery system is used and do not describe the stimulus variables. Generally this type of surface stimulation with its high-current density and transcutaneous resistance causes a noxious sensation, as well as a local sensory paresthesia provided that the amplitude is advanced to the upper-tolerance level of the patient. Commercial devices such as Neuroprobe* offer stimulus variables that, when applied to body or auricular acupuncture points through a metal probe electrode, produce sensations similar to those just described, which may be accompanied by rhythmic muscle contractions, depending on the proximity of the probe

---

*Physiotechnology, Inc., 1925 West 6th Street, Topeka, KS 66606.

electrode to a motor point. There is some evidence that noxious but tolerable stimulation combined with pulsing muscle contractions may be critical factors associated with beta-endorphin-mediated pain suppression.[39-41] This stimulation approach to electroanalgesia corresponds to the acupuncturelike mode of traditional TENS and is best suited for aching, deep, pain of a chronic nature. Empirically derived clinical protocols for this approach often recommend the application of direct or pulsed current through the probe electrode to acupuncture or trigger points for 15 to 90 seconds. Pulsed or burst currents may be applied at fixed rates ranging from 1 to 99 pps or between 0.1 and 10,000 bps.[42] Generally, pulse and burst rates between 1 and 5 pulses or bps are selected because these correspond to the manual rate of twirling inserted acupuncture needles.

Numerous experimental and clinical studies are reported in the literature related to the use of traditional TENS and acupuncture point stimulation devices to stimulate body and auricular acupuncture points for elevation of pain threshold. In two controlled experimental studies on healthy subjects, electrical stimulation of auricular points significantly increased the threshold of cutaneous pain produced by noxious electrical stimulation of the skin of the ipsilateral wrist.[43,44] In other experimental studies in which the analgesic effects of needle and surface stimulation of acupuncture points was compared, outcomes were similar, with surface stimulation being more effective in some cases and needle stimulation more effective in others.[45,46] Clinically, analgesia induced by these methods has been shown to produce pain relief lasting for several hours and sometimes for days.[47,48] Eriksson and Sjolund[49] compared analgesia produced by traditional and acupuncturelike TENS in 30 patients with trigeminal neuralgia; 22 of the 30 patients had previous surgical procedures that provided good but temporary pain relief. Traditional TENS was successful in only four of the 22, and acupuncturelike TENS was successful in eight other patients. Other clinical studies have reported positive treatment outcomes following surface electrical stimulation of body and auricular acupuncture points in combination.[50,51] Paris, Baynes, and Gucker[50] found that combined stimulation of auricular and ankle acupuncture points in patients with second degree ankle sprains, significantly improved ankle range of motion and reduced rehabilitation time compared with patients who received conventional physical therapy consisting of cryotherapy, compression wrapping, and elevation of the ankle. However, no significant difference in reduction of pain or edema was found among groups. In a single case study, Leo[51] stimulated bilateral auricular and upper extremity acupuncture points in a child with severe hyperesthesia, foot edema, and pain due to reflex sympathetic dystrophy of the left-lower extremity. Following two treatments, the patient was reported to be completely asymptomatic and able to perform all activities of daily living with full range of motion and strength without pain. The analgesic efficacy of auricular-point stimulation is based primarily on anecdotal reports.

Some acupuncture point stimulation devices also provide subliminal (microcurrent) stimulation which may be applied through probe or pad electrodes. To date there is no clinical documentation published in peer reviewed journals that supports the concept or practice of using subliminal electrical stimulation to relieve pain.

Impulse Currents

Several IFC devices have the capability to produce monophasic, amplitude-modulated direct current (impulse current) as shown in Figure 6–3. This current is delivered to the patient through two electrodes, one positive and the other negative. As with IFC,

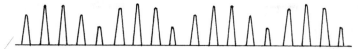

FIGURE 6–3. Amplitude-modulated impulse current is pulsed direct current that may produce charge accumulation in the tissues sufficient to cause undesirable electrochemical changes.

impulse current is applied to the skin at frequencies between 4 and 5 kHz and then modulated to select rhythmical frequencies similar to rhythmical IFC modes.[33] The accumulated charge delivered to the tissue through the anode and cathode is capable of producing a total current that may cause undesirable electrochemical irritation of the skin and, therefore, must be modulated at 100 pps and delivered at a comfortable sensory level to induce safe, temporary analgesia similar in effect to that produced by conventional mode TENS.

Diadynamic Currents

Diadynamic currents (from the Greek, dia = through and dynamis = force) were first described and used in clinical practice in 1950 by Bernard, a French dental surgeon.[4] These currents are delivered transcutaneously through anode and cathode as monophasic, half-wave, or full-wave pulses rectified from 50 Hz AC. Individual pulses have a duration of 10 ms. When successive pulses are combined with sufficient millamperage the effects produced correspond to those of galvanic current. As with impulse current, diadynamic current holds the potential for accumulation of an undesirable quantity of residual charge in the tissues, which may produce skin irritation. Devices that produce diadynamic currents allow selection of four current forms as shown in Figure 6–4. Each of the different pulse variations is assigned a French name coined by Bernard,[4] which, when translated, describes the repetition of pulses over different time periods.[52,53] The first variation of diadynamic current called diphase fixe (DF) is the preferred current for pain modulation.[52] DF produces a vibrating, prickling sensation which subsides gradually as sensory accommodation occurs in response to the constant amplitude stimulation. It is especially recommended for pain conditions of sympathetic origin.[52] Monophase fixe (MF) produces a strong vibratory sensation and much slower sensory accommodation occurs because of the 10-ms delay between successive pulses. It is more suitably used to elicit muscular contraction and is generally not used for isolated pain conditions.[53] Courtes periods (CP) combines MF and DF currents so that each one alternates at intervals of 1 s to prevent sensory accommodation. CP produces a fine tingling sensation during each DF period followed by a strong vibratory sensation during each MF period. Use of CP usually follows the DF mode previously described and is recommended for treatment of pain states associated with sprains, strains, contusions, sciatica, and radiculopathy.[53] Longues periods (LP) also combines the MF and DF current modes such that during 5-s periods MF and DF occur together but out of phase, with DF being amplitude modulated. This is followed by 10 s of MF current. LP produces a nonaccommodating stimulus, which produces a sensation similar to that produced by CP, although the alternation from fine-to-strong tingling paresthesia is less abrupt.[52] Following initial treatment with DF, this form of current is recommended for providing longer-lasting pain relief in acute-pain conditions.[53]

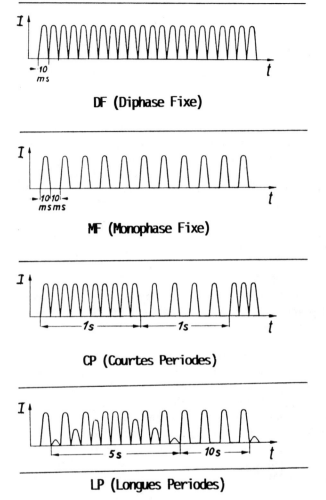

DF (Diphase Fixe)

MF (Monophase Fixe)

CP (Courtes Periodes)

LP (Longues Periodes)

FIGURE 6–4. Diadynamic currents are rectified from sine wave AC.

DF 50-Hz, full-wave rectified AC. Usually preceeds application of MF, CP or LP currents for analgesia.

MF 50-Hz, half-wave rectified AC. Generally used for muscle-stimulation application.

CP For analgesia. Current types DF and MF alternate repeatedly every second during the treatment period.

LP For analgesia. Current types DF and MF are phase shifted for 5 seconds, during which time DF is amplitude modulated. MF current then follows for 10 seconds. This alternation repeats during the treatment period.

(From Petersmann,[53] p 15, with permission.)

It is noteworthy that impulse and diadynamic currents are generally perceived as very harsh forms of electrical stimulation by most individuals. Undoubtedly, the harshness of these currents is produced by the accumulation of excessive charge in the tissues secondary to application of thousands of successive long-duration pulses. Lack of sufficient charge dissipation during and following application of these currents results in undesirable electrochemical changes similar to those produced by continuous direct current.

Alternating Currents

Griffin and Karselis[54] reported that the use of electrical stimulation for treating patients with chronic pain has been taught as part of physical therapy curricular since the 1930s. A review of the literature reveals only one report in which AC (sine waves) was used in the management of patients with acute pain. Ganne[55] reports using uninterrupted sinusoidal current to treat 100 patients with pain and other symptoms caused by trauma. Although she did not describe the stimulus frequency or amplitude, she did report that in most cases only one to four treatments, averaging 2- to 4-minutes duration, were required to produce anesthetic paresthesia followed by pain relief. Out of 100 patients, 27 were completely symptom free, 49 reported that they had experienced between 50 and 90 percent pain relief, and 24 had no pain relief at all or only a few hours of relief. There was no control or placebo group with whom to compare treatment outcomes. Additional controlled clinical studies are needed to substantiate the use of alternating current as a viable approach to pain treatment.

During the past 5 years, neuromuscular electrical stimulation devices that utilize AC at a carrier frequency ranging between 2500 and 10,000 Hz have become available in the marketplace. At 2500 Hz, the individual pulse durations are 400 μs. These devices deliver lower total current by modulating the carrier frequency into 50 bursts per second with each burst and each interburst interval having a duration of 10 ms (Fig. 6–5). Devices of this type are capable of producing anesthesia to pinpricks of the skin between electrodes separated by 4 to 5 cm in pain-free individuals. However, this level of analgesia only occurs concurrently with electrically elicited, very vigorous isometric muscle contractions. It appears that the short-term analgesia may be induced by nerve blocking and/or by spinal gating mechanisms. No clinical studies have specifically evaluated these devices for efficacy in producing pain relief.

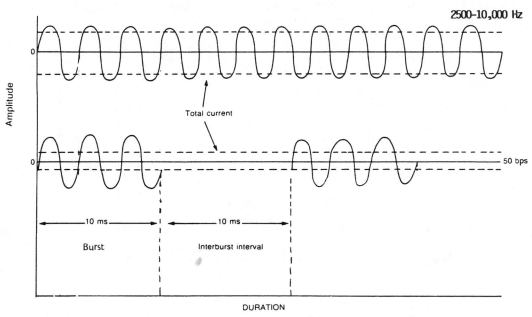

FIGURE 6–5. Alternating currents at carrier frequencies that may range between 2500 and 10,000 Hz that are modulated into bursts, produce analgesia concurrently with production of vigorous isometric muscle contractions. Total (average) current is the absolute quantity of current delivered to the tissue per second and is dependent on pulse amplitude, frequency, and pulse and phase duration. (From Alon,[56] p 52, with permission.)

HIGH VOLTAGE PULSED CURRENT (HVPC)

Alon[56,57] has clearly indicated that HVPC stimulation should be considered monophasic pulsed TENS. High voltage devices deliver impulses with very short phase durations ranging from 5 to 65 μs at a very high peak-current amplitude (2000 to 2500 mA). With such short phase durations, a high-driving voltage (up to 500 V) is required to produce adequate peak-pulse charge for eliciting physiologic effects. This relationship between stimulus duration and amplitude demonstrates the classic strength-duration relationship. Because the interval between paired pulses generated by HVPC devices make up as much as 99 percent of each second that the current flows (Fig. 6–6), the total current (average) delivered to the tissue per second does not exceed 1.2 to 1.5 mA.[15] This is the quantity of total current delivered only if the amplitude is set at 500 V which is not realistic in terms of patient tolerance. At a more clinically realistic amplitude such as 100 V, the paired pulse charge may be only 3.0 to 3.5 μC, and if the pulse rate is set at 100 pps, the total pulse charge accumulation would not exceed 350 μC/s. Apparently this very small current charge at microamperage amplitude, delivered to the tissue over time (i.e., 20 to 45 minutes), is rapidly dissipated and does not remain in the tissue as residual charge after the current is turned off. Indeed, Newton and Karselis[58] were unable to demonstrate alteration of human skin pH and subsequent irritation following 30 minutes of stimulation with this current. Thus, when pulse rate and amplitude variables for HVPC and traditional TENS stimulation are compared, charge from HVPC will often be lower than for traditional TENS because of the very short pulse duration inherent in the HVPC waveform. When HVPC is used for electroanalgesia and applied through pad electrodes for 20 to 30 minutes, it will likely be most effective for relieving acute, superficial pain as is conventional mode TENS. In some

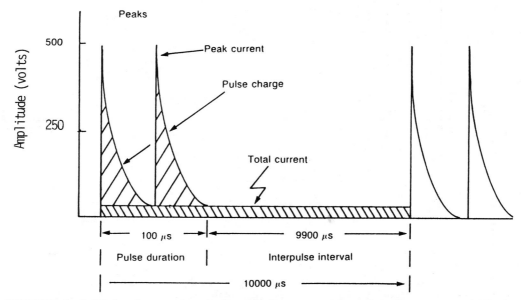

FIGURE 6–6. High voltage, monophasic, pulsed current produces low-charge accumulation in the tissues at clinically tolerated voltages and, therefore, is well tolerated by most individuals. (From Alon,[56] p 53, with permission.)

cases, however, this current may also suppress chronic, deep, aching pain, if delivered at 80 to 120 pps with the amplitude adjusted to produce a comfortable tingling electrical paresthesia without muscle contraction. This is because the inherent (fixed) short phase duration (5 to 65 μs) combined with the other variables make this form of stimulation consistent with the conventional TENS modes.

In as much as HVPC devices deliver pulses with fixed, short durations when applied through pad electrodes at a comfortable level of stimulation, these pulses are not likely to be as effective as longer duration pulses from other TENS devices in suppressing pain by excitation of A-delta and C fibers. These nerve fibers not only require longer pulse durations but also higher amplitude for excitation. However, noxious stimulation of A-delta and/or C fibers may be achieved by applying HVPC to trigger and/or acupuncture points. By delivering 1 to 5 pps[39,59] or 15 to 200 pps[60-62] through a 1- to 5-mm-diameter probe electrode to these points for 15 to 90 seconds per site, relief of chronic, deep, localized or referred pain may occur by activation of an inhibitory serotonergic mechanism.[63-65] When transcutaneous application of HVPC to acupuncture points at 1 to 4 pps elicits intense rhythmic muscle contraction without electrical paresthesia, the resulting analgesia corresponds to pain suppression produced either by the acupuncturelike mode or the high-amplitude burst mode of classical TENS.

Only two studies were found in the literature in which HVPC was used to treat pain. Sohn, Weistein, and Robbins[66] report achieving complete relief of pain in 55 of 80 patients with levator ani syndrome following three treatments with HVPC. These findings are corroborated by Morris and Newton[67] who, using a descriptive research design, treated 28 patients with levator ani syndrome using HVPC at 120 pps and negative polarity for two 60-minute treatment sessions per week. They reported that 21 (75 percent) of the patients reported pain relief or other symptom reduction after 7.5 treatments. Additional clinical studies utilizing control groups are needed to establish high-voltage stimulation as an efficacious method for electroanalgesia.

CLINICAL DECISION MAKING

After the patient has been evaluated and the goals and plan of care are established, a transcutaneous stimulation device must be selected that is appropriate for administering electroanalgesia treatments. Selection of the device should be based on the patient's pain profile, that is, the device should be capable of delivering stimulus characteristics that will effectively reduce the reported pain, whether the pain is determined to be acute, chronic, superficial, or deep, or occurs concurrently with administration of a therapeutic procedure. Other factors that should also be considered when selecting a TENS device include the anatomic site or area of the body to be treated, and the presence of metal or electronic devices or accessories implanted in the tissues.

Acute, superficial pain of musculoskeletal origin such as pain associated with acute epicondylitis may respond favorably to treatment with either IFC or HVPC. IFC applied at 2 bps with a primary carrier frequency of 4000 Hz would provide 2000 pulses per beat with each of the 2000 pulses having a duration of 5 μs. HVPC could be applied at 50 to 100 pps with the duration of each pulse pair lasting 5 to 65 μs. The amplitude for both types of current should be adjusted to provide only a comfortable tingling electrical paresthesia without muscle contraction, which corresponds to the conventional mode of traditional TENS.

A patient with cervical osteoarthritis and a history of chronic, deep, aching pain originating from the suboccipital area may be treated successfully with either HVPC, IFC, or diadynamic current. With each device the fact that the pulse/beat duration is preset is inconsequential, since the primary goal is to produce the strongest tolerated rhythmical muscle contractions. The amplitude must be adjusted accordingly with the frequency set at 1 to 5 pulses, beats, or cycles per second, respectively. These stimulus variables would produce stimulation similar to the acupuncturelike-mode TENS described in Chapter 5.

Debridement of a decubitus ulcer can be a painful procedure. The patient may benefit from analgesia provided by passing current from an IFC, HVPC, or AC device through the wound or adjacent tissue during the procedure. A mode of stimulation similar to brief, intense TENS can be produced with these devices by eliciting mild tetanizing muscle contractions concurrently with tingling electrical paresthesia for short periods of time. Pulse and beat durations are usually not adjustable; however, pulse and beat frequencies may be adjusted as shown in Table 6–2, to produce analgesia during an acute painful procedure. Table 6–2 summarizes the stimulus variables for five different types of current and their alternative uses for acute pain, chronic pain, and pain associated with therapeutic procedures.

CONTRAINDICATIONS AND PRECAUTIONS FOR ELECTRICAL STIMULATION FOR PAIN CONTROL

Generally, the same contraindications and precautions that apply to the use of traditional TENS also apply to the use of the alternative, low and high voltage TENS devices discussed in this chapter. Although documented reports of adverse effects are not identified in the literature, the use of TENS in any of its forms is contraindicated in four instances:[68,69]

1. In a patient with a demand-type cardiac pacemaker who would be vulnerable to cardiac arrest or arrhythmia[69]
2. Over the carotid sinus, which, if stimulated with electrical impulses, may result in a hypotensive response
3. Over thrombotic or embolic blood vessels particularly when rhythmical muscle contractions will be elicited
4. Over tissues or blood vessels that are vulnerable to hemorrhage

Precaution is advised when any form of TENS is considered for treatment of pain in the following conditions:[68]

1. Over the lumbar and abdominal areas of pregnant women, except during labor or delivery that is not accompanied by complications
2. On individuals who have epilepsy or who are confused, combative, or intellectually incompetent
3. Transthoracic application in very asthenic individuals, particularly children who may be more vulnerable to cardiac arrhythmia or arrest if electric current reaches the pericardium or the vagus nerve
4. Over the anterior, lateral, and posterior chest walls of patients with histories of cardiac problems unless clearance is given by the cardiologist
5. Over the eyeball (however, tissues around the orbit may be stimulated)

TABLE 6-2 Suggested Stimulus Variables for Electroanalgesia from Five Alternative TENS Sources

	Interference Current	High-Voltage Pulsed Current	Impulse Current	Diadynamic Current	Alternating Current
Acute/superficial pain	f:1–2 bps* d:250 μs* a:Comfortable tingling paresthesia without muscle contraction*	f:50–100 pps d:5–65 μs a:Comfortable tingling paresthesia without muscle contraction	f:100 pps d:250 μs a:Comfortable tingling paresthesia without muscle contraction		
Chronic, deep, aching pain	f:1–5 bps d:250 μs a:Highest comfortable, tolerated, rhythmical muscle contraction	f:1–5 pps d:65 μs a:Highest comfortable, tolerated, rhythmical muscle contraction		f:10 Hz d:10 μs a:Highest comfortable, tolerated, rhythmical muscle contraction	
Acute painful procedure (debridement, friction massage, mobilization)	f:50–100 bps d:250 μs a:Highest tolerable level of paresthesia with tetanizing muscle contraction	f:50–100 pps d:65 μs a:Highest tolerable tingling paresthesia with tetanizing muscle contraction			f:2.5 kHz d:400 μs a:Highest tolerable level of paresthesia with tetanizing muscle contraction

*f = frequency; d = duration; a = amplitude.

6. Over or immediately adjacent to wounds that are vulnerable to or in the process of dehiscence, particularly when TENS is used to produce muscle contractions
7. On skin of the head, face, and neck of individuals who have suffered a cerebrovascular accident (CVA) or are subject to transient ischemic attacks or seizures

A LOOK TOWARD THE FUTURE

Since the early 1970s when Long[8,9] and Shealy[10,11] found that TENS was almost as effective in ameliorating pain as direct stimulation of the dorsal columns, there has been a steady increase in the number and use of low voltage, portable (traditional) TENS devices. These devices, with a variety of pulse modulations have often been marketed as having some unique ability to diminish one's perception of pain. Despite the abundance and variety of traditional TENS devices that are available, many clinicians have elected to use alternative TENS devices such as IFC and HVPC to treat patients who report pain and sensory dysfunction.

As technological refinements and discoveries in electronics and electrophysiologic delivery systems advance in the future, steady improvements will be made in TENS devices that will allow clinicians to select specific stimulation variables most appropriate for meeting the needs of the patient. One of the important variables that not only influences patient perception of and compliance with electrical stimulation but also dictates the type of response produced is the quantity of electrical charge delivered to the tissues. In the future, we should begin to see both traditional and alternative TENS devices offering the clinician the ability to select specific charge quantities delivered to treatment electrodes and measured in microcoulombs. Being able to select the total charge along with the type of current, and time and amplitude-dependent characteristics and modulations, allows the clinician to administer treatment and document outcomes more accurately, as well as replicate treatments when favorable outcomes are achieved.

In addition to improvements in TENS devices that only deliver electrical charge to the tissues for pain management, improvements will also be forthcoming in iontophoretic devices and their drug-delivery systems for the treatment of musculoskeletal and myofascial pain. As microprocessors continue to undergo miniaturization it appears likely that TENS devices such as IFC and HVPC will also become smaller and perhaps even portable, much like the present traditional TENS devices. In conclusion, as the health care professionals and consumers of tomorrow become increasingly aware of the many available electrical-stimulation alternatives, and recognize that adverse side effects associated with electroanalgesia are minimal, when compared with those associated with other methods of pain control, all forms of transcutaneous electrical stimulation will be more widely accepted and universally used as efficacious analgesic alternatives.

SUMMARY

This chapter reviews a variety of electrical waveforms that have been used for the relief of pain. Electrophysiologic principles of pain perception and modification are reviewed. The application of various electrical waveforms, including interference current, transcutaneous electrical stimulation of acupuncture points, impulse currents, diadynamic currents, alternating currents, high voltage pulsed currents, and modes of stimulation are compared with regard to electrical stimulus parameters, biophysical effects, and treatment considerations. Clinical evidence of treatment efficacy is critically reviewed and examples of specific applications are suggested. Finally, the advancement of electroanalgesia is predicted as technological development and critical evaluation of treatment outcomes continue to grow.

REFERENCES

1. Stillings, D: A survey of the history of electrical stimulation for pain to 1900. Med Instrum 9:255, 1974.
2. Stillings, D: A short history of electrotherapy in England to about 1800. Bakken Museum of Electricity in Life, Minneapolis, 1974.
3. Barcalow, DR: Electreat relieves pain. Electreat Mfg. Co., Peoria, 1919.
4. Bernard, PD: La therapie diadynamique. Les Editions Naim, Paris, 1950.
5. Nemec, H: Electromedizinischer Apparat patent number 163979. Patent document number 165657. Published by the Austrian Patent Office, April 11, 1950.
6. Melzack, R and Wall, PW: Pain mechanisms: A new theory. Science 150:971, 1965.
7. Shealey, CN, Mortimer, JT, and Reswick, JB: Electrical inhibition of pain by stimulation of the dorsal column: Preliminary clinical reports. Anesth Analg (Cleveland) 45:489, 1967.
8. Long, DM: Recent advances in the management of pain. Minn Med 56:705, 1974.
9. Long, DM: External electrical stimulation as treatment of chronic pain. Minn Med 57:195, 1974.
10. Shealy, CN: Transcutaneous electroanalgesia. Surg Forum 23:419, 1973.
11. Shealy, CN: Six year's experience with electrical stimulation for control of pain. Adv Neurol 4:775, 1974.
12. McNeal, DR: 2000 years of electrical stimulation. In Hambrecht, F, and Reswick, J, (eds): Functional Electrical Stimulation: Applications in Neural Prostheses. Marcel Dekker, New York, 1977, p 3.
13. Electrotherapeutic Terminology in Physical Therapy: Report of the Electrotherapy Standards Committee of the Section on Clinical Electrophysiology of the American Physical Therapy Association, Washington, DC, 1990.
14. Binder, SA: Application of low and high voltage electrotherapeutic currents. In Wolf, SL (ed): Electrotherapy, Churchill-Livingstone, New York, 1981, p 1.
15. Alon, G: High voltage stimulation: An integrated approach to clinical electrotherapy. Chattanooga Corp, Chattanooga, TN, 1987, pp 39, 54, 65.
16. Geddes, LA: A short history of the electrical stimulation of excitable tissue. Physiologist (Suppl) 27:1, 1984.
17. Alon, G, Allin, J, and Inbar, GE: Optimization of pulse duration and pulse charge during transcutaneous electrical stimulation. Aust J Physiother 29:195, 1983.
18. Crago, PE, et al.: The choice of pulse duration for chronic electrical stimulation via surface, nerve and intramuscular electrodes. Ann Biomed Eng 2:252, 1974.
19. Sinclair, D: Mechanisms of Cutaneous Sensation. Oxford University Press, Oxford, 1981.
20. Witters, D: Center for Devices and Radiological Health, FDA. Personal Communication, 1988.
21. Miller, BA, et al.: A comparison of modulated rate and conventional TENS. Phys Ther 64:744, 1984.
22. Leo, K: Perceived comfort levels of modulated versus conventional TENS current. Phys Ther 64:745, 1984.
23. Mannheimer, JS: Electrode placement for transcutaneous electrical nerve stimulation. Phys Ther 58:1455, 1978.
24. Mannheimer, JS: Optimal stimulation sites for TENS electrodes. Hibbert Co., Trenton, NJ, 1980.
25. Mannheimer, JS and Lampe, GN: Electrode placement sites and their relationships. In Mannheimer, JS and Lampe, GN (eds): Clinical Transcutaneous Electrical Nerve Stimulation. FA Davis, Philadelphia, 1984, p 249.
26. Mannheimer, JS: Transcutaneous electrical nerve stimulation: Its uses and effectiveness with patients in pain. In Echternach, JL (ed): Pain. Churchill Livingstone, New York, 1987, p 220.
27. Selkowitz, D: Improvement in isometric strength of the quadriceps femoris muscle after training with electrical stimulation. Phys Ther 65:186, 1985.
28. Eriksson, E and Haggmark, T: Comparison of isometric muscle training and electrical stimulation supplementing isometric muscle training in the recovery after major knee ligament surgery. Amr J Sports Med 7(3):169, 1979.
29. Laughman, RK, et al.: Strength changes in the normal quadriceps femoris muscle as a result of electrical stimulation. Phys Ther 63:494, 1983.
30. Walker, DC, Currier, DP, and Threlkeld, AJ: Effects of high voltage pulsed electrical stimulation on blood flow. Phys Ther 68:481, 1988.

31. Tracy, JE, Currier, DP, and Threlkeld, AJ: Comparison of selected pulse frequencies from two different electrical stimulators on blood flow in healthy subjects. Phys Ther 68:1526, 1988.
32. Kloth, LC: Interference current. In Nelson, R and Currier, D (eds): Clinical Electrotherapy. Appleton/Lange, Norwalk, CT, 1987, p 183.
33. DeDomenico, G: New Dimension in Interferential Therapy. A Theoretical and Clinical Guide. Reid Medical Books, Lindfield, NWS 2070, Australia, 1987, pp 14, 35, 36.
34. Bueche, F: Principles of Physics. McGraw Hill, New York, 1965, p 278.
35. DeDomenico, G: Pain relief with interferential therapy. Aust J Physiother 28:14, 1982.
36. Burghart, W: Behandlung mit dem Nemectron. Wiener Medizinische Wockenschrift 101(51–53):999, 1951.
37. Nicolova-Troeva, L: Surgical conditions. In Nikolova, L (ed): Treatment with Interference Current. Churchill Livingstone, New York, 1987, p 95.
38. Taylor, K, et al.: Effects of interferential current stimulation for treatment of subjects with recurrent jaw pain. Phys Ther 67:346, 1987.
39. Sjolund, BH, Terenius, L, and Eriksson, MBE: Increased cerebrospinal fluid levels of endorphin after electro-acupuncture. Acta Physiol Scand 100:382, 1977.
40. Sjolund, BH and Eriksson, MBE: Electro-acupuncture and endogenous morphine. Lancet 2:1035, 1976.
41. Akil, H, et al.: Appearance of beta-endorphinlike immunoreactivity in human ventricular cerebrospinal fluid upon analgesic electrical stimulation. Proc Natl Acad Sci USA 75:5170, 1978.
42. Castel, C: Personal Communication, April, 1989.
43. Oliveri, AC, et al.: Effects of auricular transcutaneous electrical nerve stimulation on experimental pain threshold. Phys Ther 66:12, 1986.
44. Noling, LB, et al.: Effect of transcutaneous electrical nerve stimulation at auricular points on experimental cutaneous pain threshold. Phys Ther 68:328, 1988.
45. Holmgren, E: Increase of pain threshold as a function of conditioning electrical stimulation: An experimental study with application to electroacupuncture for pain suppression. Am J Chin Med 3:133, 1975.
46. Andersson, SA and Holmgren, E; Pain threshold effects of peripheral conditioning stimulation. In Bonica, J and Albe-Fessard, D (eds): Advances in Pain Research and Therapy, Vol 6. Raven Press, New York, 196, p 761.
47. Melzack, R: Prolonged relief of pain by brief intense transcutaneous electrical stimulation. Pain 1:357, 1975.
48. Melzack, R: Myofascial trigger points: Relation to acupuncture and mechanisms of pain. Arch Phys Med Rehabil 62:114, 1981.
49. Eriksson, MBE and Sjolund, BH: Pain relief from conventional versus acupuncture-like TNS in patients with chronic facial pain. Pain Abstracts. Second World Congress on Pain, IASP, Montreal, 1978, p 128.
50. Paris, DL, Baynes, F, and Gucker, B: Effects of the Neuroprobe in the treatment of second-degree ankle inversion sprains. Phys Ther 63:35, 1983.
51. Leo, KC: Use of electrical stimulation at acupuncture points for the treatment of reflex sympathetic dystrophy in a child: A case report. Phys Ther 63:957, 1983.
52. Schmid, F: Diadynamic current. In Siebler, WH (ed): Stimulatory Current Practice. Robert Bosch, Berlin, 1982, p 19.
53. Petersmann, K: Practical hints for treatment with diadynamic currents according to Bernard. Siemens Aktiengesellschaft, Erlanger, West Germany, 1979, pp 3, 15.
54. Griffin, JE and Karselis, TC: Physical Agents for Physical Therapists, ed 2. Charles C Thomas, Springfield, IL, 1982, p 91.
55. Ganne, JM: Report on the results of treatment of pain with sustained sinusoidal current on 100 patients during 1964 and 1965. Aust J Physiother 14(2):47, 1968.
56. Alon, G: Principle of electrical stimulation. In Nelson, RM and Currier, DP (eds): Clinical Electrotherapy. Appleton and Lange, Norwalk, Connecticut, 1987, pp 52, 53.
57. Alon, G: High voltage stimulation: A monograph. Chattanooga Corp, Chattanooga, TN, 1984, p 8.
58. Newton, RA and Karselis, TC: Skin pH following high voltage pulsed galvanic stimulation. Phys Ther 63:1593, 1983.
59. Eriksson, MBE, Sjolund, BH, and Neilzen, S: Long term results of peripheral conditioning stimulation as analgesic measure in chronic pain. Pain 6:335, 1979.
60. Strassburg, HM, Krainick, JV, and Thoden, U: Influence of transcutaneous nerve stimulation on acute pain. J Neurol 217:1, 1977.
61. Melzack, R: Prolonged relief of pain by brief, intense transcutaneous somatic stimulation. Pain 1:357, 1975.
62. Fox, EJ and Melzack, R: Transcutaneous electrical stimulation and acupuncture: Comparison of treatment for low back pain. Pain 2:141, 1976.
63. Proudfit, HFK and Anderson, EC: Morphine analgesia: Blockade of raphe magnus lesions. Brain Res 98:612, 1975.
64. Simator, R, Juhar, MJ, and Uhl, GP: Opoid peptide enkephalin: Immunohistochemical mapping in the rat central nervous system. Proc Natl Acad Sci USA 74:2167, 1977.

65. Basbaum, AI, Clanton, CH, and Fields, HL: Three bulbospinal pathways from the rostral medulla of the cat: An autoradiographic study of pain modulating systems. J Comp Neurol 178:209, 1978.
66. Sohn, N, Weinstein, MA, and Robbins, RD: The levator ani syndrome and its treatment with high voltage electrogalvanic stimulation. Am J Surg 144:580, 1982.
67. Morris, L and Newton, RA: Use of high voltage pulsed galvanic stimulation for patients with levator ani syndrome. Phys Ther 67:1522, 1987.
68. Mannheimer, JS and Lampe, GN: Some limitations of TENS. In Mannheimer, JS and Lampe, GN (eds): Clinical Transcutaneous Electrical Nerve Stimulation. FA Davis, Philadelphia, 1984, pp 57, 58.
69. Eriksson, MBE, Schuller, H, and Sjolund, BH: Letter. Hazard from transcutaneous nerve stimulators: In Patients with pacemakers. Lancet 1:1319, 1978.

CHAPTER 7

Neuromuscular Electrical Stimulation (NMES) in Rehabilitation

Julie DeVahl, M.S., P.T.

Neuromuscular electrical stimulation (NMES) is the application of electrical current to elicit a muscle contraction. Use of NMES for orthopedic and neuromuscular rehabilitation has grown significantly in recent years. The neurophysiologic principles on which the treatment is based are reviewed in Chapter 1. This chapter will review the origin of NMES as a clinical modality. Principles of application and specific indications will be discussed and applied to a specific case study. Finally, a look toward future technologic advances will help to describe the role of NMES in clinical practice for years to come.

HISTORICAL PERSPECTIVE

The earliest use of electrical "devices" in medicine was described by Hippocrates in about 420 B.C. He recommended that the torpedo fish, a species which has special organs that produce an electrical charge to shock its prey, be boiled and included as part of breakfast for asthmatic patients.[1] The torpedo fish's properties were used by Scribonius Largus, a Roman physician, in 46 A.D. to treat painful conditions; placement of the fish over the ailing body part was recommended for headache and gout.[1]

The torpedo fish was not a convenient modality for application of electrotherapy. It was not until electricity could be generated and stored that this type of treatment could be used on a regular basis. The Leyden jar, invented in 1745, is a glass jar that is coated inside and out with metal foil[2] and is able to generate and store static electricity (Fig. 7–1).

The first recorded medical treatment using a similar device dates back to 1744 in Germany.[3] Christian Gottlieb Kratzenstein claimed to have restored function to a para-

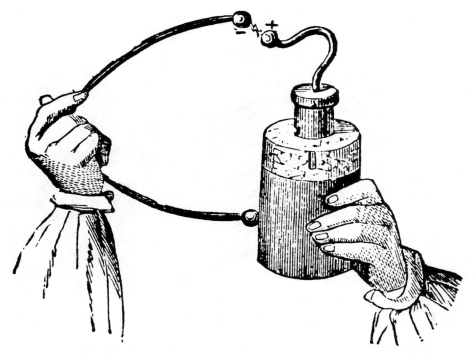

FIGURE 7–1. The Leyden jar, made of glass with a coating of tinfoil inside and out. (Courtesy of the Bakken, a Library and Museum of Electricity in Life, Minneapolis, Minnesota.)

lyzed small finger of a female patient by applying electricity for less than one quarter of an hour. Subsequent reports include Benjamin Franklin's use of electricity to cure a 24-year-old female suffering from convulsive fits.[4] Although many treatments for paralysis of extremities were reported in the 1700s, other therapeutic applications of electricity included treatment for kidney stones, sciatica, and angina pectoris.[5]

Luigi Galvani and Alessandro Volta[6] investigated the effects of electricity on animal muscle and nerve in the late 1700s. Galvani believed that muscle had an inherent "animal electricity," whereas Volta attributed the source of electricity to the metal rod used in the experiment, rather than the animal's muscle.

Advances in electricity-generating devices and animal experimentation continued in the 1800s. In 1831, Michael Faraday invented an electric generator that produced a current when a metal wire was rotated in a magnetic field. This device was the forerunner of the electric motor; the current produced in this manner was termed faradic current.[6] By the middle of the century, D. B. Duchenne[7] began to publish his work. Often called the "father of electrotherapy," Duchenne was interested in the physiology underlying electrotherapy. He is known for identification of motor points and muscle actions. In his research, he expressed a preference for faradic (biphasic) current over galvanic (monophasic) current because it avoided the electrolytic and heating actions of galvanic current. Figure 7–2 illustrates stimulation of the hand muscles with one of Duchenne's early stimulators.

Electrodiagnostic devices were introduced in the mid-1800s. Investigators noted

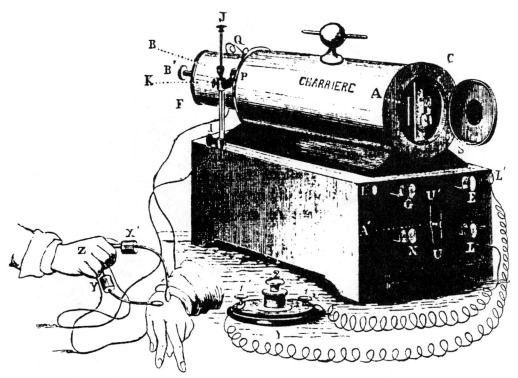

FIGURE 7–2. Stimulation of the hand with Duchenne's stimulator. (Courtesy of the Bakken, a Library and Museum of Electricity in Life, Minneapolis, Minnesota.)

that paralyzed muscle responded to galvanic but not faradic current. The duration of current flow was found to be an important factor in eliciting a muscle contraction. The terms *rheobase* and *chronaxie* were coined by Louis LaPicque[8] in 1909 to describe the relationship between amplitude and duration of current flow required to excite muscle or nerve. By 1916, the strength-duration curves for healthy and diseased human muscle illustrating this relationship were documented by Adrian.[9]

Once the battery and induction coil were invented and readily available, the golden age of medical electricity began.[6] Most physicians used some form of electrotherapy in their practices on a regular basis. The early 20th century electrical devices, although greatly refined since the days of the Leyden jar, were cumbersome. Figure 7–3 illustrates one device in which the physician became a part of the circuit by handling a sponge electrode. In this way, the proper dosage of current could be monitored by the physician's response to the current. Electrodes were typically made of brass or chrome-plated brass covered with felt or sponge. Water provided the conductive medium for current transmission. Treatment of peripheral nerve injuries grew during World War II with the development of a clinical stimulator able to generate stimuli capable of exciting both denervated and partially innervated muscles.[10]

The concept of NMES to provide functional use of limbs was demonstrated by Liberson in 1961.[11] Using a single channel of stimulation, ankle dorsiflexion was triggered with a foot switch during the swing phase of gait, thus correcting the patient's foot drop. The stimulator used by Liberson was about the size of a cigar box and was worn

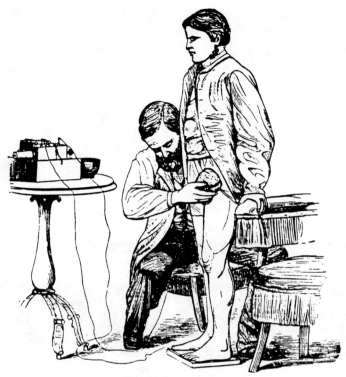

FIGURE 7–3. Application of electrical stimulation to the lower extremities with a sponge electrode. The return path for the current is provided by a metal plate under the patient's feet. (Courtesy of the Bakken, a Library and Museum of Electricity in Life, Minneapolis, Minnesota.)

on the patient's belt. Conductive rubber electrodes were secured to the lower limb by straps. Liberson also noted a transient carryover of function in the tibialis anterior following peroneal nerve stimulation in hemiplegic patients. Details of this type of clinical application are described later in this chapter.

The NMES devices of today are, for the most part, portable, adaptable, comfortable, and reliable. Figure 7–4 illustrates several commercially available stimulators. Microcircuitry and programmable electrical outputs allow considerable flexibility of application. The units can be adjusted by the clinician and some may be used by patients at home as well as in the clinical setting. A major benefit of integrating NMES into a treatment program is the reduction of total time for rehabilitation, thus reducing health care costs and returning the patient to gainful employment or independent living.

NEUROPHYSIOLOGIC EFFECTS OF NMES

A nerve action potential may be elicited by a "command" originating in the motor cortex of the brain or by an electrically induced stimulus at the periphery. In either case, the mechanism of action potential propagation and release of synaptic transmitter substance is the same. A fundamental difference between the two mechanisms and the

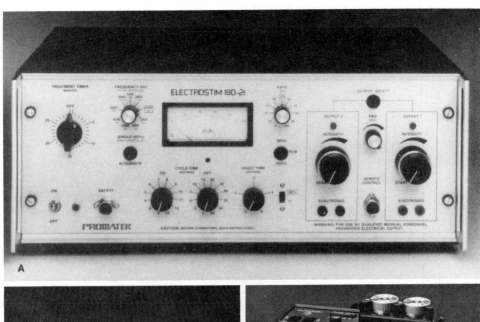

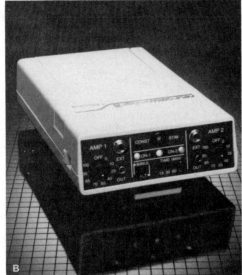

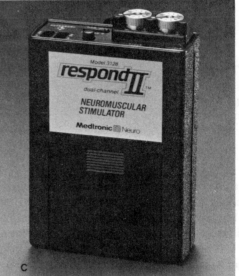

FIGURE 7–4. A variety of commercially available NMES devices. ([A] Courtesy of Electrostim® USA LTD, Joliet, Illinois. [B] Courtesy of Medical Devices, Inc., St. Paul, Minnesota. [C] Reproduced with permission from Medtronic, Inc., © Medtronic, Inc., 1991.)

resultant muscle contraction exists in the recruitment order of individual motor units.[12] Recruitment order based on intracellular versus extracellular excitation is described in detail in Chapter 1.

During a voluntary muscle contraction, smaller motor units composed of primary Type I, fatigue-resistant fibers tend to be recruited first. Different motor units are recruited asynchronously. As some are relaxing, others are contracting, and constant tension of the muscle is maintained.[13] Composed primarily of Type II, readily fatigable fibers are recruited first because their (large diameter) motor nerves have low thresholds to electrical excitation.[12] Motor units of similar threshold lying superficially beneath the stimulating electrodes will be recruited simultaneously. As they begin to fatigue, tension in the muscle will begin to decrease unless the intensity of the stimulus is increased, recruiting additional motor units with higher thresholds or with similar thresholds, but at more remote locations.[14] Excessive fatigue can be minimized during electrically induced muscle contractions by limiting the frequency at which the stimulus is applied and the duration of the contraction. Adequate rest periods between contractions will increase the likelihood that subsequent muscle contractions will be sufficiently strong.

PHYSIOLOGIC CHANGES IN MUSCLE FOLLOWING STIMULATION

Changes in properties of skeletal muscle following repetitive electrical stimulation have been studied in animal and human subjects.

Animal Studies

Salmons and Henriksson,[15] and Hudlicka and associates[16] observed increased capillary permeability in the muscles of rats and rabbits less than 1 week after initiation of stimulation delivered at 10 Hz. The investigators found an increase in the activity of enzymes of aerobic metabolism as well as a decrease in the enzymes of anaerobic metabolism. As stimulation continued, properties of the Type II, fast-twitch muscle fibers began to resemble those of the Type I, slow-twitch fibers. Other investigators,[17,18] using higher stimulation frequencies such as 60 and 2500 Hz carrier frequency, demonstrated similar fast-to-slow transformation when analyzing histochemical and morphologic changes.

Human Studies

The studies of human muscles through biopsy have also shown net changes in fiber characteristics and metabolism following electrical stimulation. Munsat, McNeal, and Waters[19] implanted electrodes to isometrically stimulate the quadriceps muscles of five patients with knee flexion contractures. In four patients the proportion of Type I fibers increased, and both Type I and Type II muscle fibers increased in size. The fifth patient showed a decrease in the number and size of Type I fibers, but had undergone more of an isotonic contraction of the quadriceps muscles due to a surgical release of the rectus femoris to correct a hip flexion contracture. Conclusions cannot be drawn from this small sample size, but it appears that the type of contraction elicited influences the type of physiologic changes that NMES can induce.

Eriksson and Haggmark[20] studied eight patients whose legs were immobilized after repair of the anterior cruciate ligament in the knee. Each subject had muscle biopsies of the quadriceps femoris muscle performed prior to surgery and at 1 and 5 weeks postoperatively. All patients performed volitional isometric quadriceps contractions. Four patients participated in a NMES program. The electrically stimulated group had significantly higher levels of succinate dehydrogenase (SDH), an enzyme indicative of mitochondrial oxidative capacity, than the control group, indicating that the stimulated group's quadriceps muscles had a greater capability for aerobic metabolism.

In the study by Stanish and associates[21] of 12 patients who had undergone major knee surgery, muscle biopsies were used to evaluate levels of adenosine triphosphatase (ATPase) and glycogen. Six subjects received NMES in addition to standard physical therapy exercises. The "exercise only" group showed a significant decrease in ATPase during the 6 weeks of immobilization whereas the NMES group did not. Higher ATPase levels suggested higher levels of muscle activity, and in this example, less disuse atrophy during immobilization. Glycogen levels did not change significantly.

A number of studies have been conducted using measurements of force, muscle cross-sectional area, and limb girth to evaluate changes in muscular performance rather than specific physiology. These investigations will be discussed in the section of this chapter on the application of NMES.

PRINCIPLES OF APPLICATION

Principles of physics and physiology provide a basis for selecting stimuli that are efficient and effective in eliciting the desired motor response.

Electrode Systems

TYPES OF ELECTRODES

Early electrodes were made from conductive metal and a sponge or felt pad moistened with water. This system served its purpose well by reducing skin-electrode impedance,[22] but the electrodes were not flexible enough to contour to body parts and were difficult to secure during patient movements. Carbon-impregnated silicon-rubber electrodes have replaced metal in most cases and are available in a range of shapes and sizes. They are very flexible and can be trimmed to fit different locations. They require a conductive interface to transmit the current from the electrode to the patient's skin. Conductive gel, karaya pads (a natural conductive gum), and synthetic copolymer gel pads are examples of interfaces used today (Fig. 7–5). Some systems secure the rubber electrode in place with tape strips or patches. Synthetic copolymers are usually conductive and adhesive, eliminating the need for tape,a possible source of skin irritation. Effective electrode systems should meet the following criteria:

1. Promote low skin-electrode impedance.
2. Conduct current uniformly.
3. Maintain uniform contact with skin.
4. Allow desired movement of body part.
5. Avoid skin irritation.
6. Be cost effective.

ELECTRODE SIZE AND PLACEMENT

The optimal size of the electrode is based on the desired muscular response, the size of the target muscle or muscles, and the electrode placement chosen. Larger electrodes will be effective in generating torque from large muscles or groups of muscles that contract together.[23] For example, two 5.08- by 10.16-cm or 7.62- by 15.24-cm electrodes may be used to stimulate the quadriceps or hamstring muscles. When small, individual

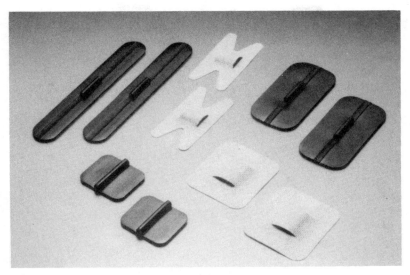

FIGURE 7–5. A variety of electrodes for surface electrical stimulation. (Reprinted with permission from Medtronic, Inc., © Medtronic, Inc., 1991.)

muscle stimulation is desired, a small electrode that increases the current density is placed over the motor point of that muscle. Current density is the amount of current delivered per unit area of the electrode.[14] A second, larger reference electrode is placed distally, often over the tendinous portion of the muscle. The second electrode acts to provide a return path for the current but has insufficient current density to cause significant depolarization of excitable tissue under this electrode. Figure 7–6 illustrates electrode placement to stimulate the extensor digitorum for finger extension. The active electrode is about 2.54 cm in diameter and is placed over the extensor digitorum motor point, midway between the lateral epicondyle and the ulnar styloid. The reference electrode is about 5.08 cm in diameter or 5.08 cm² placed distally on the forearm, but proximal to the ulnar styloid. Intensity of the stimulation should be limited because a strong contraction of the extensor digitorum with its distal insertion will result in wrist extension.

In general, electrodes should be no smaller than the size of a dime if used for prolonged stimulation periods to avoid concentration of current, sensory discomfort, and possible burns. A smaller electrode may be used for individual motor-point stimulation when generating twitch contractions. Effects of positive and negative polarity will be discussed under waveform descriptions.

As previously mentioned, an individual muscle contraction may be generated with placement of the active electrode over a motor point (refer to the Appendix for illustration of the motor-point locations of the major muscles). A motor point may be defined as a point on the skin overlying a concentration of terminal motor nerve branches where they infiltrate the muscle fibers they innervate.[24] When one electrode is placed over a motor point and the other is placed at a site remote from that area, the term monopolar stimulation is used. Bipolar stimulation describes placement of both electrodes to the muscle or muscle group to be activated.[24]

The patient's tolerance of stimulation and the quality of the muscle contraction are related to the amount of current needed to produce the desired response. Carefully

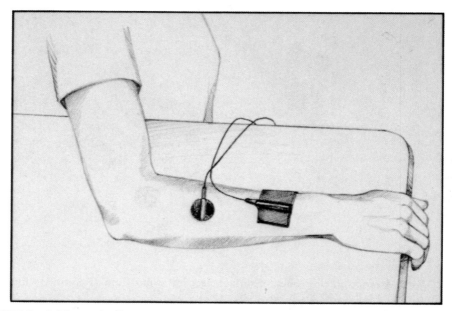

FIGURE 7–6. Electrode placement used to elicit finger extension. (Reprinted with permission from Medtronic, Inc., © Medtronic, Inc., 1991.)

positioning electrodes over motor points will assist in delivering effective, well-tolerated stimulation, as a minimal amount of current may be effective.[25] Bipolar placements tend to be used most often in NMES because, for a given intensity of stimulation, more current reaches the muscle to be stimulated.[24] The stimulation tends to be more efficient and the cutaneous sensation more comfortable because of the lower current density under each electrode.[25]

Placement of the active electrode should be avoided over scar tissue and bony prominences because impedance is increased compared to normal skin and muscle. Conductivity is related to water and ion content of the tissues. Muscle is a good electrical conductor, especially when current flow is parallel to the direction of its fibers.[10] For example, one electrode is usually placed proximally and the other distally in long muscles like the biceps brachii or the quadriceps femoris.

Close spacing of electrodes encourages superficial passage of current, whereas increased spacing of electrodes farther apart promotes deeper penetration of current.[14] If deep penetration causes recruitment of undesired muscle, the electrodes may be moved closer to one another. For example, stimulation of the anterior tibialis is desired to produce ankle dorsiflexion. If plantar flexion occurs, current may be reaching the deeper-lying posterior tibialis. Repositioning the reference electrode close to the active electrode may limit the current penetration and yield the desired response.

The Electrical Stimulus

POLARITY

By convention, electric current is described as flowing in the direction opposite to movement of electrons. Electrons travel from a region of high concentration (the *cathode*

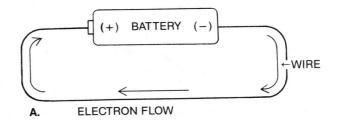

A.   ELECTRON FLOW

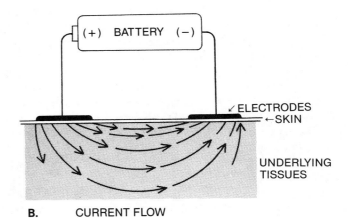

B.   CURRENT FLOW

FIGURE 7–7. (*A*) Electrons traveling along a wire conductor. Arrows indicate the direction of electron flow. (*B*) Current traveling through a tissue interface. Arrows indicate the direction of current flow.

or *negative* electrode) to one of lower concentration (the *anode* or *positive* electrode). At the cathode, negative ions are repelled and positive ions are attracted. At the anode, positive ions are repelled and negative ions are attracted. The net result is electron flow from cathode to anode (Fig. 7–7*A*) and current flow from anode to cathode (Fig. 7–7*B*). Once the current reaches the electrode-tissue interface, the current continues through the tissue as the movement of both negatively and positively charged ions.

Pfleuger's law[26] indicates that, under normal physiological conditions, less current is required from a cathodal (negative) stimulus to evoke a muscle contraction of given strength than from an anodal (positive) stimulus. Therefore, the negative electrode is often used to evoke the muscle contraction and is termed the *active* electrode, because depolarization of the biologically excitable tissue is most easily accomplished at the cathode. Excitable tissue under the positive electrode is less prone to depolarization and thus, the anode is often termed the *inactive, reference,* or *dispersive* electrode. A charge through either electrode is capable of eliciting a muscle contraction, but the anode is not usually as effective in doing so, unless the stimulus amplitude is increased. In one study[25] using a monophasic waveform, the strength of a muscle contraction produced by the inactive electrode (anode) was about 70 percent of the contraction produced by the active electrode (cathode) at a given current amplitude.

WAVEFORMS

Although a variety of waveforms are available in electrical devices, two waveforms have been used traditionally for NMES: the asymmetrical biphasic square (rectangular) and the symmetrical biphasic square (rectangular) waveforms (see Figs. 3–21 and 3–24). Both waveforms allow an equal amount of current to flow in either phase, thus avoiding undesirable electrochemical effects and possible skin irritation. The square wave is characterized by a fast-rising leading edge of the pulse, flat plateau at peak, and rapid return to zero at the end.

The asymmetrical biphasic square wave allows selective recruitment of smaller muscles by allowing the clinician to identify the anode and cathode, and choose the most effective direction of current flow for depolarization. When the current flows from the positive to the negative poles, depolarization occurs under the cathode (stimulating phase). (See Fig. 1–5B.) When current flows in the reverse direction, it flows at low amplitude so depolarization generally does not occur under the anode (balancing phase). The stimulating phase acts much as a monophasic current would, with the balancing phase merely reducing the likelihood of untoward polar effects.

The symmetric biphasic square wave dictates that the current flows equally "hard and fast" in both phases, thus allowing both electrodes to act as active electrodes. This waveform is preferred for stimulation of large muscle groups. McNeal and Baker[25] reported that the symmetric biphasic square wave can generate 20 to 25 percent greater force in a muscle at a given intensity than a monophasic waveform. In Bowman and Baker's study[28] of 23 female subjects, the symmetric biphasic square wave was preferred in terms of comfort over an asymmetric biphasic wave for generating a preselected torque output (27 Nm) from the quadriceps muscle. In another study by Baker, Bowman, and McNeal,[27] the asymmetric biphasic wave was perceived as more comfortable by 43 female subjects for quadriceps muscle stimulation when compared to monophasic-paired spike and modulated sine, or sine and square medium-frequency waveforms. It appears then that biphasic waveforms are preferred to monophasic or sine wave forms when applied at intensities sufficient to elicit muscle contractions. When symmetric and asymmetric biphasic waveforms were compared for comfort, the symmetric biphasic waveform was preferred. Tissue irritants can accumulate under one of the electrodes if the asymmetric biphasic waveform is unbalanced, and an accumulation of charge occurs, resulting in a burning or itching sensation under the electrode. The application of a balanced, symmetric biphasic waveform eliminates this accumulation of charge and the associated noxious sensations. The characteristics of various waveforms are discussed in Chapter 3.

AMPLITUDE (INTENSITY)

The intensity or amplitude of current is measured by the height of the waveform as it deviates from the isoelectric line. Most devices have a maximum output of 100 mA. As amplitude is increased there is an increase in the number of motor units recruited, thus, an increase in the muscle force developed (Fig. 7–8).

PHASE DURATION

Many NMES devices have a fixed-phase duration of between 0.2 and 0.4 ms. If the phase duration is fixed at 0.3 ms, for example, the development of muscle force can be adjusted from the point at which a muscle contraction just begins to near maximal force

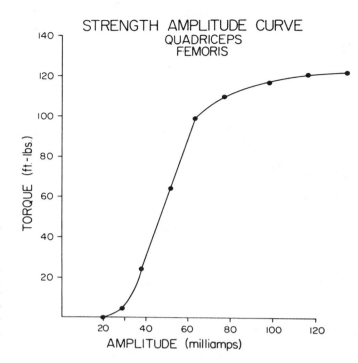

FIGURE 7–8. An increase in amplitude produces greater torque from the quadriceps femoris muscle (From Baker, LL: Neuromuscular electrical stimulation in the restoration of purposeful limb movements. In Wolf, SL (ed): Electrotherapy. Churchill Livingston, New York, 1981, p 36, with permission.)

by merely varying current amplitude.[14] During electrically induced muscle contractions, a phase duration of 0.3 ms was preferred for comfort over a narrower (0.05 ms) or wider (1.0 ms) phase duration.[28,29] A waveform with a phase duration of 0.05 ms requires that a greater amplitude of current be used to produce a pulse charge sufficient to generate a muscle contraction. The increased amplitude also is sufficient to recruit small diameter afferent fibers that elicit a painful sensation when stimulated. Similarly, a waveform with a phase duration of 1.0 ms generates a pulse charge sufficient to recruit both motor and pain-sensitive axons, at an amplitude sufficient to produce a muscle contraction. The basis for generating an electrical stimulus that produces a muscle contraction without eliciting pain is still being evaluated.

FREQUENCY (PULSE RATE)

The rate at which the individual pulses are delivered to the nerve is called the frequency and is measured in pulses per second (pps) or Hz. The effect of frequency on muscle contraction forces is illustrated in Figure 7–9. Low frequencies (1 to 5 pps) generate twitch contractions, allowing little sustained tension to develop in the muscle. Low frequency stimulation may be used to locate motor points since the twitching muscle may be readily visualized or palpated and little fatigue or discomfort occurs. Higher frequencies (10 to 20 pps) cause a "vibration" or fasciculating contraction of the muscle termed *incomplete tetany*. In healthy muscle at frequencies of approximately 30 pps, the muscle contractions usually become fused or tetanized, so that a smooth contraction is apparent. This type of contraction allows the most force to be generated in the muscle. In denervated muscle, tetany may occur at lower frequencies.[10]

Clinically, it is often desirable to limit the frequency to create a tetanic contraction,

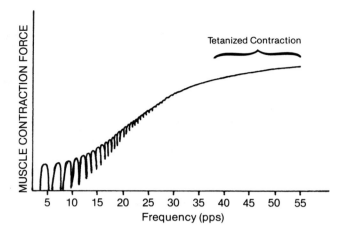

FIGURE 7–9. Wave summation and tetanization as a function of frequency of stimulus pulses. (Figure 9–12 from *Human Physiology and Mechanisms of Disease* by Arthur C. Guyton, copyright © 1982 by Saunders College Publishing, a division of Holt, Rinehart and Winston, Inc., reprinted by permission of the publisher.)

because neuromuscular fatigue at the level of the neuromuscular junction is more likely to occur at higher stimulation frequencies.[14,30]

DUTY CYCLE

As discussed previously, an electrically elicited muscle contraction recruits motor units with similar thresholds that are superficially located in the area of the stimulating current. To ensure that the muscle does not fatigue excessively and to effectively "exercise" the target muscle, the electrical stimulus may be automatically turned on and off. This mimics the contraction and relaxation of the voluntarily controlled exercise. In most NMES units, contraction time is simply labeled as "on time," measured in seconds. The relaxation time is labeled as "off time," also measured in seconds. Figure 7–10 illustrates this definition. The on and off times are often expressed as a ratio. The example in Figure 7–10 of 10 seconds on and 20 seconds off can be noted as a ratio of 1:2.

The ratio of contraction to relaxation time is mathematically related to the duty cycle. The duty cycle is expressed as a percentage derived by the following equation:

$$\text{Duty cycle} = \frac{\text{Pulse-train duration} \times 100}{\text{Total cycle time}}$$

According to this equation the duty cycle for the example in Figure 7–10 is 33 percent.

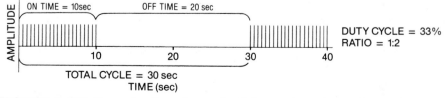

FIGURE 7–10. Example of on time and off time expressed as ratio and duty cycle.

The patient's diagnosis and degree of muscle weakness should be considered when selecting the preferred duty cycle for initiation of a NMES program. A 1:5 ratio (17-percent duty cycle) may be an appropriate starting point for a patient with hemiparesis. In Packman-Braun's study[31] of 18 patients with hemiparesis, the 1:5 ratio (5 seconds on and 25 seconds off) appeared to be best suited for stimulation of the wrist extensor muscles compared to a 1:1 or 1:3 ratio. A 1:3 ratio is commonly used for patients with orthopedic problems. As muscle strength or endurance improves, the ratio of on-to-off times may be decreased, approaching a 1:1 ratio. The number of muscle contractions per unit time increases with a lower ratio, providing a more aggressive program for the patient.

Frequency and duty cycle must be considered together when adjusting parameters for an optimal NMES program. In a study by Cole and associates[32] of 10 healthy female subjects, the quadriceps muscles were stimulated with various duty cycles and quadriceps torque output was measured over time. Stimulation of the quadriceps muscles at 30 pps and the 1:3 duty cycle did not provide statistically different torques from stimulation at 50 pps and a 1:7 or 1:10 duty cycle. Increasing off times and/or reducing frequencies are recommended when muscle fatigue is evident.

RAMP TIME

Most commercially available NMES devices offer a preset or adjustable period of time that the stimulus takes to reach the peak intensity and also to return to zero intensity. The times may be labeled as ramp, rise or surge time, and fall, or ramp down, respectively, and are measured in seconds. The ramp time is used to produce a "soft start," allowing the patient to become accustomed to the stimulation as it rises from nonperceptible levels to sensory and finally motor thresholds. At the cessation of the train of pulses, the fall time allows the muscle contraction to gradually relax, producing a contraction that may more closely mimic some voluntary contractions. Figure 7–11 illustrates how the ramp time relates to the on and off times.

Patient Safety Guidelines

Like all therapeutic modalities, NMES should be applied with sound clinical judgment. Precautions governing both the use of electricity and exercise should be considered prior to the application of NMES.

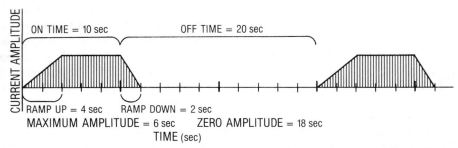

FIGURE 7–11. Example of the relationship between ramp times and on/off times. Each division on horizontal axis equals 2 seconds. Note that the ramp-up time is considered part of the on time, while the ramp-down time is considered part of the off time.

NMES may interfere with the output of demand-type cardiac pacemakers. Demand-type cardiac pacemakers are set to stimulate the cardiac muscle to contract at a specific minimum rate. If the patient's oxygen demand increases, as with aerobic exercise, and the patient's heart responds with an increased firing rate, the demand-type pacemaker normally shuts off, in order not to interfere with the heart's own increased rate of firing in response to increased activity. In contrast, an asynchronous (constant) cardiac pacemaker fires at a specific (minimum) rate *all the time*, without regard to the patient's activity level or autogenous myocardial excitability.

NMES applied at frequencies of less than 10 to 15 pps can interfere with the firing frequency of demand-type cardiac pacemakers, resulting in a decreased rate of firing. This inhibition of pacemaker activity may generate cardiac output insufficiency and can be fatal. Conversely, NMES applied at frequencies of greater than 30 pps can cause *reversion* of a demand-type pacing mode to an asynchronous mode. In this case, the pacemaker would stimulate the myocardium to contract even in the presence of an autogenously generated rapid heart rate and may produce potentially fatal ventricular dysrhythmias.

In closely monitored studies using NMES[33] and TENS (transcutaneous electrical nerve stimulation) devices,[34,35] interference of pacemaker output was not demonstrated. However, because of the possibility of dire consequences, use of NMES with patients who have demand-type cardiac pacemakers is not recommended, except under closely monitored conditions. In addition, NMES should be applied with caution to patients with known or suspected cardiac conditions such as arrthymias or conduction disturbances. More research is necessary to determine the safety of using NMES on patients with pacemakers or cardiac disease. All cardiac patients should be closely monitored for signs of dizziness, shortness of breath, palpitations, or syncope, during and immediately following application of NMES.

The effect of NMES on fetal development and health has not been defined. Therefore, the application of NMES to the abdominal perineal or lumbar region during pregnancy is not recommended. The effect of NMES on levels of circulating hormones has not been determined; therefore, NMES should be applied with caution to pregnant patients.

Electrode placement must be considered as a factor in patient safety. Avoid placement of electrodes over the anterior neck. Currents delivered to the vagus or phrenic nerves may cause spasm of the laryngeal or pharyngeal muscles and diaphragm, respectively, or interfere with normal function of the carotid sinus. Placement over or close to an incision site, causing resultant muscle activity should be avoided so that wounds will not be stressed or healing impaired. Scar tissue has a higher impedance than normal skin tissue and stimulation over scar tissue should be avoided, especially if part of the electrode is over a significant amount of scar and the remainder is over normal tissue. This consideration is important because the differences in impedance between the scar tissue and healthy tissue surrounding the scar would allow current to concentrate along the border of the scar, possibly resulting in skin irritation and an electrochemical burn. Electrode placement over significant adipose tissue is not contraindicated but may prohibit the stimulation program from being effective, because adipose tissue impedes current flow. Thus, stimulation usually becomes uncomfortable on the skin before underlying muscles can be effectively stimulated. If electrodes are placed over an area devoid of sensory innervation, such as may occur after spinal-cord injury, strict instructions for observation of the site and regular skin care are necessary.

Skin irritation may be caused by electrical, chemical, or mechanical factors. Electrical burns are not commonly associated with the balanced, biphasic waveforms used in most NMES devices. However, an improper electrode-skin interface is a potential source of irritation. To decrease the possibility of irritation from electrical factors, a larger stimulating surface should be used and uniform contact with a conducting medium should be maintained between the electrode and skin.[36] Chemical irritation is caused by allergic reactions from conductive gel or adhesive materials.[37-39] Selecting a different type of electrode usually overcomes this problem and is easy to accomplish given the wide variety of electrodes now commercially available. Mechanical irritation is generally caused by shear forces between the skin and adhesive material during movement. Placing the limb in the position of maximum skin stretch when applying electrodes will decrease the incidence of irritation. In addition, the patient or assistant should be instructed to separate gently the edges of the electrode from the patient and remove it slowly. Trimming excessive body hair from the area and removing the electrode in the direction that the hair grows will also lessen the mechanical stresses.

After orthopedic surgery NMES may be used as an adjunct to voluntary exercise to minimize disuse atrophy in muscle groups uninvolved with the surgical procedure. In this case, no special considerations are necessary, and general exercise guidelines apply. However, if the muscle, tendon, or structures influenced by that muscle's contraction were involved in the surgery, the surgeon must approve active muscular exercise prior to initiation of NMES. Specific level of strength of contraction or range of motion limitations within which the patient may exercise may be recommended by the physician. The amplitude of the NMES device can be regulated to produce an appropriate strength of contraction based on limitations dictated by the surgical procedure and stage of rehabilitation. Lower intensities produce weak contractions that avoid joint movement, similar to a "poor" or "grade 2" active muscle contraction. Higher intensities may be used when the surgeon allows active motion at the joint through a greater range.

All patients should be medically stable prior to initiation of a NMES program, as is the case for an active exercise program. In spinal cord injured patients, there is no evidence that dysreflexia is more prevalent following NMES treatments[14] but the therapist should be aware of the possibility of such an occurrence.

CLINICAL APPLICATIONS

NMES is a versatile modality that can be integrated into treatment plans for a variety of patient problems. The Food and Drug Administration has approved NMES devices as safe and effective for the following applications:[40]

1. Treatment of disuse atrophy
2. Increase and maintenance of range of motion
3. Muscle re-education and facilitation.

Other areas of clinical use include:

4. Spasticity management
5. Orthotic substitution
6. Augmentation of motor recruitment in healthy muscle.

Each of the major clinical applications will be discussed separately with examples of treatment protocols for specific diagnoses.

Disuse Atrophy

Disuse atrophy refers to changes in the muscle after a period of immobilization or reduced activity. This atrophy may occur as a result of immobilization (e.g., after fracture or ligament reconstruction) or as a result of central nervous system trauma, such as a stroke or spinal cord injury. The most obvious change following prolonged immobilization is a decrease in muscle cross-sectional area (i.e., reduction of muscle mass).

Several investigators[41,42] have reported greater atrophy of Type I, slow-twitch muscle fibers than Type II, fast-twitch fibers in humans following immobilization. There was no change in the number of fibers, but rather a decrease in the mean fiber cross-sectional area. Haggmark, Jansson, and Eriksson[43] studied patients who were placed in long leg casts after major knee surgery and observed selective atrophy of Type I fibers after several weeks of immobilization even though patients were instructed to perform isometric contractions inside the cast. Type I fibers also showed a decrease in SDH, an oxidative enzyme, indicative of aerobic metabolism. Concentrations of these enzymes decreased significantly within the first week of immobilization. Baugher and associates[44] studied patients with unrepaired anterior cruciate ligaments in their knees for an 18-month period following injury and found predominantly Type-II fiber atrophy, despite the patients' return to relatively normal function and some athletic competition. It is possible that atrophy of Type II fibers is a more gradual process and only observed months after immobilization has occurred. Haggmark, Jansson, and Eriksson[43] only followed patients for 6 to 8 weeks following injury.

The cross-sectional area of the muscle is related to its ability to generate force. The level of oxidative enzymes is related to aerobic muscle performance with good endurance. Thus, atrophied muscle is weak and has poor endurance when compared to healthy muscle. NMES has been used to overcome the deleterious effects of disuse atrophy. While NMES has not been successful in preventing atrophy, NMES may be used to retard the effects of immobilization.[45-52] Most of the published research concerning disuse atrophy in human subjects has assessed the ability of NMES to delay or reduce disuse atrophy in immobilized quadriceps femoris muscles. After injury, surgery, or prolonged immobilization, patients have difficulty contracting the quadriceps muscle voluntarily, perhaps because of reflex inhibition and lack of coordination.[45,46] NMES is an effective way to induce exercise in muscles during the initial phase of rehabilitation (Fig. 7–12). Smaller decreases in muscle mass, as measured by limb girth and computerized tomography of quadriceps muscle occurs when NMES is used.[20,47-51] Muscle torque measurements before and after immobilization show less strength loss following the use of NMES than without NMES.[47,48,51,52]

Morrissey and associates[52] reported that NMES could significantly minimize the loss of strength after anterior cruciate ligament (ACL) repair, but no differences were found in limb girth.

Bouletreau and associates[53] measured by-products of muscle catabolism (break down of protein) during immobilization of patients in an intensive care unit to further investigate the effects of NMES on immobilized muscles. A decrease in two types of by-products associated with changes in muscle catabolism during immobilization was seen following the application of NMES, suggesting that NMES can abate some deleterious metabolic effects of immobilization.

Patients who have not had an acute injury or surgery may also benefit from NMES programs. Patients with chondromalacia patellae and subluxing, or dislocating patallae have difficulty exercising to strengthen the quadriceps because of pain. NMES can be

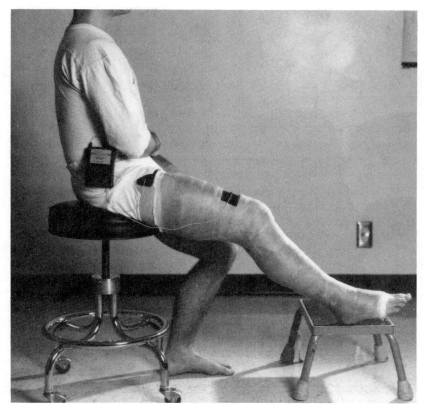

FIGURE 7–12. NMES applied during cast immobilization to reduce disuse atrophy of the quadriceps femoris muscles. (Reprinted with permission from Medtronic, Inc., © Medtronic, Inc., 1991.)

used to minimize weakness associated with disuse atrophy by facilitating passive exercise in the presence of pain.[54,55] Emphasis on strengthening of the vastus medialis obliquus (VMO) muscle, whose function is critical to dynamic patellar alignment, can be accomplished by placing the active electrode over the VMO or by using two channels of NMES, with electrodes from one channel specifically placed for optimal facilitation of the VMO (Fig. 7–13) and electrodes from the other channel applied to stimulate the remaining quadriceps musculature.

Treatment protocols reported to decrease the effects of disuse atrophy vary considerably. The patient's diagnosis and preinjury condition will influence the initial parameter settings and rate of progression. Table 7–1 illustrates suggested parameters for initiating a NMES program for patients with various degrees of atrophy. A patient with a long-standing neurological insult may experience severe disuse atrophy. Appropriate treatment is directed toward reinnervated muscle following peripheral nerve injury or recovery of some function following spinal cord decompression surgery. Moderate atrophy is observed in a postoperative total knee replacement patient with pre-existing atrophy associated with osteroarthritis or in a patient who began NMES after several weeks of cast immobilization rather than during the immobilization period. A lesser degree of atrophy is observed in the patient who experiences an acute injury and for whom NMES is initiated within the first week postinjury.

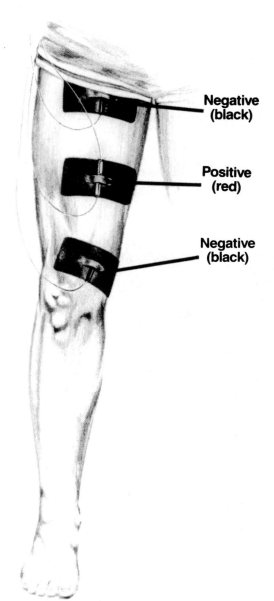

Negative (black)

Positive (red)

Negative (black)

FIGURE 7–13. Electrode placement for the quadriceps femoris muscles, emphasizing the vastus medialis obliquus for patellar tracking. Both channels share a common reference electrode. (Reprinted with permission from Medtronic, Inc., © Medtronic, Inc., 1991.)

TABLE 7–1 Suggested Treatment Parameters for Patients with Disuse Atrophy

	Severe Atrophy	Moderate Atrophy	Minimal to No Atrophy
Frequency (pps)	3–10	10–30	30–50
On time (s)	5	5–10	10–15
Off time (s)	25–50	20–30	10–30
Session length (min)	5–10	15	15
Number of sessions per day	3–4	3–4	1–2

Guidelines for voluntary exercise programs may also be appropriate for NMES. For example, a patient may begin treatment with frequent, but short sessions. As muscular endurance improves, the length of each session can be increased up to 4 to 6 hours.[14] In a NMES program, the off time between contractions can also be shortened, thus allowing more contractions to occur within a given session.

In programs designed to delay the effects of disuse atrophy, the patient's activities should also be considered. A patient who has undergone a major knee ligament reconstruction, whose leg is in a cast, and who ambulates nonweight-bearing on the affected limb will require more stimulation time to deter disuse atrophy than a patient who has had a partial meniscectomy under arthroscopy and is allowed to bear weight and perform active range-of-motion and isometric exercises within a short time after surgery, because the former patient provides less voluntary activation of his quadriceps muscle than does the latter.

The decision to discontinue a NMES program for disuse atrophy should be based on the patient's recovery of function of the involved limb. As mentioned, pain and swelling may prevent the patient from optimally exercising the involved leg. When the patient has recovered from the initial trauma and is able to voluntarily exercise *effectively* against resistance, NMES may be discontinued. In other cases, the use of NMES should be continued until the functional goals previously established are achieved or modified. For example, a patient who has recently undergone surgical repair of the flexor tendons in the hand may have regained the range of motion and grip strength necessary to be considered functional and ready to return to work. But if the patient is a bricklayer, the patient requires exceptional endurance of the wrist extensors as well as the finger flexors. NMES can be used to increase endurance of the wrist extensors, even though the patient is capable of working on voluntary finger flexion activities independently.

Range of Motion

Patients who are weak or experience pain and joint swelling have difficulty moving a joint through its available range of motion. In the absence of a fracture involving the joint itself, early motion is desirable to accelerate rehabilitation and prevent loss of motion. NMES may be used for patients with orthopedic or neurologic dysfunction to promote full return of joint mobility.[48,56-62]

If range of motion (ROM) is limited in only one direction, a single channel of NMES is sufficient. A patient who has moderate flexor spasticity in the hand secondary to a cerebrovascular accident (CVA) tends to lose full extension of the wrist and fingers. Passive ROM exercises can be augmented by stimulation with electrodes placed over the wrist and finger extensor muscle bellies and near the tendinous insertion of the wrist extensors. By positioning the upper extremity so that the forearm rests on its volar surface, gravity provides the return to the flexed or neutral position after stimulation extends the wrist and fingers against gravity, if wrist flexors are also weak.

Two channels of stimulation may be useful when ROM is limited in two directions (e.g., flexion and extension.) Figure 7–14A, 7–14B, and 7–14C illustrates wrist ROM by alternate stimulation of flexors and extensors. The forearm is positioned to allow motions to occur in a horizontal plane so that gravity is not a major factor in the movements. Electrode placement should be adjusted so that balanced wrist flexion and extension occur without ulnar or radial deviation. A dual-channel NMES device with

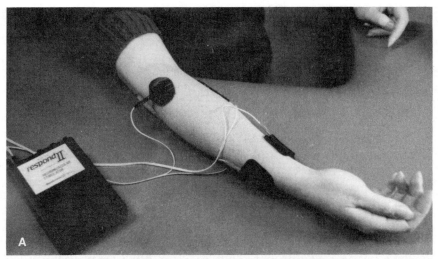

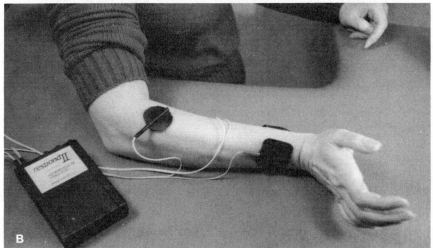

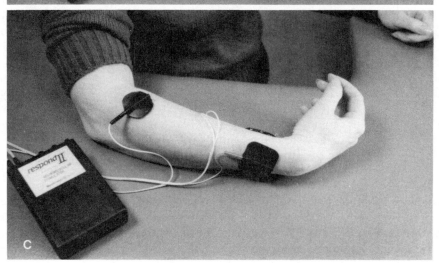

the ability to select a reciprocal or alternating mode of stimulation would permit this type of application. A patient who has lost wrist range of motion and strength in both flexion and extension secondary to a Colles fracture of the distal radius would be an appropriate candidate for this type of treatment.

Frequency and duty cycle selection have been discussed with regard to disuse atrophy. Most patients who have difficulty regaining or maintaining ROM have been immobilized or have significant weakness and disuse atrophy, thus similar guidelines for selecting frequency and duty cycle parameters may be followed.

A 30-minute session of NMES daily is generally adequate to maintain ROM,[14] but longer and more frequent periods of stimulation may be required to increase ROM by overcoming soft-tissue contractures and swelling. Treatments of up to 4 hours of stimulation have been reported to be effective in overcoming soft-tissue contractures.[58,60,62]

NMES is ideally suited as an adjunct to active ROM exercises because of its cyclic, repetitive nature. The patient need not participate actively during the entire session, but it should be noted that NMES is not intended to replace passive stretching, active, or active-assisted ROM exercises. During a portion of the treatment session, (e.g., 10 minutes of a 30-minute session), a patient should exercise to the end range of motion, thus working on increasing his or her functional range.

Muscle Re-education and Facilitation

The goal of therapeutic exercise for muscle re-education and facilitation is to re-establish voluntary control of body positions and movements after injury or disease has affected the motor control mechanism. Motor control may be affected by damage to either or both the afferent and efferent neural pathways, as well as to central control centers in the motor and premotor cortex. Animal studies have shown that interrupting afferent fibers at the dorsal roots may result in paralysis, even though the ventral roots (efferent pathway) are intact.[63] This may be due to the absence of tonic influences from afferent to efferent pathways that normally maintain a state of "readiness" for motor activity to occur.

Although exact mechanisms are not clear, the nervous system is continually adapting to environmental stimuli. This reorganization is termed *neural plasticity.*[64] The peripheral and central nervous systems (CNS) are capable of remarkable recovery in response to injury, through the processes of collateral sprouting and synaptic reclamation.[65] However, complete spontaneous recovery is the exception rather than the rule in the presence of significant nervous system trauma. Neural plasticity is critically important to return of function using muscle re-education and facilitation applications.

The effects of electrical stimulation on the damaged peripheral nervous system are discussed in Chapter 8. This section will address the application of NMES for muscle re-education in the presence of CNS trauma, when the peripheral pathways remain intact. The electrical stimulation of a muscle through its peripheral nerve appears

FIGURE 7–14. Electrode placement used to facilitate range of motion of the wrist. (*A*) Wrist in neutral position, (*B*) wrist extension — electrodes are placed on the muscle bellies and tendinous insertions of the wrist extensors, (*C*) wrist flexion — electrodes placed on the muscle bellies and tendinous insertions of wrist flexors (not shown). (Reprinted with permission from Medtronic, Inc., © Medtronic, Inc., 1991.)

adequate to enhance neuromuscular plasticity.[66] Function-induced plasticity is evident based on changes in skeletal muscle as a result of prolonged stimulation: A more fatigue-resistant muscle is produced.[15]

NMES can be used as a tool to establish new strategies for motor control. An electrical stimulus applied transcutaneously at an intensity sufficient to evoke a perception analogous to "light touch" or "tapping" is presumed by clinicians to activate sensory nerve fibers, including the A-beta (Group II) fibers.[67] NMES used at a sensory level only may behave similarly to facilitation techniques that involve light stroking, tapping, or touch in handling the involved limb. Electrodes are placed over the impaired muscle, and current amplitude is adjusted to sensory threshold. The patient should be able to detect a sensation, but a muscle contraction is neither visualized nor palpated. A low-pulse rate (3 to 10 pps) or a higher tetanizing pulse rate (30 to 100 pps) may be used. It is hypothesized that sensory stimulation increases awareness of the involved extremity and may promote improved function. A study by Teng and associates[68] in which implanted electrodes provided electrical stimulation of hemiplegic patients' affected muscles suggested that NMES with implanted electrodes was less effective than electromyographic (EMG) biofeedback in increasing voluntary motor control. It may be that sensory input from the electrical stimulation was minimized with the implanted electrodes and is a necessary component of successful NMES programs for some patients.

Improvement in motor control following NMES used at a current intensity sufficient to evoke a muscle contraction (motor threshold) has been documented by several researchers.[56,60,69,70] In addition to the direct muscle contraction, afferent activity from the muscle spindles and Golgi tendon organs may provide additional information to the central nervous system, thus contributing to the processes of inhibition and facilitation. Gracanin[70] theorized that NMES helps to establish a more "normal" pattern of movement that can be integrated by supraspinal mechanisms and that its repetitive nature assists the CNS in adapting this new pattern as the motor engram of choice.

When using electrical stimulation for muscle re-education and facilitation, the patient should attempt to perform the desired movement or contraction along with the stimulation. Patients generally prefer to practice functional activities during NMES, if possible. Figure 7–15A and 7–15B illustrates the retraining of a grasp and release pattern of the finger flexors and extensors. A remote hand switch is used to override the stimulator's duty cycle, allowing the stimulation to be synchronized with verbal commands and voluntary effort. This movement pattern requires reciprocal activity of the flexors and extensors which can be facilitated by most dual-channel NMES devices. A remote hand switch may be used to trigger the stimulation only as needed by an individual patient. For example, NMES may be used briefly to initiate a movement by an apraxic head-injured patient, complete an arc of motion, or sustain a contraction in a quadriplegic patient with an incomplete spinal cord injury, who has weak function of the prime mover. Figure 7–16 illustrates use of the remote hand switch to activate the quadriceps to a greater degree than the patient's voluntary effort to complete terminal knee extension. In this way, NMES is used to augment the patient's voluntary effort, not to replace it.

The therapist may also trigger electrical stimulation using a heel switch. (Specific use of this accessory for gait training will be discussed in the orthotic substitution section.) This switch overrides the stimulator's duty cycle in the same manner as the hand switch but allows the therapist to activate the switch with pressure from the foot, freeing both hands to assist the patient. This technique is beneficial, especially when

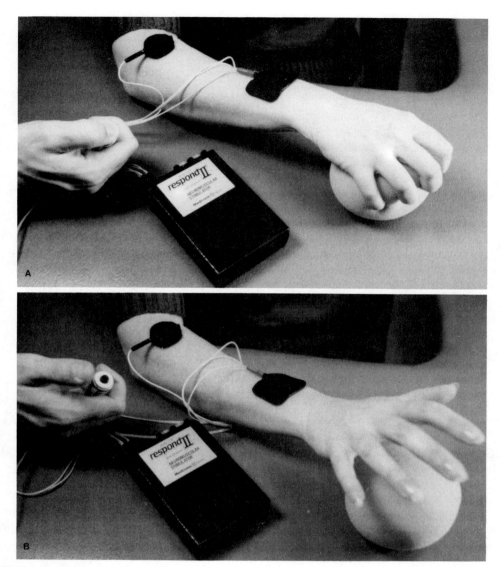

FIGURE 7–15. Re-education of grasp (*A*) and release (*B*) function of the hand, using dual-channel NMES. (Reprinted with permission from Medtronic, Inc., © Medtronic, Inc., 1991.)

performing preambulation skills in the parallel bars. The therapist may safely support and guide the patient during weight shifting and lower extremity placement drills. Stimulation of the affected muscles, such as the gluteus medius and quadriceps for stance stability, may be triggered as needed by the therapist applying foot pressure to the heel switch. The patient may wear the heel switch in his or her own shoe, at which time the correct performance of the task (e.g., weight bearing) consistently triggers the switch. Other activities, such as balance drills in the "all-fours" position on a mat, may require significant assistance from the therapist. This position is used to provide upper-extremity weight bearing and facilitation of shoulder stability and elbow extension.

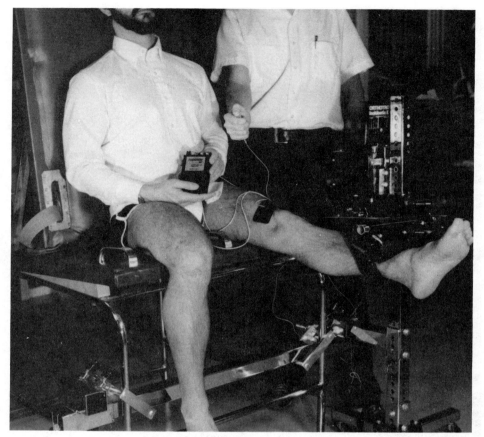

FIGURE 7–16. Facilitation of terminal knee extension, with single-channel NMES. (Reprinted with permission from Medtronic, Inc., © Medtronic, Inc., 1991.)

NMES of the deltoid and/or triceps muscles may facilitate activation of this function. The heel switch can be activated by pressure from the therapist's knee or foot, while he or she assists the patient in maintaining balance during this activity.

Use of NMES as a facilitation tool is limited only by the therapist's creativity. Combining NMES with other facilitation techniques, such as positional feedback[61,62] and EMG biofeedback,[71] appears to augment the effects of either facilitation technique alone.

Spasticity Management

Spasticity is a condition associated with hyperreflexia, including resistance to passive movement, hyperresponsive deep tendon reflexes, and clonus.[72] Spasticity interferes with recovery of function after CNS trauma. The spastic muscle may inhibit a weak agonist, prohibiting the patient from using the extremity correctly. Moderate to severe spasticity interferes with good posture and proximal stability, making coordinated movements impossible.

For many years, NMES has been used to manage the problems associated with spasticity, but optimal treatment techniques have not been established. Levine, Knott, and Kabat[73] applied a biphasic current at 100 pps to create a tetanic contraction in the muscle antagonistis to the spastic muscle. They reported the results of such treatment in patients with hemiplegia, paraplegia, or multiple sclerosis. Patients demonstrated relaxation of the spastic muscles as measured by increased range of motion and improved function. The authors hypothesized that the decrease in spasticity was due to reciprocal inhibition, in which an increase in activity of the antagonist muscle results in a relative inhibition of the agonist. Others have used this technique to reduce spasticity in patients with CVA, head trauma, and cerebral palsy with positive results as measured by increases in force output from the agonist, improved function, and a transient carryover period of decreased spasticity following treatment.[69,70,74-77] Treatment sessions of 10 to 45 minutes resulted in decreased spasticity varying in duration from 10 minutes to several hours.[14,75,76] During periods of diminished spasticity, therapeutic exercise can be performed to elongate soft-tissue contractures and facilitate return of voluntary function in the agonist muscles.

The management of spasticity following a spinal cord injury varies somewhat from the management of spasticity resulting from a more centrally located injury. A classic study by Dimitrijevic and Nathan[78] reported that repetitive cutaneous stimulation applied to the plantar surface of the foot in 10 paraplegic patients decreased the flexion reflex, an indicator of spasticity. The authors hypothesized that a mechanism of habituation to a cutaneous stimulus occurs at the level of the spinal cord. Walker[79] studied the effects of electrical stimulation on ankle clonus in nine patients with multiple sclerosis and four with postlaminectomy neuromuscular irritability. Clonus is the repetitive contraction of a hyperactive muscle in response to a quick-stretch. Subcutaneous stimulation of the radial, median, and saphenous nerves in a double-blind manner suppressed clonus observed at the ankle for up to 3 hours. A mechanism of segmental or supraspinal inhibition was proposed since stimulation of nerves remote to those supplying the ankle musculature was also effective in suppressing clonus. These studies formed the basis for further investigations of spasticity in spinal cord injured patients.

Electrical stimulation was applied to the spastic quadriceps muscle of 12 spinal cord injured patients by Robinson, Kett, and Bolam.[80] Strong contraction of the muscles was obtained with a current intensity of 100 mA, a frequency of 20 pps, a phase duration of 0.5 ms, and short on and off times of 2.5 seconds each. The stimulation session lasted 20 minutes. The results showed an immediate decrease in quadriceps spasticity as measured by a pendulum drop test (allowing the leg to swing freely and measuring the oscillatory knee motion). The greatest decrease in spasticity was noted in patients with the greatest initial levels of spasticity. There was no carryover effect after 24 hours. When similar patients participated in a long-term stimulation program (twice per day, 6 days per week, 4 to 6 weeks), these authors observed a tendency toward *increasing* spasticity.[81] These studies suggest that it may be desirable to stimulate the spastic muscles in patients with spinal cord injury for short periods when immediate effects are desired but that prolonged stimulation of the spastic muscles should be avoided.

Efforts to determine the preferred protocol for stimulation to inhibit the spastic quadriceps of spinal cord injured patients have not been conclusive. Vodovnik, Stefanovska, and Bajd[82] observed that a frequency of 100 pps was more effective than 10 or 1000 pps in inhibiting spasticity. Phase duration appeared to be a less critical variable, but the results favored 0.1 ms. Although the rationale underlying these preferred stimulus settings is unclear, the authors propose a relationship between mechanisms subserving spasticity and those subserving pain. These stimulus settings are often effective for the management of pain, as discussed in Chapter 5.

While a specific protocol for the management of spasticity is not available, it appears that attempts to "fatigue" spastic muscles with strong, prolonged stimulation may cause habituation of the spinal mechanisms with inconsistent outcomes. Electrical stimulation of the antagonist to the spastic muscle may be a preferred technique, because the stimulation is directed toward the weak agonist, facilitating return of function. Joint motion that is obtained may assist in lengthening soft-tissue contractures which may be present. The probability of reciprocally inhibiting the spastic muscle exists, further improving the functional outcome. Stimulation parameters are comparable to those appropriate for disuse atrophy and range-of-motion programs.

Orthotic Substitution

Neuromuscular electrical stimulation may be used to enhance the function of a patient's paralyzed or weak muscles, thus eliminating the need for a brace or orthosis. Sophisticated computerized systems to assist gait will be discussed at the end of this chapter. This section will focus on applications currently in clinical use.

GAIT TRAINING

In 1961 Liberson and associates[11] reported on the use of a pressure-sensitive switch to trigger electrical stimulation of the muscles innervated by the peroneal nerve during gait. Specifically, this stimulator assisted in ankle dorsiflexion during the swing phase of gait. Figure 7–17 illustrates a similar type of heel switch and a NMES unit with electrodes. The heel switch is a pressure-sensitive contact switch arranged to open the circuit (i.e., stop stimulation) when the heel is in contact with the floor, and provide stimulation when the heel leaves the floor during the swing phase of gait. NMES has been used to increase torque output from the ankle dorsiflexors and reciprocally decrease spastic reflexes in the plantarflexors, which improved the gait pattern of hemiplegic patients.[11,69,70,74,83,84] Carnstam, Larsson, and Prevec[69] noted improved function from the calf muscles at push-off and extension of the knee during stance associated with stimulation of the ankle dorsiflexors during the swing phase of gait.

Prior to using NMES as an electrical orthosis, the patient should build up endurance in the muscles to be stimulated during the gait cycle. This "pregait" program has the benefit of minimizing any pre-existing disuse atrophy.[74,85,86] Actual gait training with stimulation can be initiated when the patient has sufficient balance to require minimal to moderate assist from an assistive device and the target muscles can consistently generate strong contractions over approximately 30 minutes. A reliable contraction is necessary every time the muscle is stimulated before the patient will feel confidence in this method of assistance.

Facilitation of ankle dorsiflexion is the most common application for orthotic assist in hemiplegic patients, but NMES may also be applied to the gluteals and/or quadriceps muscles to enhance stability during the stance phase of gait. Plantarflexors or hamstring muscles can be facilitated during the brief period of the gait cycle (push off and late swing phase, respectively) in which they function if the therapist uses a handheld switch to synchronize the desired muscle contraction to the correct portion of the gait cycle. Figure 7–18 illustrates placement of electrodes to facilitate both ankle dorsiflexion

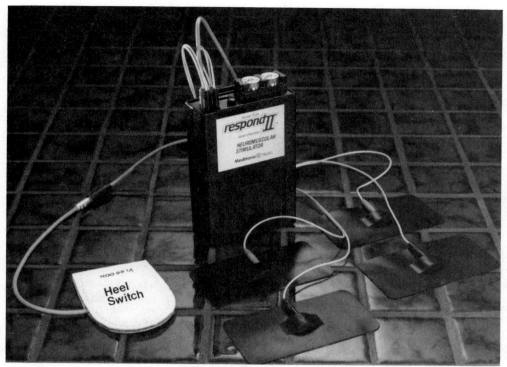

FIGURE 7–17. A heel switch is used to trigger NMES appropriately during the gait cycle. (Reprinted with permission from Medtronic, Inc., © Medtronic, Inc., 1991.)

during the swing phase and knee extension during the stance phase of gait. Additional applications of NMES for the hemiplegic patient are presented in Chapter 12.

Stimulation of the flexion reflex may be a facilitation tool suitable for the swing phase of gait for patients who have disabilities, such as hemiplegia or incomplete paraplegia, resulting in the involvement of several muscle groups in the lower extremity. The flexion reflex is facilitated by stimulating the sole or dorsum of the foot, or the lower posterior thigh.[85,87] Because the optimal response will vary with electrode placement, several placements should be considered during the evaluation phase of treatment.

IDIOPATHIC SCOLIOSIS

Scoliosis is an abnormal lateral curvature of the spine. It may develop secondary to muscle imbalances from neuromuscular disease or congenital spinal deformities. Idiopathic scoliosis describes a condition for which the cause is unknown and patients are generally healthy, young, and active. The usual form of treatment for a progressive scoliosis curve consists of bracing the spine for 23 hours per day. For most patients bracing is undesirable in that the brace may be uncomfortable, restrictive, and may adversely affect self-image[88] and coping skills.[88] Patients are often reluctant to wear the brace as prescribed and poor compliance may cause the treatment to fail.

In the 1970s the use of NMES as an electrical orthosis was initiated. Research of systems using implanted electrodes and antennae and a radio-frequency transmitter

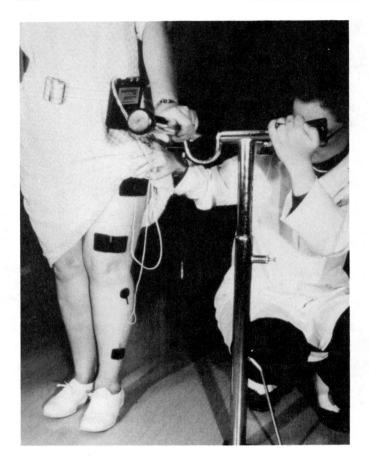

FIGURE 7-18. Electrode placement used to elicit knee extension during stance (electrodes placed on the quadriceps femoris muscle) and ankle dorsiflexion during the swing phase of gait (electrodes placed on the tibialis anterior muscle). (Reprinted with permission from Medtronic, Inc., © Medtronic, Inc., 1991.)

suggested that electrical stimulation could be used to stabilize or limit the progression of spinal curvature found in children and adolescents with idiopathic scoliosis.[89-91] Although the implanted system was an effective treatment modality, it required a surgical procedure with some inherent risks, such as infection, migration of the electrodes, electrode breakage, and a second surgery to remove the components after treatment was concluded. The use of surface electrodes and an externally powered device as an alternative to implanted electrodes was suggested.

Application of the external system involves placing surface electrodes on the convex side of the curve. Single- or dual-channel stimulation may be used, based on the individual patient's curve. Contraction of the spinal musculature produces a force to reduce the lateral curvature.[92,93] The electrodes are placed superior and inferior to the apex of the curve in either a paraspinal, intermediate, or lateral array (Fig. 7-19). Some controversy exists as to the preferred placement, but x-rays taken with the patient prone and the stimulation active, can confirm the location that results in the best acute correction.

Stimulation is applied during nighttime hours when the patient is sleeping, totaling 8 to 10 hours of treatment compared to the nearly 23-hour regimen recommended by most bracing programs (Fig. 7-20). The stimulation parameters (Table 7-2) are adjusted to generate strong contractions but avoid fatigue during the entire treatment. The

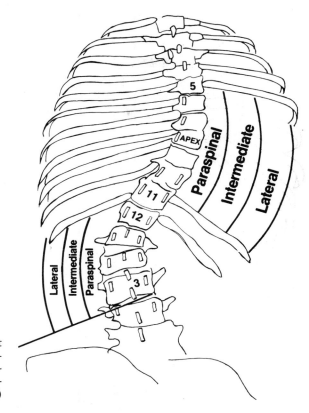

FIGURE 7–19. Electrode placement for idiopathic scoliosis may be paraspinal, intermediate, or lateral. (Reprinted with permission from Medtronic, Inc., © Medtronic, Inc., 1991.)

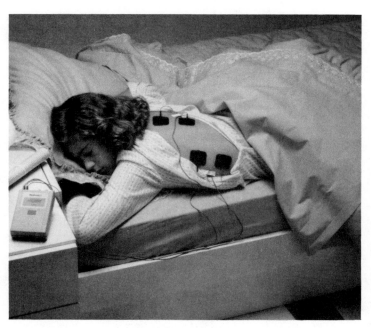

FIGURE 7–20. NMES for treatment of idiopathic scoliosis is applied during the night as the patient sleeps. (Reprinted with permission from Medtronic, Inc., © Medtronic, Inc., 1991.)

TABLE 7–2 Stimulus Parameters Used for Treatment of Idiopathic Scoliosis

Type of Stimulator	Amplitude (mA)	Frequency (pps)	Phase Duration (ms)	On Time (s)	Off Time (s)	Ramp Up (s)	Ramp Down (s)
Rancho Los Amigos Rehabilitation Engineering Center Research Prototype*	60–80	25	0.2	6	6	1.5	0.8
Medtronic Scoliosis System (Model 3100-2)†	60–80	35	0.225	6	25	1.5	0
EBI Scolitron (Model 601-03)‡	60–80	24.4	0.22	6.4	4.1	1.3	1.0

*Rancho Los Amigos Hospital Rehabilitation Engineering Center, Downey, CA.
†Medtronic Nortech Division, San Diego, CA.
‡EBI Medical Systems, Inc., Fairfield, NJ.

treatment is continued until skeletal maturity is reached, when the patient is gradually weaned from the stimulation.

Results have generally shown the NMES system to be as effective as bracing in arresting or decreasing the degree of curvature.[94-100] Patient characteristics such as location and degree of curve, skeletal and chronologic age, and compliance with treatment affect the success of this treatment. Generally, curves of greater than 20° but less than 40°, with documented progression, are considered appropriate for treatment. Patients with larger curves or more immature skeletal systems have greater risk of progression and appear less responsive to treatment with NMES.[101,102] In addition, a recent study by O'Donnell and associates[103] indicated that treatment with NMES may not have an effect on altering the natural history of the idiopathic curve, based on the size of the curve at initial evaluation and the percentage of curves that increased 5° or more. Poor outcome may also be related to poor compliance or inadequate stimulation.[104]

Effects of long-term NMES on the skeletal muscles of scoliosis patients have been examined.[104-106] There appears to be an increase in the Type I (aerobic) characteristics of muscle fibers and evidence of an adaptive process toward greater fatigue resistance. No damage to muscle tissue has been noted. Some patients have difficulty with skin irritation because of sensitivity to gels and adhesives used in the electrodes. An alternate electrode type and brand usually corrects the problem. Rarely must a patient discontinue NMES treatment because of irritation that persists because electrodes are worn in the same location every night to ensure proper correction of the curve.

SHOULDER SUBLUXATION

Shoulder subluxation is a problem associated with severe weakness or flaccidity of the muscles supporting the glenohumeral joint. Subluxation may be found in patients with CVA, quadriplegia or Guillain-Barré syndrome. The stability of the glenohumeral joint is compromised when the supporting muscles, primarily the supraspinatus and posterior deltoid, are unable to contribute.[107,108] The weight of the upper extremity in an unsupported position, and traction that may inadvertently be applied during assisted transfers, can stretch the joint capsule. Subluxation at the glenohumeral joint may be accompanied by pain localized in the shoulder or radiating into the elbow and hand.[109] Edema of the wrist and hand may also be present, interfering with finger motion. In a series of 219 hemiplegic patients reviewed by Van Ouwenaller, Laplace, and Chantraine,[110] subluxation seemed to be responsible for the greatest number of painful complications of the shoulder in patients with either spastic or flaccid muscles.

Shoulder subluxation may be treated by a variety of orthotic supports or slings.[108-111] However, this type of treatment often inhibits the patient from using the involved upper extremity, even when some distal function exists. Furthermore, use of slings and supports can facilitate the flexion synergy because the arm is frequently held in an adducted position with the elbow flexed.

A protocol for application of NMES to provide stability with the glenohumeral joint yet allow freedom of movement and alternative positioning of the limb has been suggested.[112] If applied early in the rehabilitation process, capsular stretch and subsequent subluxation can be reduced or, in some cases, prevented.

Baker and Parker[56] studied 63 CVA patients who displayed a minimum of 5 cm of subluxation at the glenohumeral joint. The patients were treated either with hemislings, wheelchair arm supports, or a NMES program consisting of an electrical stimulus with

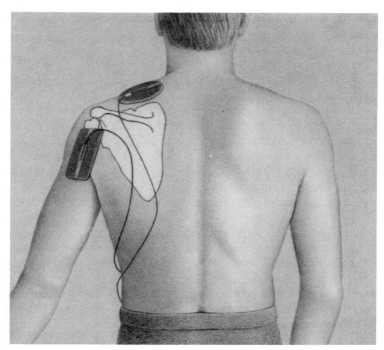

FIGURE 7–21. Electrode placement on the supraspinatus and posterior deltoid muscles for the reduction of shoulder subluxation. (Reprinted with permission from Medtronic, Inc., © Medtronic, Inc., 1991.)

an asymmetric biphasic waveform applied to the supraspinatus and posterior deltoid muscles, as illustrated in Figure 7–21. The reference electrode was placed over the supraspinatus muscle to minimize undesirable activation of the overlying upper trapezius muscle, which can result in shoulder elevation. An aggressive increase in stimulation time was selected in order to build endurance in these muscles so that a sustained contraction is tolerated and functional glenohumeral alignment can be maintained during the patient's waking hours. At the end of 5 days of NMES treatment, patients tolerated 6 to 7 hours of stimulation with a 1:3 on:off ratio. Over the next 5 weeks, stimulus on times were increased and off times were decreased, so that, for each stimulus cycle the stimulus was on for 24 seconds, and off for 2 seconds, resulting in correction of subluxation the majority of the time.

The results of this study demonstrated that NMES significantly decreased the amount of shoulder subluxation, as indicated by x-ray. The slings and wheelchair arm supports did not result in any change in the degree of subluxation measured. There was no relationship between the degree of subluxation and the amount of pain reported by the patient in this study, suggesting that factors other than subluxation may contribute to reports of shoulder pain in CVA patients. These factors can include circulatory aberrations or a heightened perception of pain (hyperalgesia) because of diminished use of the arm. To date the magnitude of successful shoulder subluxation reduction reported by Baker and Parker[56] has not been replicated by other investigators. Additional clinical evaluation of the efficacy of NMES for reduction or prevention of shoulder subluxation is warranted.

NMES may be used as an orthotic tool early in rehabilitation programs and discontinued when the patient has regained sufficient voluntary function of the supraspinatus and deltoid muscles to support glenohumeral alignment and function. NMES may continue to be used as an electrical orthosis when flaccid paralysis and subluxation persist. A patient may find the use of NMES cosmetically preferable to the donning of slings or wheelchair-mounted arm supports.

Augmentation of Motor Recruitment in Healthy Muscle

The goal of improving human performance in sport and exercise has been a fascinating topic for coaches, athletic trainers, physical therapists, exercise physiologists, and athletes alike. Based on basic science research that shows anatomic and physiologic changes in muscle following NMES, ongoing research is directed toward discovering how NMES can be used to optimize rehabilitation and training programs in injured and healthy clients. In 1977, a Russian physician, Yakov Kots,[113] presented his theories and results of training protocols at a Canadian-Soviet Exchange Symposium. He reported a 30 to 40 percent increase in strength of the quadriceps femoris muscles following electrical stimulation in elite athletes. Although Dr. Kots's research is not well documented or replicated in western literature, his report led to a flurry of research activity in this country. Stimulation protocols for traditional NMES devices, as well as those specifically based on Kots's work are reviewed below. The positive training effects of exercise alone, however, can obscure any effects that NMES may contribute to the augmentation of motor-unit recruitment in healthy muscle.

LOW VOLTAGE, LOW FREQUENCY NMES

Several researchers have compared the effects of NMES plus exercise to exercise or NMES alone on muscle strength in healthy subjects.[114–122] Since the training protocols are all very similar, their parameters may be generally summarized here. The quadriceps femoris muscle was electrically stimulated to produce isometric contractions, with the knee flexed at angles of 60° to 90°, as shown in Figure 7–22. Sustained contraction times varied from 4 to 10 seconds, with rest times of 4 to 50 seconds. Training sessions were conducted 3 to 5 times per week for 2 to 6 weeks. All stimulators produced a tetanic contraction of the quadriceps muscle, using frequencies of 25 to 200 pps. The maximum amplitude tolerated by the subjects was used. Most investigators concluded that NMES alone improved isometric strength of the quadriceps muscles but that the gains were not significantly different from those obtained with voluntary exercise alone or NMES plus simultaneous voluntary contractions.

In studies by Hartsell[119] and Nobbs and Rhodes,[120] when patients trained their quadriceps muscles isometrically with NMES, isokinetic strength gains were identified both in terms of muscular power and endurance at rotational velocities of 180° per second. Other investigators[115,121] confirmed these isokinetic strength gains at velocities of contraction, up to 180° per second.

Wolf and associates[123] studied the benefits of NMES during a resistive squatting exercise and found that the results from the addition of NMES to voluntary efforts did not differ significantly from those of voluntary exercise alone, although the NMES group showed greater, absolute strength gains over time. Most researchers[115,119,120,123] have concluded that augmentation of voluntary muscle contractions with low voltage,

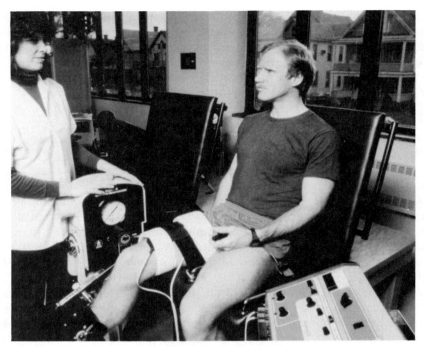

FIGURE 7–22. Sample set-up for training the quadriceps femoris muscle with NMES. (Reprinted with permission from Medtronic, Inc., © Medtronic, Inc., 1991.)

low frequency NMES is probably most beneficial for patients with weakened muscles who cannot contract these muscles optimally with voluntary effort alone. Healthy subjects, able to maximally contract their muscles voluntarily during training appear not to benefit from the addition of NMES to their training protocols.

MEDIUM FREQUENCY NMES

More recently investigators have studied whether NMES plus exercise produces results superior to exercise or NMES alone using the medium frequency stimulation (2500 Hz) previously described by Kots[113] (Fig. 7–23). The stimulus output is inter-

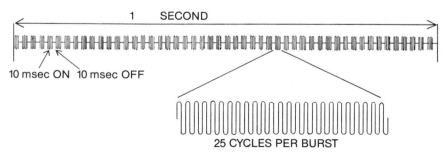

FIGURE 7–23. Medium frequency waveform with timing sequence.

rupted every 10 ms to create 50 "bursts" of stimulation every second. The 10-ms off period is not detectable by the subject. Kots believed that this type of waveform was preferred because the high carrier frequency "blocked" the afferent nerve supply in the area, creating an anaesthetic effect and enabling maximum recruitment of large diameter efferent fibers. A total of 10 maximal contractions sustained for 10 seconds each, with a 50-second off time defined a treatment session. These treatment parameters are confirmed in a technical discussion by Moreno-Aranda and Seirig.[124]

Protocols proposed by several investigations[125-128] to train the quadriceps femoris muscle in healthy subjects using medium frequency current were similar to those described previously for low voltage, low frequency NMES. Isometric contractions were generated by voluntary efforts, medium frequency (MF) NMES or a combination of voluntary effort superimposed on MF NMES. The knee was secured at an angle of 60° to 65° of flexion. The MF stimulators had a ramp-up time of 5 seconds, thus a total on time of 15 seconds provided 10 seconds of stimulation at maximum intensity, with a 50 second off time as proposed by Kots.[113] Training sessions occurred two to five times per week, for 4 to 5 weeks. To ensure that the maximum amplitude tolerated was used, the amplitude was increased periodically during treatment sessions, as the patient's pain tolerance increased.

These researchers[125-128] concluded that MF NMES alone appeared to have a beneficial isometric strengthening effect, but this effect was equivalent, not superior, to voluntary exercise alone or to a combination of electrical stimulation and voluntary exercise. In a related study, Delitto and Rose[129] evaluated 20 subjects' preferences for one of three different MF waveforms. They reported that no preference for the relative comfort of one waveform over another was expressed by these healthy subjects. Apparently the type of MF waveform does not effect the maximum amplitude tolerated by the individual.

Training Intensity

The intensity of training [stimulated, or voluntary contraction force, expressed as a percent of an individual's maximum voluntary isometric contraction (MVIC)] appears to influence the effects of MF NMES. For most persons MF NMES alone is able to generate 60 to 70 percent of a MVIC. The intensity of training that produced improved strength with MF NMES alone is much lower than the training intensity required for voluntary exercise to produce similar effects.[125,126] Selkowitz[130] increased the off time from 50 seconds to 2 minutes (presumably to allow complete recovery of the phosphagens used during muscle contraction). The average training intensity tolerated using NMES alone was 91 percent of MVIC, higher than the intensity reported in other studies. He found that the mean training intensity and mean contraction duration were related to strength gains. Soo, Currier, and Threlkeld,[131] using NMES alone, at a minimum dosage of 50 percent MVIC and 8 contractions per session for 10 sessions, demonstrated significant strength increases in 15 healthy subjects. It appears from this study that, while higher training intensities (91 percent MVIC) using NMES alone may be well tolerated, they are not necessary for the realization of strength gains. In addition, strength gains may be achieved at lower intensities using NMES than the exercise intensity required by voluntary exercise training. Additional research is required to determine the variety of conditions under which these strength gains can be measured (e.g., isometric, isotonic, and isokinetic) as well as to determine whether training (voluntary and with NMES) in one mode produces strength gains measured in other modes.

Fatigue

Fatigue is another factor that can influence the benefits that may be gained from MF NMES. Two patterns of MF NMES were evaluated by Parker and associates[132] in an isokinetic fatigue test: a 15:50 second and 12:8 second on-to-off-time ratio. Subjects demonstrated significantly more fatigue and poorer strength gains with the shorter off time. The authors suggested that there is probably a selective recruitment of Type II, fast-twitch muscle fibers with MF NMES training, hence the improved performance with adequate rest time.

Although it is generally accepted that MF NMES can generate stronger contractions than low voltage, low frequency NMES, a study by Stefanovska and Vodovnik[133] indicated that a 25-pps rectangular waveform produced a 25 percent increase in torque while the MF NMES produced only a 13 percent increase. They also used the 10:50 second on-to-off and explained that the increased fatigue produced by MF NMES compared to low frequency NMES may have diminished the strengthening effects anticipated of the MF NMES.

Effects of MF NMES on Patients

The benefit of MF NMES appears to be the increase in muscle strength at lower training intensities that those required by voluntary contractions. Delitto and associates[134] suggest that this application may be useful when it is desirable to begin strengthening early in the rehabilitation program. For example, in a case study reported by Nitz and Dobner,[135] a patient with a Grade II sprain of the medial collateral and anterior cruciate ligaments was immobilized for 3 weeks. During this time MF NMES was used to produce strong isometric contractions of the quadriceps and hamstring muscles in the cast. Within 3 weeks after cast removal, the patient could perform a vertical leap at 92 percent of the height obtained by the uninjured leg and returned to athletic competition. The authors suggested that the patient's early return to competition was facilitated by the early introduction of strengthening exercises using NMES.

Williams, Morrissey, and Brewster[136] studied the use of MF NMES in the rehabilitation of 21 postmeniscectomy patients. The length of time since surgery ranged from 21 to 88 days. One group of patients performed isometric and isotonic resistive exercises of the quadriceps and hamstring muscles three times per week. The experimental group applied MF NMES to the quadriceps muscles five times a week, in addition to the standard exercise program performed by the control group. After a 3-week training period, the MF NMES group showed significant increases in quadriceps strength at four isokinetic speeds (120°, 180°, 240°, and 300° per second). The voluntary exercise group showed increased strength only at the two slower speeds (120° and 180° per second). The investigators suggested that the improvement of muscular performance at higher speeds may be due to the selective training of Type II fast-twitch muscle fibers with NMES.

Twenty patients who had undergone anterior cruciate ligament reconstructive surgery participated in a study by Delitto and associates.[137] A rehabilitation program, consisting of cocontractions of the hamstring and quadriceps muscles elicited either voluntarily or by MF NMES, was implemented. The exercise sessions, consisting of 15 contractions of 15 seconds duration with 50 seconds of rest, were performed 5 days per week for 3 weeks. All the patients finished the training period within the first 6 postoperative weeks. Greater gains in isometric strength of both the quadriceps and hamstring muscles were seen in the MF NMES group than in the voluntary exercise group. The investigators believed that the voluntary cocontraction of two opposing muscle groups is a difficult exercise to perform compared to a single muscle group contraction. They suggested that the use of MF NMES to facilitate cocontraction reduces the time required for motor learning. They also suggested that if Type II muscle-fiber atrophy was the predominant obstacle to recovery of function in patients with ACL reconstruction, then MF NMES would be expected to produce better results than voluntary exercise alone.

Effects of NMES on Muscles of the Trunk

The application of NMES for correction of scoliosis has been discussed previously. Several investigators have evaluated the effect of NMES on trunk muscles in healthy subjects. Alon and associates[138] evaluated the effects of training abdominal muscles with voluntary exercise, NMES alone, or a combination of NMES superimposed on voluntary contractions. Contraction and relaxation times began at 5 seconds each and were increased to 12.5 seconds each by the fourth week of training. The number of repetitions was also increased, based upon the subject's original performance during the testing period. The subjects exercised three times per week for 4 weeks. NMES plus exercise produced the greatest gains in endurance, as measured by the number of repetitions performed in the testing period. NMES alone produced the second best gains in endurance. No training group showed improvement in duration of time an isometric contraction could be sustained.

Kahanovitz and associates[139] reported significant increases in endurance with NMES alone, but not with voluntary exercise alone, in training the back extensors in women. In this study, two types of NMES waveforms (symmetrical biphasic square and monophasic triangular waveforms) were compared to voluntary extension exercises. The NMES groups received 25 seconds of isometric stimulation-induced contractions of the lumbar paraspinal muscles followed by 8 seconds of rest for 20 minutes. An additional 5 minutes of sensory threshold stimulation was used as a "warm-up" period to accustom the subject to the stimulation prior to achieving the motor threshold. The session ended with a 5-minute sensory level stimulation "cool down." The exercise group followed a similar time sequence with the warm up and cool down consisting of stretching rather than sensory level stimulation, but performed 20 minutes of prone-trunk extension, prone leg and arm lifts, and arm-leg lifts in the "all fours" position. Isokinetic (30° to 60° per second), but not isometric strength was significantly increased in one of the NMES groups (symmetrical biphasic waveform) and the exercise group. Only the NMES groups showed an improvement in endurance. While these studies were conducted on healthy subjects, the results suggest that NMES may be a valuable treatment adjunct for patients with acute or subacute back pain, who could benefit from extensor strengthening, before a voluntary exercise and conditioning program is feasible.

Although studies suggest that NMES can *augment* muscle recruitment and strength in normal muscle, the goals of such treatment should be clearly defined. If an individual is able to exercise voluntarily under optimal conditions, that is probably the best method. "Toning salons" or programs advertising "no-sweat exercise" are not as effective over time as a well-designed and executed voluntary exercise program.[140] Further research must be done to substantiate the effects of NMES on the performance of elite athletes when selective muscle-fiber-type training may be beneficial.

Considerations for NMES in Pediatric Patients

Little has been published about the use of NMES for children. However, the problems associated with the rehabilitation of the neurologically involved pediatric patient are very similar to those of the adult patient. Muscle re-education, spasticity management, correction of contractures, and gait training are some examples of indications of NMES in pediatric patients with cerebral palsy (CP) or head trauma.

The most extensive report concerning the use of NMES with patients with CP was published in 1978. Gracanin[70] used electrical stimulation of the peroneal nerve to facilitate the dorsiflexion and eversion of the foot and evaluated changes in gait and posture. The specific protocol is not described by the author. Two children were under 1 year of age, 128 were between 1 and 5 years, and 151 were older than 5 years. A total of 190 children continued with a therapeutic program at home or at a rehabilitation institute. One hundred and fifty were described as showing "some improvement" in gait and posture with 42 of these children described as "markedly improved." Criteria for improvement were not clearly described. The author suggests that NMES may enhance the development of underdeveloped motor function in some children with CP.

Other researchers[141,142] have reported that NMES can facilitate improvement of lower-extremity function by increasing muscle strength and endurance, improving gait and decreasing spasticity. Leyendecker[143] compared electrical stimulation combined with neurodevelopmental therapy to neurodevelopmental therapy alone in 20 patients with CP. The ages of the patients were not specified. The treatment course was 4 months long, divided into two 1-month intervals with a 2-month rest interval. The group using electrical stimulation combined with neurodevelopmental therapy progressed more rapidly than the group using neurodevelopmental therapy alone during the first phase, but by the end of the second phase, both groups were equally successful.

Pediatric patients with neuromuscular disorders often develop joint contractures secondary to muscle strength or tone imbalances. Severe contractures often require surgical release. After surgery, it is important to concentrate on function of the antagonist to the spastic muscle, or in time, the contracture may recur. NMES is an ideal tool to facilitate return of function through a program designed to counter the effects of existing disuse atrophy and spasticity.

Improvement of stance stability and gait patterns may involve surgical release of the Achilles [tendon Achilles lengthening (TAL)], or lengthening of the hamstring or hip-adductor muscles. NMES can facilitate restoration of muscle function following these surgeries. Kieklak and DeVahl[144] described a protocol for use following the TAL procedure. The leg is often immobilized in a short leg cast or rigid splint. Electrodes are placed prior to casting to obtain optimal ankle dorsiflexion. The active electrode is placed over the peroneal nerve just distal to the fibular head. The reference electrode is placed distally over the peroneal muscles several inches proximal to the lateral malleolus (Fig. 7–24). The current amplitude required to evoke an isometric contraction is recorded so it can be duplicated after the cast is applied. Markers are placed at the electrode site and the cast is applied. Cast windows are cut out at the marker site so the electrodes can be changed regularly and skin integrity observed. The windows are closed and secured with tape or ace wrap after the electrodes are in place. Initial stimulation parameters are designed to initiate muscle contraction of the ankle dorsiflexors but avoid excessive tension development in the muscles to allow healing and proper positioning of the ankle inside the cast. The frequency is set at 3 pps with a gradual ramp-up time of 8 seconds and a total on time of 15 seconds. Ten seconds off

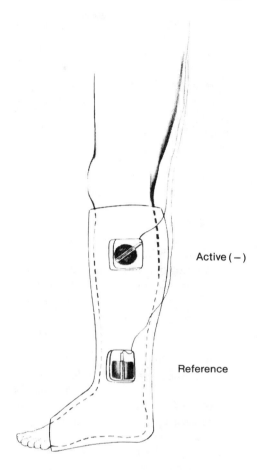

Active (–)

Reference

FIGURE 7–24. Electrode placement to elicit isometric contraction of the ankle dorsiflexors during cast immobilization following lengthening of the Achilles tendon. (Reprinted with permission from Medtronic, Inc., © Medtronic, Inc., 1991.)

time usually provides sufficient recovery time. Treatment sessions are brief (15 minutes) but are applied several times per day. As the muscle becomes accustomed to the electrical stimulus, the frequency is increased to 30 to 50 pps and the on-to-off cycle is increased to 20 and 10 seconds. Treatment sessions are increased to 1 hour, three times per day. When the cast is removed, the patient is ready for the gait training program as described previously in the orthotic substitution section.

Patients with Duchenne muscular dystrophy (DMD) experience progressive, debilitating weakness. There is evidence suggesting that the muscle properties of patients with DMD resemble those of immature muscle with prolonged contraction and relaxation times.[145] The application of low-frequency (5 to 10 pps) NMES was studied by Scott and associates[146] in 16 boys with DMD, ages 5 to 12 years. Stimulation was applied to the anterior tibialis muscles for three, 1-hour sessions daily. Patients participated in the study from 7 to 11 weeks. There was a significant increase in the mean maximum voluntary contraction force of the stimulated leg compared to each subject's unstimulated leg. The authors concluded that the muscles affected by DMD can benefit from chronic low frequency stimulation, provided that the child is not yet severely debilitated, and has the ability to generate some voluntary muscle activity.

NMES can be integrated into a variety of traditional therapy programs for pediatric patients as described in clinical protocols by Kieklak and DeVahl.[144,147]

GUIDELINES FOR THE PEDIATRIC PATIENT

1. NMES is a new and unusual sensation, therefore parameters should be adjusted slowly.
2. It may take several sessions before the child will accept intensity levels that produce a strong tingling sensation; it may take up to 1 week to develop a functional muscle contraction.
   a. For the first session, apply electrodes, but do not turn the stimulator on.
   b. At the next session, start with the stimulation at a low frequency (3 to 10 pps) and tell the child that he or she will feel a "tapping" sensation. Lightly tap the electrode with your finger to simulate the sensation before turning on the unit.
   c. Start with the stimulation intensity at a sensory level only, then increase as tolerated until a twitch contraction is seen or palpated.
   d. When an amplitude sufficient to get a muscle contraction is tolerated, increase the frequency to cause a tetanized contraction and a "tingling" sensation.
   e. If the child has adequate comprehension and coordination skills to adjust the amplitude, allow him or her to do so.
3. Electrodes should be trimmed so that stimulation is focused over the target muscle without causing overflow to other muscles. Never trim electrodes smaller than 1.5 cm in diameter, or the stimulation may become uncomfortable or injure the skin. The reference electrode is often larger than the active electrode in a monopolar placement design.
4. If overflow to the antagonist occurs, move the reference electrode closer to the active one to keep the current flow more superficial.
5. Start with brief (10-minute) sessions.
6. When the desired response is obtained and easily reproduced, family members may be taught to apply electrodes and adjust the stimulator for use in home treatment.
7. In children, when muscle-surface area is limited in size, two muscle groups that act synergistically may be stimulated simultaneously using only two electrodes. One electrode is placed over each muscle belly. For example, to facilitate wrist and elbow extension as a protective reaction, place one electrode over the muscle bellies of the dorsal forearm and the other electrode over the triceps.
8. In children it is especially important to watch for nonverbal signs that the stimulation is being felt, such as changes in facial expression, behavior, breathing, or heart rate.
9. Use of a remote hand or heel switch allows the therapist to trigger stimulation during functional activities when needed. For example, the therapist may use a heel switch to trigger the stimulation while keeping both hands free to stabilize or guide the child's actions on a balance board, bolster, or therapy ball.

A LOOK TOWARD THE FUTURE

NMES has tremendous potential for improving the function of patients with a variety of neurologic and musculoskeletal conditions, as well as for enhancing athletic performance. Additional research is needed to determine the specific doses required to obtain optimal treatment or training goals. Additional information is needed regarding the long-term physiologic effects of short- and long-term NMES programs.

One of the areas that has been extensively pursued in the laboratory setting, but is not yet a part of common clinical practice, is the computer-controlled NMES programs for improving function of paralyzed muscle, specifically in spinal cord injured patients. This application is appropriately called functional electrical stimulation (FES) because the goal is to provide the patient with return of a functional skill, such as walking or voluntary grasp and release. Microcircuitry enables the use of multiple channels of stimulation to recruit muscles in appropriate synergistic order in response to a control signal. The control signal can be triggered manually by a button on an assistive device, or by an automatic mechanical signal on a bicycle pedal. It also may be a physiologic signal generated by changes in muscle activity or the voice.

Ambulation can be facilitated in paraplegic patients using a variety of methods. A four-channel FES system can produce a primitive walking pattern with surface stimulation of the quadriceps femoris muscles bilaterally for the double-stance phase of gait, unilateral quadriceps stimulation for the single-stance phase, and cutaneous stimulation of the flexion-withdrawl reflex in the lower extremity for the swing phase.[148-151] Such a system can be triggered with manual controls on the patient's walker or crutches. EMG signals from the intact thoracic erector spinae muscles bilaterally have also been used as a control signal. Two additional channels of stimulation applied to the gluteus medius and tensor fascia latae or gluteus maximus have been suggested to provide better control of the pelvis.[152,153] Patients using these FES systems have been able to stand, transfer, and ambulate on a limited basis in a supervised environment.[151] However, a patient may not be safe in an unsupervised environment; in the event of a malfunction of the electrical system, the patient would be unable to control his or her lower limbs and could sustain a serious injury.

Petrofsky and associates[154] designed a system that combines orthotics and FES to allay the concern for injury in case of electrical failure. Six channels of stimulation plus the use of a Louisiana State University reciprocating-gait orthosis (RGO) provides postural support and stability in case of an electrical-system failure. The FES increases the efficiency and speed of movement, allowing the patient to ambulate with less energy consumption than with the RGO alone.

Additional research is being conducted to study the feasibility of implanted FES systems for ambulation. These are meant to address concerns over the durability and reliability of equipment and the amount of time needed to apply multichannel external systems. Up to 26 channels of stimulation have been used to control the lower extremity muscles through percutaneous intramuscular electrodes.[155,156] Complex patterns of movement can be programmed, allowing the patient to ascend and descend stairs (with the skilled use of a walker or crutches) in addition to ambulating on level surfaces.[157] This research has shown that FES with implanted electrodes is feasible, but patient safety remains a concern. A closed-loop system that provides feedback to the computer to make automatic changes in the program is necessary. For example, in an open-loop system, if a patient caught a foot on the walker, the computer would continue to send signals to the muscles to continue the ambulation pattern. This continuation without modification might cause a fall and possible injury. A closed-loop system would provide feedback of such an incident to the computer and trigger modifications of computer signals, thus halting progress and allowing proper positioning of the limbs to avoid a fall.[157-160]

Computer control has been incorporated into exercise equipment for the spinal cord injured patient. Bicycle ergometers can be powered by paralyzed muscles given appropriately timed electrical stimulation. The primary goal of this form of exercise is to improve the patient's cardiovascular strength by exercising the large muscles of the body.[161] In addition, increases in muscular strength and endurance have been observed, contributing to the conditioning that is necessary for FES ambulation programs. An enhanced self-image may also be associated with muscle hypertrophy and improved physical fitness. Additionally, improved fitness may decrease the incidence of urinary tract infections, decubitus ulcers, pneumonia, and osteoporosis.

Functional control of the muscles of the upper limb is also possible using multiple-channel NMES. Implanted electrodes with an internally or externally placed power supply can provide input from four to eight channels of stimulation for C-5– and C-6–level quadriplegic patients.[162,163] Stimulation of various combinations of muscles in the hand and forearm enable the patient to use the paralyzed upper limb in several functional grasp patterns. Control may be provided by voluntary changes in shoulder position of the contralateral extremity. These systems use advanced microprocessors and microcircuitry to provide reliability and require low maintenance. Research continues to evaluate the response of muscle tissue to implanted electrodes over extended periods of stimulation.

Voice-controlled signals have been used to control upper-limb stimulation for functional tasks.[164,165] Instructions for movement patterns and the muscles necessary to carry out the movement are preprogrammed into the computer controller. A verbal command is recognized by the computer which activates the specific program designed to carry out the task. Cooper and associates[165] have shown that 2 to 3 months of NMES can significantly increase the force output of paralyzed muscles in C-5– and C-6–level quadriplegic patients. "Vocabularies" of 10 to 25 words can be used to produce upper-extremity motor control with stimulation provided by surface electrodes imbedded in a custom-plastic orthosis. The benefit of this system is that the patient simply "thinks aloud" to control the paralyzed extremity.

Computer technology can assist clinicians and individuals involved in training elite athletes to analyze human performance and disability to a greater degree than current techniques allow. The use of NMES to initiate and reinforce proper movement as analyzed and controlled by the computer system should allow precise and efficient motor retraining to occur. Exciting new treatment options will be possible with the advancement of bioengineering capabilities and ongoing basic and clinical research.

CASE STUDY

The following case presentation is designed to demonstrate the use of NMES as part of a comprehensive rehabilitation program to facilitate improved function for a patient with left hemiparesis following a CVA. A 63-year-old woman sustained a right CVA 3 weeks previously. The infarct occurred in a branch of the right-middle cerebral artery, leaving her alert, oriented, and cognitively functional, but with significant neuromuscular deficits in her left limbs. Initially, she was unable to voluntarily move her left arm or leg, although deep tendon reflexes were present. She could not turn herself in bed or sit up without assistance. She demonstrated neglect of the left side of her body.

Three days following the CVA she began a physical rehabilitation program and made steady progress. She now is able to move about in bed independently, although she occasionally turns onto her left side and unwittingly lies on her left arm unaware that she is doing so. She demonstrates impaired cutaneous sensation and proprioception throughout her left arm. She is able to assume and maintain a functional sitting position independently, and is able to stand with supervision and ambulate with assistance, using a quadriped cane.

TABLE 7–3 Results of Manual Muscle Test for Case Study

Muscle	Grade Prior to NMES Program	Grade Following 2 Weeks of NMES
Upper trapezius	Good	Good+
Deltoid (all portions)	Poor–	Fair (limited range)
Rhomboid major/minor	Poor	Fair
Infraspinatus/teres minor/subscapularis	Poor–	Fair
Pectoralis major	Fair	Good
Biceps brachii	Poor+	Good
Triceps brachii	Trace	Fair
Pronator teres	Poor	Good
Supinator	0	Poor
Extensor carpi radialis	0	Poor–
Extensor carpi ulnaris	0	Poor–
Extensor digitorum	0	Poor
Flexor carpi radialis	Trace	Fair
Flexor carpi ulnaris	Trace	Fair
Flexor digitorum profundus	0	Poor+
Extensor pollicis longus	0	Poor–
Flexor pollicis longus	0	Poor
Opponens pollicis	0	Poor

Voluntary control of the patient's left arm has not progressed as rapidly. She can shrug her left shoulder and flex her left elbow minimally. This lack of independent function of her left arm is particularly distressing to the patient, since she is the organist in her church and enjoys gardening and handicrafts. The patient expresses a strong desire to regain the functional use of her left arm, commensurate with the return of neuromuscular control that she now perceives in her left leg.

Following a strength evaluation of the patient's left arm (Table 7–3), an NMES program was initiated to facilitate function in the proximal muscles in order to attain proximal stability and prevent shoulder subluxation. It is recognized that some clinicians prefer to evaluate strength in terms of function in patients with central nervous system dysfunction. However, a single, objective functional assessment of strength for patients with this kind of deficit is not widely accepted by clinicians, whereas the manual muscle test provides an often-used and generally accepted determination of strength.

Surface electrodes were applied over the left supraspinatus and posterior deltoid muscles, as shown in Figure 7–21. A portable NMES device delivering an asymmetric biphasic square wave was connected to the electrode lead wires, and stimulation parameters were initially set as described in Table 7–4.

The patient has a history of cardiac arrythmias, so her heart rate and blood pressure were monitored prior to, during, and after stimulation sessions in physical therapy for 2 days. No adverse effects were noted. The stimulation program was initiated while the patient was still in the hospital. Because the sessions in physical therapy were well tolerated, the NMES program was expanded to four times per day. Electrodes were applied during the morning therapy session and the first session was completed while she participated in gait training activities. The NMES device provided her with sufficient support of the shoulder musculature to allow

TABLE 7–4 Suggested Stimulus Settings for Initial NMES Program
to Reduce Shoulder Subluxation: Case History

Stimulus Parameter	Suggested Setting
Frequency	30 pps
Phase duration	0.3 ms
Amplitude	30–35 mA (sufficient to generate "poor" grade contraction of the stimulated muscles while avoiding shoulder elevation)
Ramp-up/ramp-down time	4/2 s
Total on time	10 s
Total off time	20 s
Treatment duration	15 minutes; two times daily

her left arm to remain freely by her side, resulting in improved balance. She independently turned on the stimulator at lunch and dinner time—an easy time schedule for the patient to remember. An additional treatment was carried out during the afternoon physical therapy session.

The stimulation program progressed with the goal of building endurance of the supraspinatus and posterior deltoid. Sessions were increased to 30 minutes, and after 1 week of stimulation, 60-minute treatments were tolerated easily. At that time, the stimulus on time was increased to 15 seconds and the off time shortened to 15 seconds. The amplitude was increased to 45 mA, which provided a strong visible contraction, but did not cause abduction or extension of the humerus.

The patient began to complain that her shoulder ached in the evening when she went to bed. Two possible causes were considered. First, the timing cycle did not provide adequate time for recovery of the working muscles, and the aching was due to fatigue and possible build up of metabolites. The second possibility was that the increased strength of the muscle contraction caused some compression of the head of the humerus against the glenoid fossa or capsular structures. The program was modified by increasing the off time to 20 seconds and decreasing the amplitude to 40 mA. Mobilization of the glenohumeral joint and scapula with passive range-of-motion exercises also assisted in eliminating any complaints of pain.

After the patient had received the shoulder-stimulation program for 2 weeks her strength improved substantially, as shown in Table 7–3. She was able to use her left arm to secure a piece of paper while writing with her right hand. She was able to touch the top of her head and to reach out for a door knob. Her grip strength was insufficient to pick up items independently, although she was able to hold an item, such as a rolled-up washcloth, if it was positioned in her hand. Fortunately, the patient demonstrated only slight hypertonicity in the finger and elbow flexors.

During the third week of rehabilitation, stimulation of the shoulder musculature was continued to increase strength and endurance for functional activities that required overhead motions, such as washing her hair. The middle or anterior deltoid was stimulated instead of the posterior deltoid. In addition, NMES was used to facilitate muscle re-education of the wrist extensors and finger flexors. Initially, the wrist extensors and finger flexors were stimulated independently, in combination with her therapeutic exercise program. Later, these two muscle groups were stimulated simultaneously, with a slightly shorter ramp time for the wrist extensors, to adequately position the wrist prior to eliciting flexion of the fingers. The patient continued to work on this skill at home after discharge. She practiced diligently, three to four times a day. As the stimulator began to cycle on, she attempted to grasp objects of varying sizes and weights. She gripped the object and reached across the table, releasing the object when the stimulation cycled off.

The patient continued outpatient physical therapy twice a week for a total of 3 months. At discharge she was able to hold the material of her blouse with her left hand while she manipulated the button into the buttonhole with her right hand. She was able to use both hands to put away dishes on a shelf at shoulder height. She could dress and bathe independently. She required assistance for heavy housework, but could perform light activities, such as dusting, independently. She is beginning to practice simple drills on the organ as her prime therapeutic activity and has discontinued the use of the NMES device.

The patient's prognosis and recovery after stroke were based on several factors, such as her general health, the type and location of the CVA, emergency care, motivation, and therapeutic interventions. It is impossible to define the specific role played by NMES, but this modality provides the clinician with a tool toward obtaining many of the goals of rehabilitation.

SUMMARY

Neuromuscular electrical stimulation offers a treatment adjunct to therapeutic exercise, traditional orthotics, and functional training for the management of a variety of orthopedic and neuromuscular conditions. Clinical research continues to substantiate the benefits of NMES for the deterence of disuse atrophy, maintenance and improvement of mobility, muscle re-education, spasticity reduction, and augmentation of motor-unit recruitment to enhance training in healthy individuals and elite athletes. NMES offers versatility, enabling the clinician to customize a neuromuscular facilitation program to an individual client's capabilities, needs, and goals. Additional suggestions for the integration of NMES in a comprehensive rehabilitation program are provided for orthopedic and neurologic patients, in Chapters 11 and 12, respectively.

REFERENCES

1. Kellaway, P: The William Osler Medal essay: Part played by electric fish in early history of bioelectricity and electrical therapy. Bull Hist Med 20:112, 1946.
2. Roberts, B: Medical Electricity: A Practical Treatise on the Applications of Electricity to Medicine and Surgery. Lea Brothers & Company, Philadelphia, 1887.
3. Aberti, CL: DeVi Electrica in Amenorrhea. Gottinger, 1764. In Licht, S: History of electrotherapy. In Stillwell, GR (ed): Therapeutic Electricity and Ultraviolet Radiation. Williams & Wilkins, Baltimore, 1983, p 6.
4. Evans, C: Medical observations and inquiries by a society of physicians in London, I:83, 1757.
5. Wesley, J: The Desideratum: Or Electricity Made Plain and Useful. Bailliére, Tindall, & Cox, London, 1759.
6. McNeal, DR: 2000 years of electrical stimulation. In Hambrecht, FT and Reswick, JB (eds): Functional Electrical Stimulation: Applications in Neural Prostheses. Marcel Dekker, New York, 1977, pp 12, 15, 16.
7. Duchenne, DB: Physiologie des Mouvements. Baillie're et Fils, Paris, 1867.
8. LaPicque, L: Definition experimental de l'excitabilite. Compte Rend Soc Biol 67:28, 1909.
9. Adrian, ED: The electrical reactions of muscles before and after injury. Brain 39:1, 1916.

10. Shriber, WJ: A Manual of Electrotherapy. Lea & Febiger, Philadelphia, 1975, pp 144, 178.
11. Liberson, WT, et al.: Functional electrotherapy: Stimulation of the peroneal nerve synchronized with the swing phase of gait of hemiplegic patients. Arch Phys Med Rehabil 42:101, 1961.
12. Jack, JJB, Noble, D, and Tsien, RW: Electric Current Flow in Excitable Cells. Clarendon Press, Oxford, 1983.
13. Guyton, AC: Human Physiology and Mechanisms of Disease. WB Saunders, Philadelphia, 1982, p 98.
14. Benton, LA, et al: Functional Electrical Stimulation: A Practical Clinical Guide. Rancho Los Amigos Engineering Center, Downey, CA, 1981, pp 30, 31, 33, 34, 37–41, 42, 54, 57, 62, 69.
15. Salmons, S and Henriksson, J: The adaptive response of skeletal muscle to increased use. Muscle and Nerve 4:94, 1981.
16. Hudlicka, D, et al: Early changes in fiber profile and capillary density in long-term stimulated muscles. Am J Physiol. 243:H528, 1982.
17. Sreter, FA, et al: Fast to slow transformation of fast muscles in response to long-term phasic stimulation. Exp Neurol 75:95, 1982.
18. Greathouse, DG, et al: Effects of short-term electrical stimulation on the ultrastructure of rat skeletal muscles. Phys Ther 66:946, 1986.
19. Munsat, TL, McNeal, D, and Waters, R: Effects of nerve stimulation on human muscle. Arch Neurol 33:608, 1976.
20. Eriksson, E and Haggmark, T: Comparison of isometric muscle training and electrical stimulation supplementing isometric muscle training in the recovery after major knee ligament surgery. Am J Sports Med 7:169, 1979.
21. Stanish, WD, et al: The effects of immobilization and electrical stimulation on muscle glycogen and myofibrillar ATPase. Can Appl Sport Sci 7:267, 1982.
22. Nelson, HE, et al: Electrode effectiveness during transcutaneous motor stimulation. Arch Phys Med Rehabil 61:73, 1980.
23. Alon, G: High voltage stimulation. Effects of electrode size on basic excitatory responses. Phys Ther 65:890, 1985.
24. Griffin, JE and Karselis, TC: Physical Agents for Physical Therapists. Charles C Thomas, Springfield, IL, 1978, pp 58, 59, 73, 74.
25. McNeal, DR and Baker, LL: Effects of joint angle, electrodes and waveform on electrical stimulation of the quadriceps and hamstrings. Ann Biomed Eng 16:299, 1988.
26. Pfleuger, EFW: Ueber die tetanisierende Wirkung des Constanten Stromes und das Allgemeingesetz der Reizung. Virchow's Arch 3:13, 1858.
27. Baker, LL, Bowman, BR, and McNeal, DR: Effects of waveform on comfort during neuromuscular electrical stimulation. Clin Orthop 233:75, 1988.
28. Bowman, BR and Baker LL: Effects of waveform parameters on comfort during transcutaneous neuromuscular electrical stimulation. Ann Biomed Eng 13:59, 1985.
29. Gracanin, F and Trnkoczy, A: Optimal stimulus parameters for minimum pain in the chronic stimulation of innervated muscle. Arch Phys Med Rehabil 56:243, 1975.
30. Jones, DA, Bigland-Ritchie, B, and Edwards, RHT: Excitation frequency and muscle fatigue, mechanical responses during voluntary and stimulated contraction. Exp Neurol 64:401, 1979.
31. Packman-Braun, R: Relationship between functional electrical stimulation duty cycle and fatigue in wrist extensor muscles of patients with hemiparesis. Phys Ther 68:51, 1988.
32. Cole, KE, et al: Muscle fatigue during electrically induced isometric contractions at varying duty cycles (abstr). Phys Ther 67:792, 1987.
33. Volosin, KJ, et al: Use of external muscle stimulation in a patient with a unipolar DDD pacemaker. PACE 10:958, 1987.
34. Shade, SK: Use of transcutaneous electrical nerve stimulation for a patient with a cardiac pacemaker. A case report. Phys Ther 65:206, 1985.
35. Rasmussen, MJ, et al: Can transcutaneous electrical nerve stimulation be safely used in patients with permanent cardiac pacemakers? Mayo Clin Proc 63:443, 1988.
36. Balmaseda, MT, et al: Burns in functional electrical stimulation: Two case reports. Arch Phys Med Rehabil 68:452, 1987.
37. Zugerman, C: Dermatitis from transcutaneous electric nerve stimulation. J Am Acad Dermatol 6:936, 1982.
38. Fisher, AA: Dermatitis associated with transcutaneous electrical nerve stimulation. Cutis 21:24, 1978.
39. Castelain, P-Y and Chabeau, G: Contact dermatitis after transcutaneous electrical analgesia. Contact Dermatitis 15:32, 1986.
40. Food and Drug Administration Compliance Policy Guidelines. Guide Number 7124.26, Chapter 24. Devices, July 1, 1982.
41. Sargeant, AJ, et al: Functional and structural changes after disuse of human muscle. Clinical Science and Molecular Medicine 52:337, 1977.
42. Edstrom, L: Selective atrophy of red muscle fibres in the quadriceps in long-standing knee-joint dysfunction. Injuries to the anterior cruciate ligament. J Neurol Sci 11:551, 1970.
43. Haggmark, T, Jansson, E, and Eriksson, E: Fiber type area and metabolic potential of the thigh muscle in man after knee surgery and immobilization. Int J Sports Med 2:12, 1981.

44. Baugher, WH, et al: Quadriceps atrophy in the anterior cruciate insufficient knee. Am J Sports Med 12:192, 1984.
45. Spencer, JD, Hayes, KC, and Alexander, W: Knee joint effusion and quadriceps reflex inhibition in man. Arch Phys Med Rehabil 65:171, 1984.
46. Almekinders, LC: Transcutaneous muscle stimulation for rehabilitation. Physician and Sports Medicine 12:118, 1984.
47. Gould, N, et al: Transcutaneous muscle stimulation as a method to retard disuse atrophy. Clin Orthop 164:215, 1982.
48. Gould, N, et al: Transcutaneous muscle stimulation to retard disuse atrophy after open meniscectomy. Clin Orthop 178:190, 1983.
49. Arvidsson, I, et al: Prevention of quadriceps wasting after immobilization: An evaluation of the effect of electrical stimulation. Orthopedics 9:1519, 1986.
50. Buckley, DC, et al: Transcutaneous muscle stimulation promotes muscle growth in immobilized patients. J Parenter Nutr 11:547, 1987.
51. Wigerstad-Lossing, I, et al: Effects of electrical muscle stimulation combined with voluntary contractions after knee ligament surgery. Med Sci Sport Exerc 20:93, 1988.
52. Morrissey, MC, et al: The effects of electrical stimulation on the quadriceps during postoperative knee immobilization. Am J Sports Med 13:40, 1985.
53. Bouletreau, P, et al: Effects of intermittent electrical stimulation on muscle catabolism in intensive care patients. J Parenter Nutr 11:552, 1987.
54. Bohannon, RW: Effect of electrical stimulation to the vastus medialis muscle in a patient with chronically dislocating patellae. Phys Ther 63:1445, 1983.
55. Johnson, DH, Thurston, P, and Ashcroft, JF: The Russian technique of faradism in the treatment of chondromalacia patellae. Physiotherapy Canada 29:1, 1977.
56. Baker, LL and Parker, K: Neuromuscular electrical stimulation of the muscles surrounding the shoulder. Phys Ther 6:1930, 1986.
57. Cannon, NM and Strickland, JW: Therapy following flexor tendon surgery. Hand Clin 1:147, 1985.
58. Haug, J and Wood, LT: Efficacy of neuromuscular stimulation of the quadriceps femoris during continuous passive motion following total knee arthroplasty. Arch Phys Med Rehabil 69:423, 1988.
59. Apfel, LM, et al: Functional electrical stimulation in intrinsic/extrinsic imbalanced burned hands. J Burn Care Rehabil 8:97, 1987.
60. Baker, LL, et al: Electrical stimulation of wrist and fingers for hemiplegic patients. Phys Ther 59:1495, 1979.
61. Bowman, BR, Baker, LL, and Waters, RL: Positional feedback and electrical stimulation: An automated treatment for the hemiplegic wrist. Arch Phys Med Rehabil 60:497, 1979.
62. Winchester, P, et al: Effects of feedback stimulation training and cyclic electrical stimulation on knee extension in hemiparetic patients. Phys Ther 63:1096, 1983.
63. Bach-y-Rita, P: Sensory substitution: The basis for a new therapy. In New Directions in Rehabilitation Medicine: Retraining Neuromuscular Function with EMG Sensory Feedback Therapy. Cordis Corp, Miami, FL, 1981, p 10.
64. Bishop, B: Neural plasticity, Part 2: Postnatal maturation and function-induced plasticity. Phys Ther 62:1132, 1982.
65. Bishop, B: Neural plasticity, Part 3: Responses to lesions in the peripheral nervous system. Phys Ther 62:1275, 1982.
66. Craik, RL: Clinical correlates of neural plasticity. Phys Ther 62:1452, 1982.
67. Howson, DC: Peripheral neural excitability: Implications for transcutaneous electrical nerve stimulation. Phys Ther 58:1467, 1978.
68. Teng, EL, et al: Electrical stimulation and feedback training on the voluntary control of paretic muscles. Arch Phys Med Rehabil 57:228, 1976.
69. Carnstam, B, Larsson, L-E, and Prevec, TS: Improvement of gait following functional electrical stimulation. Scand J Rehabil Med 9:7, 1977.
70. Gracanin, F: Functional electrical stimulation in control of motor output and movements. In Cobb, WA and Van Duijn, H (eds): Contemporary Clinical Neurophysiology (EEG Suppl). Elsevier, Amsterdam, 1978, p 355.
71. Cozean, CD, Pease, WS, and Hubbell, SL: Biofeedback and functional electrical stimulation in stroke rehabilitation. Arch Phys Med Rehabil 69:401, 1988.
72. Landau, WM: Spasticity: What is it? What is it not? In Feldman, RG, Young, RR, and Koella, WP (eds): Spasticity: Disordered Motor Control. Year Book Medical Publishers, Chicago, 1980, p 18.
73. Levine, MG, Knott, M, and Kabat, H: Relaxation of spasticity by electrical stimulation of antagonist muscles. Arch Phys Med Rehabil 33:668, 1952.
74. Merletti, KR, et al: A control study of muscle force recovery in hemiparetic patients during treatment with functional electrical stimulation. Scand J Rehabil Med 10:147, 1978.
75. Fulbright, JS: Electrical stimulation to reduce chronic toe-flexor hypertonicity: A case report. Phys Ther 64:523, 1984.
76. Alfieri, V: Electrical treatment of spasticity. Scand J Rehabil Med 1:177, 1982.

77. Vodovnik, L, et al: Spinal and cerebral spasticity: Modifications by electrical stimulation. Presented at the 9th Annual Conference of the Engineering in Medicine and Biology Society, 1987.
78. Dimitrijevic, MR and Nathan PW: Studies of spasticity in man: 4. Changes in flexion reflex with repetitive cutaneous stimulation in spinal man. Brain 93:743, 1970.
79. Walker, JB: Modulation of spasticity: Prolonged suppression of a spinal reflex by electrical stimulation. Science 216:203, 1982.
80. Robinson, CJ, Kett, NA, and Bolam, JM: Spasticity in spinal and injured patients: 1. Short-term effects of surface electrical stimulation. Arch Phy Med Rehabil 69:598, 1988.
81. Robinson, CJ, Kett, NA, and Bolam, JM: Spasticity in spinal and injured patients: 2. Initial measures and long-term effects of surface electrical stimulation. Arch Phys Med Rehabil 69:862, 1988.
82. Vodovnik, L, Stefanovska, A, and Bajd, T: Effects of stimulation parameters on modification of spinal spasticity. Med Biol Eng Comput 25:439, 1987.
83. Takebe, K and Basmajian, JV: Gait analysis in stroke patients to assess treatment of foot drop. Arch Phys Med Rehabil 57:305, 1976.
84. Merletti, R, et al: Clinical experience of electronic peroneal stimulators in 50 hemiplegic patients. Scand J Rehabil Med 11:111, 1979.
85. Cybulski, GR, Penn, RD, and Jaeger, JF: Lower extremity functional neuromuscular stimulation in cases of spinal cord injury. Neurosurg 15:132, 1984.
86. Packman, RA and Ewaski, B: Respond II Gait Training Protocol. Medtronic, Minneapolis, 1983.
87. Lee, KH and Johnston, R: Electrically induced flexion reflex in gait training of hemiplegic patients: Induction of the reflex. Arch Phys Med Rehabil 57:311, 1976.
88. Kahanovitz, N, Snow, B, and Pinter, I: The comparative results of psychologic testing in scoliosis patients treated with electrical stimulation or bracing. Spine 9:442, 1984.
89. Bobechko, WP, Herbert, MA, and Friedman, HG: Electrospinal instrumentation for scoliosis: Current status. Orthop Clin North Am 10:927, 1979.
90. Friedman, HG, Herbert, MA, and Bobechko, WP: Electrical stimulation for scoliosis. Am Fam Physician 25:155, 1982.
91. Herbert, MA and Bobechko, WP: Paraspinal muscle stimulation for the treatment of idiopathic scoliosis in children. Orthopedics 10:1125, 1987.
92. Schultz, A, Haderspeck, K, and Takashima S: Correction of scoliosis by muscle stimulation. Biomechanical analysis. Spine 6:468, 1981.
93. Schmitt, O: Electrical stimulation of intercostal muscles in idiopathic scoliosis. Artificial Organs 5 (Suppl)5:589, 1981.
94. Fisher, DA, Rapp, GF, and Emkes, M: Idiopathic scoliosis: Transcutaneous muscle stimulation versus the Milwaukee brace. Spine 12:987, 1987.
95. Axelgaard, J and Brown, JC: Lateral electrical surface stimulation for the treatment of progressive idiopathic scoliosis. Spine 8:242, 1983.
96. Axelgaard, J, Norwall, A, and Brown, JC: Correction of spinal curvatures by transcutaneous electrical muscle stimulation. Spine 8:463, 1983.
97. Axelgaard, J: Transcutaneous electrical muscle stimulation for the treatment of progressive spinal curvature deformities. Int J Rehabil Med 6:31, 1984.
98. Bradford, DS, Tanguy, A, and Vanselow, J: Surface electrical stimulation in the treatment of idiopathic scoliosis: Preliminary results in 30 patients. Spine 8:757, 1983.
99. McCollough, NC: Nonoperative treatment of idiopathic scoliosis using surface electrical stimulation. Spine 11:802, 1986.
100. Rapp, G: Idiopathic scoliosis: Transcutaneous muscle stimulation versus Milwaukee brace (abstr). Orthopaedic Transactions 11:501, 1987.
101. Sullivan, JA, et al: Further evaluation of the Scolitron treatment of idiopathic adolescent scoliosis. Spine 11:903, 1986.
102. Goldberg, C, et al: Electro-spinal stimulation in children with adolescent and juvenile scoliosis. Spine 13:482, 1988.
103. O'Donnell, CS, et al: Electrical stimulation in the treatment of idiopathic scoliosis. Clin Orthop 229:107, 1988.
104. Bylund, P, et al: Is lateral electrical surface stimulation an effective treatment for scoliosis? J Pediatr Orthop 7:298, 1987.
105. Grimby, G, et al: Changes in histochemical profile of muscle after long-term electrical stimulation in patients with idiopathic scoliosis. Scand J Rehabil Med 17:191, 1985.
106. Velazquez, RJ, et al: Histological and histochemical characteristics of skeletal muscle after long-term intermittent electrical stimulation in idiopathic scoliosis (abstr). Orthopaedic Transactions 10:613, 1986.
107. Basmajian, JV and Bazant, FJ: Factors preventing downward dislocation of the adducted shoulder joint. J Bone Joint Surg 41-A:1182, 1959.
108. Chaco, J and Wolf, E: Subluxation of the glenohumeral joint in hemiplegia. Am J Phys Med 50:139, 1971.
109. Griffin, JW: Hemiplegic shoulder pain. Phys Ther 12:1884, 1986.
110. Van Ouwenaller, C, Laplace, PM, and Chantraine, A: Painful shoulder in hemiplegia. Arch Phys Med Rehabil 67:23, 1986.

111. Hurd, MM, Farrell, KH, and Waylonis, GW: Shoulder sling for hemiplegia: Friend or foe? Arch Phys Med Rehabil 55:519, 1974.
112. Eiguren, BE and Baker, L: Respons II (TM) shoulder subluxation protocol. Medtronic, Minneapolis, 1984.
113. Kots, Y: Notes from lectures and laboratory periods. Canadian-Soviet Exchange Symposium on Electro-stimulation of Skeletal Muscles (translated by Babkin, I and Timtsenko, N). Concordia University, Montreal, Quebec, December 6–15, 1977.
114. Currier, DP, Lehman, J, and Lightfoot, P: Electrical stimulation in exercise of the quadriceps femoris muscle. Phys Ther 59:1508, 1979.
115. Eriksson, E, et al: Effects of electrical stimulation on human skeletal muscle. Int J Sports Med 2:18, 1981.
116. McMiken, DF, Todd-Smith, M, and Thompson, C: Strengthening of human quadriceps muscles by cutaneous electrical stimulation. Scand J Rehabil Med 15:25, 1983.
117. Kramer, JF and Semple, JE: Comparison of selected strengthening techniques for normal quadriceps. Physiotherapy Canada 35:300, 1983.
118. Kramer, J, et al: Comparison of voluntary and electrical stimulation contraction torques. J Orthop Sports Phys Ther 5:324, 1984.
119. Hartsell, HD: Electrical muscle stimulation and isometric exercise effects on selected quadriceps parameters. J Orthop Sports Phys Ther 8:203, 1986.
120. Nobbs, LA and Rhodes, ED: The effect of electrical stimulation and isokinetic exercise on muscular power of the quadriceps femoris. J Orthop Sports Phys Ther 8:260, 1986.
121. Fahey, TD, et al: Influence of sex differences and knee joint position on electrical stimulated-modulated strength increases. Med Sci Sports Exerc 17:144, 1985.
122. Walmsley, RP, Letts, G, and Vooys, J: A comparison of torque generated by knee extension with a maximal voluntary muscle contraction vis-a-vis electrical stimulation. J Orthop Sports Phys Ther 6:10, 1984.
123. Wolf, SL, et al: The effect of muscle stimulation during resistive training on performance parametes. Am J Sports Med 14:18, 1986.
124. Moreno-Aranda, J and Seireg, A: Electrical parameters for over-the-skin muscle stimulation. J Biomech 14:579, 1981.
125. Laughman, RK, et al: Strength changes in the normal quadriceps femoris muscle as a result of electrical stimulation. Phys Ther 63:494, 1983.
126. Currier, DP and Mann, R: Muscle strength development by electrical stimulation in healthy individuals. Phys Ther 63:915, 1983.
127. Boutelle, D, Smith, B, and Malone, T: A strength study utilizing the Electro Stim 180. J Orthop Sports Phys Ther 7:50, 1985.
128. Kubiak, RJ, Whitman, KM, and Johnston, RM: Changes in quadriceps femoris muscle strength using isometric exercise versus electrical stimulation. J Orthop Sports Phys Ther 8:537, 1987.
129. Delitto, A and Rose, SJ: Comparative comfort of three waveforms used in electrically eliciting quadriceps femoris muscle contractions. Phys Ther 66:1704, 1986.
130. Selkowitz, DM: Improvement in isometric strength training of the quadriceps femoris muscle after training with electrical stimulation. Phys Ther 65:186, 1985.
131. Soo, CL, Currier, DP, and Threlkeld, AJ: Augmenting voluntary torque of healthy muscle by optimization of electrical stimulation. Phys Ther 68:333, 1988.
132. Parker, MG, et al: Fatigue response in human quadriceps femoris muscle during high frequency electrical stimulation. J Orthop Sports Phys Ther 7:145, 1986.
133. Stefanovska, A and Vodovnik, L: Change in muscle force following electrical stimulation. Scand J Rehabil Med 17:141, 1985.
134. Delitto, A, et al: Electrically elicited cocontraction of thigh musculature after anterior cruciate ligament surgery: A description and single-case experiment. Phys Ther 68:45, 1988.
135. Nitz, AJ and Dobner, JJ: High intensity electrical stimulation effect on thigh musculature during immobilization for knee sprain: A case report. Phys Ther 67:219, 1987.
136. Williams, RA, Morrissey, MC, and Brewster, CE: The effect of electrical stimulation on quadriceps strength and thigh circumference in meniscectomy patients. J Orthop Sports Phys Ther 8:143, 1986.
137. Delitto, A, et al: Electrical stimulation versus voluntary exercise in strengthening thigh musculature after anterior cruciate surgery. Phys Ther 68:660, 1988.
138. Alon, G, et al: Comparison of the effects of electrical stimulation and exercise on abdominal musculature. J Orthop Sports Phys Ther 8:567, 1987.
139. Kahanovitz, N, et al: Normal trunk muscle strength and endurance in women and the effect of exercises and electrical stimulation, Part 2, Comparative analysis of electrical stimulation and exercises to increase trunk muscle strength and endurance. Spine 12:112, 1987.
140. Lake, DA: The effects of neuromuscular electrical stimulation as applied by "toning salons" on muscle strength and body shape (abstr). Phys Ther 68:789, 1988.
141. Solomonow, M, Laborde, M, and Soboloff, H: Evaluation of the effectiveness of electrical stimulation of the leg muscles in cerebral-palsied patients. Rehabilitation R&D Progress Reports, 1986, p 167.
142. Menkveld, SR, Quinn, JR, and Ancheta, B: Functional electrical stimulation in pediatric patients with spasticity. Orthopaedic Transactions 10:376, 1986.
143. Leyendecker, C: Electrical stimulation therapy and its effects on the general activity of motor impaired

cerebral palsied children: A comparative study of the Bobath physiotherapy and its combination with Hufschmidt electrical stimulation therapy (English Abstr). Rehabilitation (Stuttg) 14:150, 1975.

144. Kieklak, H and DeVahl, J: Respond II (TM) protocol for pediatric applications. Medtronic, Inc, Minneapolis, 1986.

145. Vrbova, G: Duchenne dystrophy viewed as a disturbance of nerve-muscle interactions. Muscle Nerve 6:671, 1983.

146. Scott, OM, et al: Responses of muscles of patients with Duchenne muscular dystrophy to chronic electrical stimulation. J Neurol Neurosurg Psychiatry 49:1427, 1986.

147. Kieklak, H: Use of neuromuscular electrical stimulation (NMES) for children with neuromuscular disorders. Totline (Newsletter of the Section on Pediatrics, American Physical Therapy Association) 13:27, 1987.

148. Bajd, T, et al: The use of a four channel electrical stimulator as an ambulatory aid for paraplegic patients. Phys Ther 63:1116, 1983.

149. Graupe, D, et al: Patient controlled electrical stimulation via EMG signature discrimination for providing certain paraplegics with primitive walking functions. J Biomed Eng 5:220, 1983.

150. Braun, Z, et al: Activation of paraplegic patients by functional electrical stimulation: Training and biomechanical evaluation. Scand J Rehabil Med (Suppl) 12:93, 1985.

151. Kralj, A, Bajd, T, and Turk, R: Enhancement of gait restoration in spinal injured patients by functional electrical stimulation. Clin Orthop 233:34, 1988.

152. Kralj, A, et al: Gait restoration in paraplegic patients: A feasibility demonstration using multichannel surface electrode FES. J Rehabil Res Dev 20:3, 1983.

153. Isakov, E, Mizrahi, J, and Najenson, T: Biomechanical and physiological evaluation of FES-activated paraplegic patients. J Rehabil Res Dev 23:9, 1986.

154. Petrofsky, JS, et al: A computer-controlled walking system: The combination of an orthosis with functional electrical stimulation. J Clin Eng 11:121, 1986.

155. Marsolais, EB and Kobetic, R: Development of a practical electrical stimulation system for restoring gait in the paralyzed patient. Clin Orthop 233:64, 1988.

156. Peckham, PH: Functional electrical stimulation: Current status and future prospects of applications to the neuromuscular system in spinal cord injury. Paraplegia 25:279, 1987.

157. Marsolais, EB and Kobetic, R: Functional electrical stimulation for walking in paraplegia. J Bone Joint Surg 69-A:728, 1987.

158. Yamamoto, T and Seireg, A: Closing the loop: Electrical muscle stimulation and feedback control for smooth limb motion. SOMA October 1986, p 38.

159. Mason, CP and Gruner, JA: EMG as force-feedback in closed-loop functional electrical stimulation (abstr). J Rehabil Res Dev 24:161, 1986.

160. Gruner, JA: Considerations in designing acceptable neuromuscular stimulation systems for restoring function in paralyzed limbs. Cent Nerv Syst Trauma 3:37, 1986.

161. Ragnarsson, KT, et al: Clinical evaluation of computerized functional electrical stimulation after spinal cord injury: A multicenter pilot study. Arch Phys Med Rehabil 69:672, 1988.

162. Keith, MW, et al: Functional neuromuscular stimulation neuroprostheses for the tetraplegic hand. Clin Orthop 233:25, 1988.

163. Smith, B, et al: An externally powered, multichannel, implantable stimulator for versatile control of paralyzed muscle. IEEE Trans Biomed Eng BME-34:499, 1987.

164. Nathan, RH: Functional electrical stimulation of the upper limb: The motor nerve prosthesis. Artificial Organs (Suppl) 5:584, 1981.

165. Cooper, E, et al: A voice controlled computer system for restoring limited hand functions in quadriplegics. Proceedings from Voice I/O Systems Applications Conference. San Francisco, Oct 4-6, 1988.

SUGGESTED READINGS

Baker, L: Neuromuscular electrical stimulation in the restoration of purposeful limb movement. In Wolf, S (ed): Electrotherapy. Churchill Livingston, New York, 1981.

Kramer, JF and Mendryk, SW: Electrical stimulation as a strength improvement technique. J Orthop Sports Phys Ther 4:91, 1982.

Lloyd, T, et al: A review of the use of electromotor stimulation in human muscles. Aust J Physiother 32:18, 1986.

Rose, SJ and Rothstein, JM: Muscle mutability, Part 1, General concepts and adaptations to altered patterns of use. Phys Ther 62:1773, 1982.

Vodovnik, L, et al: Functional electrical stimulation for control of locomotor systems. CRC Crit Rev Biomed Eng 6:63, 1981.

CHAPTER 8

Electrical Stimulation of Denervated Muscle

John P. Cummings, Ph.D., P.T.

Electricity has been used to stimulate denervated muscle for almost 100 years.[1] The rationale for electrically stimulating denervated muscle is to exercise the muscle in an effort to maintain the denervated muscle in a healthy state while the injured axons regenerate and reinnervate the muscle. It is assumed that if the denervated muscle is maintained in a fairly healthy state, and can be exercised while denervated, functional recovery is facilitated following reinnervation. The purpose of this chapter is to describe the use of electrical stimulation in the rehabilitation of denervated muscle.

CHANGES FOLLOWING DENERVATION

Following denervation, muscles undergo a number of physiologic, biochemical, and anatomic changes. The muscle fibers become atrophic,[2,3,4] neuromuscular junctions begin to degenerate,[5] and electrical properties of the membrane are altered.[6,7] Additional changes include an increase in the subsarcolemmal nuclei and lysosomes,[8] and a transient increase in the synthesis of the sarcoplasm and sarcoplasmic reticulum.[9] Also, contraction time is found to increase in denervated muscle, while the amount of tension generated by the contraction decreases.[10]

Prior to denervation, the muscle is provided with a continuous supply of trophic substances from the motoneurons that maintain the physiologic integrity of the muscle fibers. However, denervation interrupts this trophic influence, and the muscle fibers undergo progressive denervation changes until the fibers are reinnervated either by collateral axons from surviving motoneurons or by axons regenerating across the lesion site. It is generally thought that if reinnervation has not occurred within 2 years, all of the contractile elements of the muscle will have been replaced by fibrous connective tissue, and recovery of function is no longer possible.

The most obvious change observed following denervation is the muscular atrophy which is invariably a progressive process.[11] Denervation atrophy is characterized by a reduction in the diameter of individual muscle fibers, which results in a decrease in the size of the muscle.

Traditionally, two methods have been used to quantify atrophy. These methods are (1) comparing the weight of the denervated muscle with the weight of the contralateral innervated muscle (intra-animal control) and (2) microscopically contrasting the transverse diameter and/or area of denervated muscle fibers with the transverse diameter and/or area of the contralateral innervated muscle. The process of comparing the weight of the denervated and contralateral control muscles may lead to questionable results since weighing does not account for the effect that such variables as edema and presence of fibrous connective tissue may have on the weight of the muscle. However, the second method, microscopically determining fiber and total muscle diameters and/or areas, allows the investigator to quantify changes in the muscle fibers as well as changes in the connective tissue component of the muscle.

Light microscopy becomes an even more powerful technique when it is combined with histochemical techniques used to identify muscle fiber types.[3] By histochemically identifying the fiber makeup of a muscle it is possible to determine whether slow (Type I) or fast (Type II) fibers are preferentially affected by denervation or by any therapeutic intervention (e.g., electrical stimulation) following denervation. Quantifying muscle weight and microscopic histochemical analysis have been extensively used to study denervation atrophy and the effect of electrical stimulation on denervated muscle in animals.[12]

Fast- and slow-twitch muscles have been shown to atrophy at relatively the same rate in rats.[13] However, this finding has not been universally accepted, with several investigators reporting that Type II fibers undergo atrophy to a greater extent than do Type I fibers.[14,15] According to Jaweed, Herbison, and Ditunno,[16] the differences observed and reported by numerous investigators may be influenced by (1) the region of the muscle from which the biopsy was taken, (2) inherent differences in the muscles examined, and (3) the amount of time between denervation and biopsy.

Loss of muscle mass is species dependent. Animal studies have shown that approximately 50 percent of the muscle weight is lost within 2 weeks following denervation.[12,17] Knowlton and Hines,[13] in a study comparing denervation atrophy of five mammals, conclude that there was a direct correlation between the rate of atrophy and the metabolic rate of the species, as well as its average life span. Therefore, the rate of loss of muscle weight in man is slower than in such animals as rabbits and cats.

Although profound muscular atrophy is the first visible change observed following denervation, it is not the first change that occurs. The first change reported following denervation is the partial depolarization of the sarcolemma. As early as 3 hours following transection of a nerve where it enters a muscle, the normal resting potential of the sarcolemma (-80 mV) is found to decrease by 1 to 2 mV.[18] The resting potential continues to decrease until approximately 24 hours following transection it stabilizes at about -65 mV.

Another change that occurs at the sarcolemma of vertebrate skeletal muscle following denervation is the development of a sensitivity to acetylcholine (ACh) beyond the vicinity of the neuromuscular junction.[19,20] Acetycholine sensitivity occurs in denervated muscle because the ACh receptors normally present only in the end-plate region in innervated muscle become incorporated into the entire length of the sarcolemma following denervation. Some investigators suggest that increased ACh sensitivity is a stimulus for reinnervation.[21] However, other investigators suggest that ACh hypersensitivity does not contribute to the reinnervation process because the denervated end plate does not become hypersensitive to ACh.[20] This is important because reinnervation usually occurs at the denervated end-plate zone.[22] According to Lomo and Slater,[23] the membrane changes underlying increased ACh sensitivity are initiated during the first 2 days following denervation.

FACTORS INFLUENCING REINNERVATION

The microenvironment of the denervated muscle and the peripheral nervous system has been hypothesized to possess properties that may either facilitate or impede regeneration and reinnervation.[24,25] As early as 1928, Cajal[26] discussed those factors necessary for successful repair of peripheral nerves as follows:

> The nervous reunion of the peripheral stump and restoration . . . of the terminal nerve structures, are the combined effect of three conditions: the neurotropic action of the sheaths of Schwann and terminal structures; the mechanical guidance of the sprouts along the old sheaths; and, finally, the superproduction of fibers, in order to insure the arrival of some of them at the peripheral . . . regions. Of all these conditions the most essential . . . is the trophism of the peripheral stump, motor plates and sensory structures.

The mechanical guidance for regenerating axons is provided by the connective tissue matrix of the nerve distal to the site of lesion. In the case of nerve transection, the surgeon must either juxtapose the transected ends of the nerve or re-establish the continuity of the nerve through a nerve graft. The superproduction of fibers referred to by Cajal is provided by regenerative sprouting at the distal ends of the transected axons and by collateral sprouting of intact axons.

However, in Cajal's treatise his emphasis is not on the mechanical factors involved in the regeneration process, but rather on the trophic influences provided by the tissues within the distal nerve stump, particularly the Schwann cells. Cajal believed that the Schwann cells of the distal nerve stump form a matrix for the regenerating axons and provide nutritive substances critically essential for successful regeneration.

The concept of trophism, in which nerve fiber growth is dependent upon environmental substances within the periphery delivered to the growing or regenerating neuron, is well accepted by the scientific community.[27] This phenomenon has been observed in the development of the central and peripheral nervous systems and is reviewed in detail by Varon and Bunge.[27] Factors implicated as potentially trophic include nerve growth factor (NGF), products of degeneration, toxins, and inactivity.[28]

Lundborg and associates[29] introduced the silicone chamber to study peripheral nervous system regeneration in vivo. The silicone chamber has given investigators the opportunity to study axonal regeneration across the interstump gap (generally 10 mm wide) that is contained within the tube. The chamber also allows investigators to prefill the interstump gap with substances thought to influence or facilitate regeneration across the gap.[30] Interestingly, axonal regeneration across the gap has been successful only when there is a distal source of Schwann cells.[31] Perhaps, through manipulation of the intrachamber environment in vivo it will be possible to identify specific regeneration-promoting factors in the near future.

Another factor that may facilitate reinnervation and recovery is the chronic electrical stimulation of denervated muscle. Although the effects of chronic electrical stimulation of innervated muscle are well documented,[32-34] the effect of chronic stimulation of denervated muscle is not well understood.[35,36]

Chronic, low frequency, indirect electrical stimulation of innervated fast-twitch muscle, similar to that occurring in nerves of slow-twitch muscle, has been shown to transform the functional properties of a fast-twitch muscle to resemble those of a slow-twitch muscle.[32,33] In a recent study of chronic denervated muscle, low-frequency stimulation of denervated rabbit extensor digitorum longus resulted in those muscles becoming more fatigue resistant when compared to nonstimulated denervated muscle.[35] Although much work needs to be done in the area of chronic electrical stimulation of denervated muscle, the possibility exists that chronic stimulation may either facilitate reinnervation or assist in maintaining the denervated muscle in a healthy state until reinnervation occurs.

THE CONTROVERSY SURROUNDING ELECTRICAL STIMULATION OF DENERVATED MUSCLE

Historical Perspective

Following denervation, the therapeutic efforts to restore nerve continuity always involve a concern for maintaining the target tissues of nerve regeneration in the best possible physiologic state until regeneration and reinnervation are complete. Unfortunately, there are no universally accepted therapeutic measures to maintain denervated muscle in a viable state. However, electrical stimulation is one therapeutic agent that has been advocated to retard muscular atrophy.[37,38]

BASIC SCIENCE STUDIES

The potential benefits of electrical stimulation of denervated muscle were first reported by Reid in 1841.[39] Shortly thereafter, Brown-Sequard[40] claimed that daily electrical stimulation of the denervated limbs of various mammals and birds produced a gradual, but complete restoration of the muscle bulk of the limbs. Although the muscle regained its mass, the limb remained nonfunctional.

In the early 1900s Langley and Kato[41] compared the effectiveness of massage, passive exercise, and electrical stimulation in preventing weight loss in denervated muscles of rabbits. They concluded that (1) massage had little if any effect on retarding weight loss in denervated muscle, (2) rhythmic extension of the muscles had very little effect, but (3) electrical stimulation did delay muscular atrophy. Langley and Kato recognized that the electrical stimulation only retarded the atrophy and did not prevent it. They suggested three factors that might have been responsible for their findings. These factors were (1) the intensity of the stimuli may only have stimulated the most superficial muscle fibers, leaving the deeper fibers unaffected and allowing the deep fibers to atrophy; (2) the number of electrically induced contractions was not adequate; and (3) the atrophy in muscle following denervation is not simply "inactive atrophy." In 1916, Langley[42] reported results from a similar study done on two rabbits having received more prolonged stimulation. He demonstrated that neither electrical stimulation nor passive movement had any definite effect on loss of muscular weight following denervation. From this study Langley concluded that atrophy of denervation is not due solely to the absence of muscular contraction.

Following World War I, very little new information was generated until 1939, when Fischer[43] proposed an explanation for Langley's negative results. Fischer suggested that Langley's lack of success possibly could have been attributed to the use of a current that was too weak to stimulate properly all the muscle fibers. Fischer further proposed that electrical stimulation should be initiated as soon as possible following denervation. He also recommended that the strength and duration of the stimulus be modified according to changes in the excitability of the denervated muscle. From his study, Fischer concluded that although denervated muscle that has been stimulated appears to improve only slightly in "power" compared to nontreated muscle, atrophy can be retarded through electrical stimulation.

Since the early 1940s, numerous investigators have studied the effect of electrical stimulation on denervated muscle in animals[12,44–47] and in humans.[48–50] Although these studies have provided varying results, some studies indicate that direct electrical stimulation of muscle, initiated shortly following denervation, may be beneficial in delaying muscle atrophy,[51,52] maintaining the cross-sectional area of denervated muscle fibers,[15,53] and reducing the loss of contractile strength.[54]

One of the most convincing studies on the effectiveness of electrical stimulation of denervated muscle is the study by Gutmann and Guttmann[44] on denervated rabbit muscle. They concluded that electrical stimulation not only delays and diminishes muscular atrophy following denervation, but that it also accelerates the return of the muscle to its initial size following reinnervation. Gutmann and Guttmann also reported that electrically stimulated muscle shows less fibrosis, larger fibers and is more excitable than unstimulated muscle.

Another early study investigating the effectiveness of different types of electrical stimulation on denervated muscle was completed by Solandt, DeLury, and Hunter.[55] Using albino rats, these investigators demonstrated that 25-cycle *alternating* (sinusoidal) current was more effective in reducing the weight loss of denervated muscle than was 60-cycle alternating (sinusoidal) *galvanic* or *faradic* current. They also showed that the effectiveness of stimulation increased with the number of treatments per day. However, no significant differences were obtained when varying individual treatment time between 1 and 5 minutes. This study supports the suggestion by Morris[56] that a fully denervated muscle will only respond to a stimulus of "approximately" 100 ms or longer duration. The use of similar, slowly rising, exponentially progressive currents for stimulating denervated muscle was stressed by Thom in 1957,[57] and will be discussed in more detail later in this chapter.

Of the numerous animal studies reported in the literature during the past 15 years,[52,53,54,58] several are particularly important because they were well controlled and the experimental protocols were described in detail. These studies are worthy of close examination.

One such study is that of Herbison, Jaweed, and Ditunno,[58] who evaluated the effect of chronic electrical stimulation on reinnervation of rat soleus muscle following sciatic nerve crush. They examined whether the ACh hypersensitivity and fibrillatory activity persisted during reinnervation, and if they were present, whether they interfered with the process of reinnervation. Electrodes were implanted in the vicinity of the soleus muscle 2 weeks prior to crush denervation of the sciatic nerve. One week following denervation, the soleus muscles in the crush-denervated and control groups were stimulated unilaterally with a 4-mA, 4-ms duration current given continuously at 10 Hz, 8 hours every day for 5, 10, 15, 20, 25, or 30 days. At the end of each time period a group of stimulated, and a group of nonstimulated (control) soleus muscles were evaluated for muscle weight, ACh sensitivity, and fibrillation potentials. Herbison, Jaweed, and Ditunno determined that the denervated-stimulated soleus muscles were significantly heavier 10 days after the initiation of electrical stimulation and had significantly fewer fibrillation potentials between 5 and 15 days after the initiation of stimulation than the denervated controls. However, the ACh sensitivity throughout the entire study and the fibrillation activity between 20 and 30 days postcrush were similar in the denervated controls and the denervated-stimulated soleus muscles. The investigators concluded that although the chronic electrical stimulation neither enhanced nor impaired the reinnervation process, it did reduce the ultimate degree of atrophy and the number of fibrillatory potentials in the soleus muscles in the denervation stage.

Herbison, Jaweed, and Ditunno[58] acknowledged that the extent of the retardation of atrophy found in their study was considerably less than the sparing of atrophy reported by Lomo and associates.[23,59] Herbison, Jaweed, and Ditunno attributed this difference to Lomo and colleagues' use of a relatively high intensity current (25 mA), whereas Herbison's group applied a stimulus no greater than 4 mA. They assumed that the muscle fibers in the central region of the soleus may not have been activated by the 4-mA current, particularly since Gutmann and Guttmann[45] demonstrated that transcutaneous electrical stimulation maintained the muscle fiber size at the surface of denervated muscle while deeper muscle fibers lost as much bulk as nonstimulated control muscles.

In the 1970s, Lomo and associates[59-61] demonstrated that contractile parameters (i.e., isometric-twitch contraction time) and fatigue properties of denervated muscle can be affected by different patterns of electrical activity. Using 100-Hz electrical stimulation, either continuously or intermittently, they were able to transform the isometric-twitch characteristics of adult rat muscles from slow-twitch types to fast-twitch types.

In a similar study with low frequency (10 Hz), long-term (200 to 240 hours) electrical stimulation of denervated rat soleus muscle, Jaweed, Herbison, and Ditunno[62] concluded that stimulation might impair isometric-twitch development in slow-twitch muscles. These investigators also demonstrated that crush denervated stimulated muscles show a significant sparing of muscle bulk during the denervation phase (to 15 days) which suggests that the 10-Hz stimulation frequency may be effective in partially maintaining muscle mass. They did not speculate on the possible mechanisms responsible for maintaining the muscle mass. Furthermore, they did not find that low frequency electrical stimulation alters the course of self-reinnervation in muscle. This finding was corroborated by Sebille and Boudoux-Jahan[63] who demonstrated that electrical stimulation of denervated muscle does not speed the reinnervation process.

A recent animal study which demonstrates that electrical stimulation following denervation can be effective in reducing the loss of muscle mass and contractile strength following denervation was reported by Cole and Gardiner[54] in 1984. The study is particularly significant because the stimulation parameters are feasible for clinical use. Using the sciatic nerve crush paradigm in adult male rats, Cole and Gardiner[54] initiated percutaneous electrical stimulation of the denervated left gastrocnemius 1 day following sciatic nerve crush in the treatment group. During stimulation, the animals were anesthetized and the knee and ankle joints immobilized, thereby rendering the contractions nearly isometric. Impulses to the muscles were delivered in the form of trains lasting 5 seconds, with a 1-second interval between trains. Each train consisted of individual 25-ms DC square waves, delivered at 20 Hz. Frequent polarity changes were made to minimize skin irritation at the electrode sites. The pattern of stimulation produced 10 semifused (subtetanic) contractions per minute. The stimulation was maintained for 5 minutes, and carried out three times a day, with at least 30 minutes between stimulation periods. Stimulation continued daily for 8 weeks. Nonstimulated, crush-control animals and nonstimulated normals were also anesthetized daily. Eight weeks following crush, the unstimulated muscles were significantly lighter in wet weight, were tetanically weaker, and showed slower isometric contractile responses *in situ* than noncrush control animals. Denervated muscles which had been stimulated daily were heavier, and tetanically stronger (the latter not different from controls) than those in the crush, nonstimulated groups. Cole and Gardiner also showed that muscle weights from animals sacrificed at 2, 4, or 8 weeks following nerve crush indicate that the major benefit of stimulation occurred during the initial 4 weeks following denervation. The investigators emphasized that since reinnervation in this model occurred at approximately 3 weeks,[15] it is evident that the daily contractile activity imposed by the electrical stimulation, independent of innervation, played a major role in attenuating denervation atrophy during the period prior to reinnervation.

Cole and Gardiner[54] proposed that the model of electrical stimulation delivered to innervated muscles (as was the case in their study between 4 and 8 weeks following denervation) is more complex than the stimulation involving denervated muscle. They also believed that when stimulating innervated muscle, more supplementary contractile activity may be necessary to provoke a muscular adaptation and that the stimulation (treatment) parameters (duration, frequency, type of stimulation, etc.) may have profound influences. They suggested that differences in stimulation characteristics provided to the muscle following reinnervation by Herbison and associates[12] may account for the differences reported in the two studies.

To more fully appreciate the potential significance of the stimulation of denervated muscle with direct current, the reader should be aware of the stimulation (treatment) parameters used by Herbison and associates.[12] Herbison's group stimulated each denervated muscle in treatment sessions lasting 1 minute (each 1-minute treatment consisted of alternating 5 seconds of continuous stimulation and 1 second of rest), twice a day, 5 days a week, with 1 hour between sessions. All the stimulation consisted of interrupted, direct, square wave current of 10-mA intensity. Herbison and colleagues concluded that (1) with interrupted direct current of 25-ms pulse duration and frequency of 20 Hz, the weight of the treated muscle exceeded that of untreated by 2 percent; (2) with a current of 100-ms pulse duration and frequency of 2 Hz, treated exceeded untreated muscle weight by 10 percent; and (3) with a current of 25-ms pulse duration and 20-Hz frequency, treated exceeded untreated muscle weight by from 10 to 33 percent.

In summary, Cole and Gardiner[54] and Herbison and associates[12] demonstrated a significant retardation of atrophy using interrupted direct-current stimulation with stimuli of 25-ms pulse duration at a frequency of 20 Hz. The primary differences in stimulation parameters between the two studies appear to be the duration of stimulation which is longer in Cole and Gardiner's study (5 minutes versus 1 minute), and the frequency of treatment sessions, which is also greater in Cole and Gardiner's study (three times per day versus two times per day). Another, possibly significant difference in the studies is the fact that while Cole and Gardiner used a nerve crush model, Herbison and colleagues used a nerve-transection model with the cut ends of the nerves immediately approximated surgically following the nerve transection. In the nerve crush model, the anatomical continuity of the nerve is maintained, whereas the continuity is at least temporarily interrupted in the nerve-transection mode. Therefore, in the transection model the continuity of the matrix through which regenerating axons must grow is dependent upon the ability of a surgeon to reapproximate the proximal and distal nerve stumps. In the nerve crush model this matrix remains intact and may facilitate regeneration and recovery of function.

CLINICAL STUDIES

Although very few human studies have been reported, Rosselle and coworkers[37,64] evaluated potential differences in a variety of nerve lesions treated by electrotherapeutic techniques or left untreated. Rosselle and collaborators performed electromyographic evaluations of 324 individuals. Their sample included 225 persons who were treated by "electrotherapeutic techniques," and 99 individuals with untreated nerve lesions. Each electromyographic examination quantified (1) the degree of fibrillary activity as "a standard of the trophic conditions of the affected muscle" and (2) the level of "motor recuperation" as assumed on the "quality of the recordings," and the number of fibrillary potentials observed during voluntary contraction. Rosselle and associates reported that when considering motor improvement during voluntary contraction, initial recovery, as defined by the presence of fibrillar activity, was obtained 50 to 100 days earlier in the treated group. It was concluded that an electromyographically distinguishable difference existed between cases of complete denervation treated by *electrical stimulation* and cases not treated by electrical stimulation. They further emphasize that electrical stimulation of muscle is the most efficient rehabilitation method for completely denervated muscle fibers.

Although the studies by Rosselle and colleagues[37,64] were supportive of the use of electrical stimulation in the treatment of denervated muscle, the studies have weaknesses. The most apparent problem is that the investigators failed to standardize or report the electrotherapeutic techniques. The value of the studies is further limited by the absence of consideration given to the extent of the denervation (i.e., partial or complete), type of denervation injury, and site of injury relative to target muscle, and to the qualitative criteria of measurement. Although, the studies support the use of electrical stimulation, the investigators' conclusion may not be justified because of flaws in the design of the studies.

More recently, Valencic and associates[38] reported success in restoring muscular contractility of the anterior tibialis muscle in humans using an electrical stimulation training program. Nine patients, 21 to 46 years of age, with complete denervation of the tibialis anterior muscle were selected for the study. The time between denervation and initiation of electrical stimulation ranged from 2 to 40 months. The maximal range of dorsiflexion was obtained using a current at 25 Hz, having equal pulse and pause durations at 20 ms each. These parameters were used throughout the training program.

In addition to nonspecified "conventional physical therapy" Valencic and associates[38] stimulated the denervated tibialis anterior muscle for 20 minutes twice a day, 5 days a week for 3 weeks. Stimulation was applied rhythmically with a 3-second pulse train followed by a 3-second pause. The amplitude of the current ranged from 15 to 35 mA and was adjusted for each subject to a level that elicited the maximal range of dorsiflexion. Prior to initiating the stimulation program, and weekly thereafter, the maximal range of dorsiflexion obtained through electrical stimulation of the tibialis anterior muscle at varying amplitudes between 15 mA and 40 mA was recorded for each subject. Following the 3-week training period there was a significant ($p < 0.01$) increase in dorsiflexion of 15.8° when compared to the amount of electrically elicited dorsiflexion obtained prior to initiating the training period. Although there were no signs of reinnervation at the end of the training program, the electrically induced contractions of the denervated muscles were improved in all of the subjects. Valencic and associates concluded that the applied training program thus reversed the course of disuse atrophy and supported the use of electrical stimulation on patients with denervated muscles. However, since the findings reported by Valencic and colleagues are specific to stimulation of the denervated tibialis anterior muscle, the conclusion that similar stimulation programs may have a similar effect on other denervated muscles may not be valid.

Although the previously discussed clinical studies are encouraging, several investigators[23,47,65] have suggested that electrical stimulation of denervated muscle in animals may actually interfere with reinnervation and delay the subsequent recovery of function.

As early as 1939, Chor and associates[66] studied denervated monkey muscles and reported that "electrical stimulation of denervated muscle does not give as good a restoration of the bulk/contour of regenerating muscle as may be obtained by massage and passive movement." However, their protocol consisted of 10 galvanic-induced contractions, once a day, which may have been insufficient to effectively stimulate denervated muscle. Furthermore, stimulation in that study was not initiated until 2 weeks after nerve section and repair. More recently, Schimrigk, McLaughlen, and Gruniger[47] have also suggested that electrical stimulation will inhibit reinnervation following nerve crush in albino rats. Their protocol involved stimulating the crush-denervated quadriceps femoris muscle with galvanic current, for 2 minutes, three times a day, until muscle biopsy at either 3, 4, 5, 6, or 7 weeks following denervation. Stimulation was supramaximal (5 to 8 V, 4 to 6 A) and delivered at a frequency of 5 pps. Histologically, they found fewer central nuclei and a greater number of necrotic single fibers in the electrically stimulated muscles than in the nonstimulated denervated muscles. They concluded that the untreated denervated fibers showed a greater anatomical tendency toward regeneration than the electrically stimulated muscles and that electrical stimulation appeared to have a delaying effect on regeneration. Electrical stimulation was not initiated until 4 days following denervation, so it is possible that stimulation was not initiated early enough to yield a positive effect.

In another often-quoted study, Lomo and Slater[23] examined how electrical stimulation affects the formation of new ectopic neuromuscular junctions in denervated muscle. To accomplish denervation, 0.5- to 1-cm lengths of the sciatic nerves of adult male white rats were removed. The denervated soleus muscles were stimulated through implanted electrodes as follows: once every 100 s a train of 100 stimuli, each 1-ms long, at a frequency of 100 Hz was delivered (overall mean frequency of 1 burst per second). Currents of 20 to 25 mA were used. Lomo and Slater reported that direct stimulation of muscles with chronically implanted electrodes from the time of denervation prevented the formation of functional neuromuscular junctions. However, if stimulation began 2 to 4 days after denervation, some functional neuromuscular junctions were formed which were detected histologically 7 to 9 days after denervation, though not as many as in the absence of stimulation. One of the conclusions of these investigators was that a period of inactivity, immediately following denervation and lasting up to 48 hours, is required to allow neuromuscular junction formation. In considering these findings one must be aware that this research involved the study of ectopic junctions formed between the superficial fibular nerve and the soleus muscle. Therefore, the conclusions drawn from this study involved reinnervation (neuromuscular junction formation) between a muscle and a nerve that did not normally innervate that muscle. This fact may severely limit the clinical application of the findings of this study.

Evidence Supporting a Role for Electrical Stimulation of Denervated Muscle:

1. Appropriate electrical stimulation can cause a denervated muscle to contract.
2. Contraction of a denervated muscle may help limit edema and venous stasis within the muscle, and therefore delay muscle-fiber degeneration and fibrosis.
3. Recovery time following denervation appears to be shortened with appropriate electrical stimulation.

Evidence Refuting the Use of Electrical Stimulation of Denervated Muscle:

1. Contraction of the denervated muscle may disrupt regenerating neuromuscular junctions and subsequently delay reinnervation.
2. Denervated muscle is more sensitive to trauma than innervated muscle, and electrical stimulation may further traumatize the denervated muscle.
3. Prolonged electrical stimulation until reinnervation occurs is not worth the financial and time costs involved.

Herbison, Jaweed, and Ditunno[58] have further suggested that a possible reason for lack of success in facilitating reinnervation using electrical stimulation in some studies is the intensity of the stimuli. Intense stimuli (i.e., 25 mA) may cause so much movement of the denervated muscle that reinnervation might be limited because of local trauma to the newly forming neuromuscular junctions. Evidence is summarized in Table 8-1 that both supports and refutes the benefits of electrical stimulation of denervated muscle.

APPLICATION TECHNIQUES FOR ELECTRICAL STIMULATION OF DENERVATED MUSCLE

It is apparent that the effectiveness of the electrical stimulation of denervated muscle depends upon many factors, including the type of current, duration of the stimulus, current amplitude, number of stimuli per second, type of contractions, length and frequency of treatment sessions, time between treatment sessions, and elapsed time between denervation and initiation of stimulation. This part of the chapter will discuss electrical stimulation parameters proposed for stimulating denervated muscle.

Current Amplitude

Faradic (balanced, asymmetrical, biphasic waveform) or *faradiclike* current having a short pulse duration (less than 1.0 ms) has been reported as somewhat beneficial in retarding muscular atrophy during the first 2 weeks following denervation.[67,68] Thereafter, the responsiveness (excitability) of the muscle is such that only interrupted, square-wave, direct current having a long-pulse duration (i.e., greater than 10 ms), or low-frequency (less than 10 Hz) sine wave alternating current will elicit single-twitch contractions.[46,69]

In order to elicit the optimal response when stimulating denervated muscle, the current waveform should have a pulse duration equal to or greater than the chronaxie of the denervated muscle. Therefore, a determination of chronaxie is essential in establishing the duration of the stimulus. Procedures for chronaxie determination are reviewed in Chapter 4.

The amplitude of the current should be great enough to elicit a maximal contraction of the denervated muscle fibers. This is of particular concern when a denervated muscle is stimulated transcutaneously. It is possible that muscle fibers within the deeper regions of denervated muscles may not be stimulated if the current is not of adequate amplitude.[58] Muscular atrophy should be retarded throughout the entire muscle and not only on the periphery of the muscle.

Also, when stimulating denervated muscle, the amplitude of the current coupled with the duration (pulse width) of the stimulus must be great enough to stimulate a muscle having a prolonged chronaxie. Therefore, once again, knowledge of the chronaxie of the denervated muscle is essential.

Pulse Rate (Frequency)

Solandt, DeLury, and Hunter[55] compared the effectiveness of interrupted direct current and 25- and 60-cycle sinusoidal (symmetrical, alternating current) current in retarding weight loss in denervated rat muscle. They concluded that the 25-cycle sinusoidal current was the most effective, followed by the 60-cycle sinusoidal current and then by the interrupted direct current. In a similar study using supramaximal stimuli, Kosman, Osborne, and Ivey[69] concluded that there is an optimal frequency at which electrical stimuli must be delivered in order to generate maximal muscle tension and delay denervation atrophy. This frequency was identified as 25 cycles per second. They also postulated that the criteria for optimal or ideal current for electrical stimulation of denervated muscle are (1) vigorous contractions at low current intensities and (2) selective stimulation of denervated muscle. They emphasized that a "modulating alternating current of 10 to 25 cycles per second" meets these criteria and stressed that this type of current is capable of producing vigorous muscle contractions with relatively little discomfort.

Types of Contraction

According to Wehrmacher, Thompson, and Hines[70] the most important factor in stimulating denervated muscles appears to be the *quantity* of tension developed rather than the particular type, frequency, phase pattern, or treatment time of the electrical stimuli. They suggested that the duration of an effective period of treatment can be very short if the muscles are stimulated under conditions which facilitate the development of maximal isometric tension. Wehrmacher, Thompson, and Hines also postulated that investigators who have reported negative results from electrically stimulating denervated muscles either failed to employ stimuli of sufficient intensity or did not provide optimal muscle-length conditions to develop maximal isometric tension.

Elliott and Thomson[71] in a study involving denervation and electrical stimulation of the rat gastrocnemius muscle demonstrated that muscles not allowed to shorten during stimulation showed a greater shortening velocity than did denervated untreated muscle, or muscle allowed to shorten freely (isotonic contraction) during stimulation. However, they also demonstrated that muscle that was allowed to contract isotonically during treatment showed a greater amount of shortening than did the isometrically contracted muscle. Elliott and Thomson postulated that electrically elicited isometric contractions minimized those changes in denervated muscle that are related to rates of activity of enzyme systems, for example, glycogen synthesis and the release of energy. Both isometric and isotonic contractions may have a role in the electrical stimulation of denervated muscle for functional recovery.

Treatment Schedule

Solandt, DeLury, and Hunter[55] demonstrated a linear relationship between the number of daily stimulation periods and the maintenance of denervated muscle mass. Kosman, Osborne, and Ivey[68] reported that this relationship holds true until the muscle reaches nearly normal values for weight when treated three times a day. Increasing the number of stimulation periods from three to six per day resulted in very little improvement in weight.

Wehrmacher, Thompson, and Hines,[70] using *faradic* current, reported that daily treatments of 5-seconds duration were almost as effective in delaying muscle atrophy in rats as treatments lasting 180 seconds. Kosman, Osborne, and Ivey[68] and Gutmann and Guttmann,[45] using galvanic stimulation, found no significant differences in results from treatment sessions lasting 30 seconds, 15 minutes, or 20 minutes. Kosman, Osborne, and Ivey[68] postulated that it is possible that the duration of the treatment session is not as important as other stimulation parameters, such as the amount of tension generated by the contraction.

Kosman, Osborne, and Ivey[69] demonstrated that the retardation of muscular atrophy is maximal if a rest period of at least 10 minutes is provided between treatment sessions. Rest periods of 2 and 5 minutes were not as effective in retarding atrophy as the 10-minute rest period. These findings may be attributed to the ease with which denervated muscle fatigues and to the time required for fatigued, denervated muscle to recover following contraction. Kosman, Osborne, and Ivey also stressed that continuation of the stimulation after the muscle begins to show signs of fatigue serves no useful purpose. The rest periods may minimize or delay the onset of muscle fatigue by providing the denervated muscle ample time for metabolic recovery [i.e., replenishing adenosine triphosphate (ATP) stores, removal of metabolic waste, etc.] to occur.

The elapsed time between denervation and the onset of electrical stimulation may affect the rate of axonal regeneration following nerve injury. In 1952, Hoffman[17] reported that a 1-hour period of electrical stimulation of the spinal cord or nerve roots immediately following partial denervation of the sciatic nerve significantly accelerated the process of axonal sprouting from intact axons, which normally occurs following a partial denervation. In 1985, Pockett and Gavin,[72] using the sciatic nerve crush model in rats, demonstrated that if the crush site is electrically stimulated through implanted electrodes immediately after the crush, the toe-spreading reflex is first observable at 4 days following crush. In contrast, if the nerve of the crush site is not stimulated, the toe-spreading reflex does not return until 10 days following crush. Pockett and Gavin[72] stimulated the nerve with 0.1-ms duration, square-wave pulses at 1 Hz for 15 minutes to 1 hour immediately following the crush. The intensity of the current was determined prior to induction of the nerve injury to be just great enough to cause the innervated muscles to twitch. From their study Pockett and Gavin showed that stimulation did not affect the number of regenerating axons but did significantly affect the rate of regeneration as measured by the return of the toe-spreading reflex following crush. Periods of 1 hour, 30 minutes, or 15 minutes of stimulation delivered immediately following crush reduced the time for recovery of the toe-spreading reflex to slightly less than half the time taken without stimulation. They also demonstrated that when the beginning of the stimulation period was delayed for 30 minutes or 1 hour after nerve crush, the effectiveness of the stimulation declined in a linear fashion, although stimulation begun after a 1-hour delay still produced a significantly shorter reflex recovery time than no stimulation. Pockett and Gavin postulated that the mechanism underlying the phenomenon may either involve the effect of the stimulation on the cell body or the local effect of the stimulation at the growing axonal tip. Several investigators have identified the following local factors that may be affected by stimulation: (1) the outgrowth of nerve processes, reported to be a local response to a local stimulus;[73] (2) release of trophic factors by Schwann cells;[74] or (3) degeneration of the distal axon process and removal of debris.[75] More recently, Pockett and Phillip[76] provided evidence that the mechanism responsible for the aforementioned phenomenon is a local one, at the site of nerve crush, rather than an effect on the cell bodies. Regardless of the mechanism responsible for the accelerated rate of regeneration, it appears that electrical stimulation initiated immediately following nerve crush may have the potential to facilitate recovery of function in a clinical setting.

Electrode Placement Considerations

The transcutaneous electrical stimulation of denervated muscle is accomplished through surface electrodes. The electrode configuration is usually monopolar with the active or treatment electrode positioned over the part of the denervated muscle that is most electrically excitable. The inactive or dispersive electrode is placed over a distant body part. The size of the active electrode is very small (i.e., 1 to 2 cm^2), providing for a large current density and for a more specific localization at the most electrically excitable part of the muscle. The size of the inactive or dispersive electrode is large enough that current flow under the inactive electrode is not perceived by the patient. The exact size of the dispersive electrode will vary according to each patient's perception of stimulation under the electrode and should be determined accordingly by the therapist.

An alternate configuration would be bipolar stimulation with the active electrode on the most excitable part of the muscle and the dispersive electrode over the tendon. The optimal stimulation site is that point along the muscle which is most electrically excitable and is not the conventional motor point because the nerve is not functioning. This point is the site at which a minimal amount of current will elicit a minimally visible contraction of the muscle being stimulated. This site of greatest excitability should be determined for each denervated muscle at the beginning of each stimulating session. Since the muscle being stimulated is denervated, the response of the muscle to stimulation will be a sluggish and somewhat wormlike contraction instead of the brisk contraction observed when stimulating innervated muscle. Having determined the optimal stimulation site, the stimulation session proceeds with the therapist using the cathode as the active or treatment electrode.

EVALUATION OF ELECTROTHERAPEUTIC DEVICES APPROPRIATE FOR STIMULATION OF DENERVATED MUSCLE

Prior to evaluating equipment for electrically stimulating denervated muscle, the clinician should thoroughly review the physiologic characteristics of denervated muscle and the basic principles of electrotherapy. Of primary concern when selecting a stimulation unit for use in stimulating denervated muscle is that the stimulator allows the therapist to control and modify the amplitude, frequency, and duration (i.e., pulse width) of the individual stimuli as indicated by the electrical excitability of the muscle. Since the electrical excitability of the denervated muscle will vary during the denervation-reinnervation period, the stimulation variables will be frequently adjusted to assure maximal contractions that are tolerated by the patient.

The stimulator must allow for an adequate rest period following each stimulus. As suggested by Thom,[57] the rest period between successive stimuli should be at least four to five times longer than the duration of the stimulus. Without the ability to control the time between stimuli, the therapist risks overstimulating the denervated muscle, which will prematurely fatigue the muscle and unnecessarily cut short the treatment session.

The stimulator of choice must also be capable of providing a stimulus having a duration long enough (i.e., at least 10 ms) to stimulate the muscle when the denervated muscle is least electrically excitable as is demonstrated by the prolonged chronaxie and shift in the strength-duration curve to the right (described in Chapter 4, Fig. 4–3). An electrical stimulator that provides for changes in duration as well as amplitude of the stimulus will allow the therapist to effectively stimulate the muscle with a minimal amount of current.

Additional factors that should be considered in selecting a stimulator are portability and ease of operation. Because the scientific evidence that supports the efficacy of electrical stimulation of denervated muscle suggests daily treatments, use of the stimulator by the patient at home should be considered. A home therapy program would require use of a stimulator that is portable and can be easily understood and operated by the patient on a daily basis.

A LOOK TOWARD THE FUTURE

Perhaps a more effective means by which the integrity of denervated muscle may be maintained is the "selective" stimulation of denervated muscle. Selective stimulation involves the stimulation of a denervated or a partially denervated muscle without overstimulation of the remaining innervated muscle fibers. Current forms having slowly increasing intensities are capable of selectively stimulating denervated muscle while avoiding overstimulation of innervated muscle fibers which accommodate to the slowly increasing intensity of each pulse (Fig. 8–1).

Direct-current pulses that progressively increase in intensity in either a straight line or a curve may be delivered. Kowarschik[77] has labeled those direct-current forms that consist of a series of exponential impulses as "progressive exponential currents" and reported using progressive exponential currents as a means of retarding the development of denervation muscular atrophy as early as 1940. He also reported that this type of stimulation proved clinically effective. Unfortunately, controlled basic science and clinical studies have not been reported using this current form.

The rationale for *selectively* stimulating denervated muscles seems plausible, and this type of stimulation may hold promise for effective clinical use. When stimulating denervated muscle, we are stimulating the sarcolemma of the muscle, which does not accommodate to an electrical stimulus as rapidly as the axolemma of the axon. Therefore, while the axolemma of intact axons accommodate to the stimulus, the denervated muscle will respond to the electrical stimulus of relatively low intensity having an adequate duration and sufficiently slow rise time. Selective stimulation of denervated

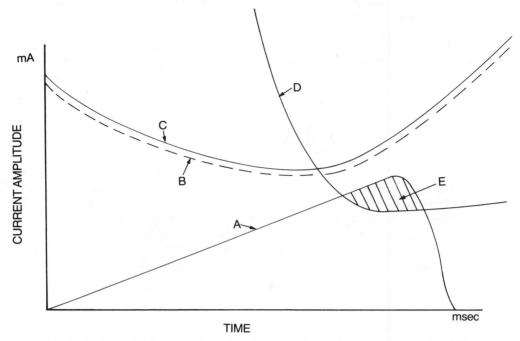

FIGURE 8–1. The selective stimulation of denervated muscle using an exponentially progressive waveform. (*A*) An exponentially progressive waveform; (*B*) and (*C*) the strength/duration curves for the intact sensory axons and innervated muscle, respectively. The intact sensory axons and innervated muscle accommodate to the gradual rise time of the exponentially progressive waveform while the denervated muscle (*D*) does not accommodate to the gradually increasing stimulus. Therefore, selective stimulation of the denervated muscle without recruitment of the sensory axons or the innervated muscle is possible at (*E*).

muscle may also be accomplished with minimal sensory stimulation since the sensory axons also accommodate to the slowly rising stimulus intensity. As stated earlier, the overstimulation of innervated muscle fibers in the vicinity of a partially denervated muscle is thereby avoided.

According to Thom,[78] denervated muscle responds best to slowly rising electrical waveforms of 150- to 600-ms duration with pauses of 3 to 6 seconds between impulses. Thom also suggested the following guidelines when selectively stimulating denervated muscle with exponentially progressive waveforms:

1. The duration of the impulse should be as short as possible, yet of long enough duration to elicit a contraction.
2. The rise should be as steep as possible but as gradual as necessary to avoid stimulation of intact axons.
3. The duration of the pause between stimuli should be at least 4 to 5 times longer than the stimulus duration to help avoid muscular fatigue.
4. The intensity of the stimulus must be sufficient to achieve a moderately strong contraction while not causing the patient unnecessary discomfort.

Current forms having the characteristics necessary for selective stimulation of denervated muscle provide the therapist with a means to stimulate a denervated or partially denervated muscle in a more effective manner while at the same time avoiding the overstimulation of innervated muscles. However, if a muscle exhibits *disuse* atrophy, and not denervation atrophy, as in the case of prolonged immobilization, the clinician should select the appropriate stimulation parameters for the electrical stimulation of innervated muscle. The reader should refer to Chapters 7 and 12 for a discussion of electrical stimulation of innervated muscle.

CLINICAL DECISION MAKING: CASE STUDIES

Electrical stimulation is only one component of a comprehensive treatment program for the rehabilitation of denervated muscle. Such a treatment program may also include progressive exercises, positioning techniques, neuromuscular re-education, the use of orthotics, and so on. Consideration of the factors presented in the previous sections are tantamount to the successful management of denervated muscle with electrical stimulation. The following case examples suggest a schema for determining optimal application techniques to retard those changes associated with denervation injuries.

CASE STUDY

A 25-year-old man received a stab wound to the right forearm 8 weeks ago. The wound partially transected the median nerve. One week following the injury, the transected ends of the nerve were surgically approximated. Physical evaluation reveals (1) normal (5/5) strength in all muscles innervated by the median nerve proximal to the wrist and (2) atrophy and no volitional activity of the intrinsic muscles of the hand normally innervated by the median nerve.

Consideration of the following questions assists in the planning of the electrical stimulation component of this patient's treatment. A suggested protocol is summarized in Table 8–2.

1. Could this patient benefit from electrical stimulation of the denervated muscles?
   The patient may benefit from electrical stimulation of the denervated muscles. Many investigators and clinicians have reported that electrical stimulation is beneficial in retarding denervation atrophy. However, electrical stimulation has not been shown to completely prevent denervation atrophy and the changes associated with denervation.

2. What type of current should be used to stimulate denervated muscle?
   The type of current selected for stimulating denervated muscle must have waveform characteristics appropriate for *direct* stimulation of the muscle.

3. How can the appropriate waveform characteristics be identified?
   To select the appropriate waveform characteristics for direct stimulation of the muscle we must know the excitability of the muscle. The excitability of the muscle is determined by plotting the strength-duration (S-D) curve and identifying the

TABLE 8–2 Suggested Stimulation Protocol for Case 1

1. Obtain a strength-duration curve for the denervated muscle, and identify the chronaxie.
2. Select the appropriate waveform (i.e., exponential progressive waveform).
3. The duration of the pulse must be greater than the chronaxie.
4. The amplitude of the current must be great enough to elicit a visible contraction.
5. Either a monopolar or bipolar electrode placement technique may be used.
6. The appropriate joints should be stabilized to assure an isometric contraction of the denervated muscle.
7. Three stimulation sessions a day, consisting of three sets of 5 to 20 isometric contractions, are recommended.
8. Avoid overfatiguing the muscle by allowing at least a 5-s rest period between contractions and a 1-minute rest period between each set of contractions.
9. Daily stimulation should continue for 4 to 6 weeks beyond the projected time for reinnervation to occur.

chronaxie for the specific muscle. The S-D curve for a denervated muscle will be shifted to the right of the S-D curve for healthy, innervated muscle. The procedure for determining an S-D curve is described in Chapter 4.

Since the position of the S-D curve will vary according to the extent of denervation, the curve should be plotted periodically (e.g., every 2 weeks). Knowledge of the S-D curve will permit the therapist to appropriately adjust the intensity and duration of the stimulus to assure adequate stimulation of the denervated muscle. For example, if the chronaxie of a denervated muscle is determined to be 125 ms, the pulse duration of the stimulating current must be at least 125 ms to effectively stimulate the denervated muscle.

4. What specific types of waveform are used to stimulate denervated muscle?

One waveform used for stimulating denervated muscle is the slowly rising exponentially progressive current. Exponentially progressive current with a slow rise time may selectively stimulate denervated muscle. A second waveform, traditionally used to stimulate denervated muscle is interrupted, square wave direct current. A third waveform capable of stimulating partially denervated muscle is low frequency (i.e., less than 10 Hz), alternating, sine wave current (Fig. 8–2).

5. Which of the three waveforms is most ideally suited to the stimulation of denervated muscle?

The exponentially progressive current is probably best suited for selectively stimulating denervated muscle. While providing for the selective stimulation of denervated muscle, this current form is quite comfortable to the patient because sensory fibers accommodate to the slowly rising stimulus. Similarly, adjacent axons to innervated muscle also accommodate to the slowly rising stimulus, so that overstimulation of nearby innervated muscle fibers is avoided. Stimulators that offer an exponentially progressive waveform usually provide a means to adjust the interpulse interval in order to avoid fatiguing the muscle by providing for adequate rest periods between successive contractions. Unfortunately this type of equipment has limited availability in the United States. One stimulator that is available in the United States is the Neuroton manufactured by Siemens.*

---

*Siemens Corporation, Erlangen, Germany.

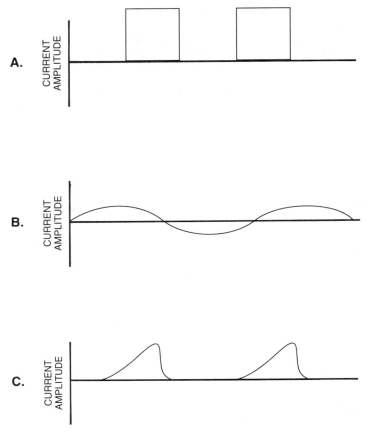

FIGURE 8–2. Representations of several waveforms used in stimulating denervated muscle. The waveforms (*A*) are pulsed, monophasic, square waveforms. The waveforms (*B*) are representative of symmetrical alternating sine-wave current, and the waveforms (*C*) are exponentially progressive waveforms.

Although interrupted, monophasic direct current has traditionally been used to stimulate denervated muscle, the waveform has limitations. Since the current is applied to the muscle instantaneously, the response of the muscle is a very sudden and rapid contraction that leads to very rapid fatigue. Also, a fairly intense stimulus is often required for this type of current, which is not only uncomfortable, but may also overstimulate any spared innervated muscle fibers. Low frequency, symmetrical alternating current (alternating sine wave current) can also effectively stimulate denervated muscle. However, one drawback with this type of current is providing for an adequate rest period following each contraction. In most stimulators that offer symmetrical alternating current, the current flow is continuous. This would require that the therapist manually interrupt the current flow after each contraction in order to provide for an adequate rest period between successive contractions.

6. When should we begin to stimulate the denervated muscle, and how often should we continue to stimulate the muscle?

A number of studies[17,72] suggest that the sooner stimulation is initiated follow-ing denervation, the better the results will be. Three stimulation sessions a day is also recommended. The number of contractions at each session will vary according to the fatigability of the muscle, but three sets of 5 to 20 repetitions should not overfatigue the muscle if an adequate rest period is provided between successive contractions, as well as rest periods of several minutes provided between sets. Such frequent sessions would require institution of a home program.

7. Are the denervated muscles stimulated as a group, or are they stimulated individually?

Each muscle is individually stimulated using either the monopolar or bipolar technique. Using the monopolar technique, the site of stimulation on each muscle is that point along the muscle that is most electrically excitable. This is the point at which a minimal amount of current will elicit a just-visible muscle contraction. This point must be determined for each muscle at each treatment session. In addition, muscles may require different pulse durations, and therefore this param-eter should be set independently for each muscle.

8. How long should electrical stimulation of the denervated muscle continue?

Stimulation should continue for 4 to 6 weeks beyond the projected time for reinnervation to occur. The projected time for reinnervation will depend upon the location and extent of the lesion. Peripheral nerves typically regenerate at approxi-mately 1.5 mm per day. Therefore, in our patient with the forearm stab wound the projected reinnervation time may be as long as 6 to 8 months.

CASE STUDY

A 55-year-old man diagnosed as having amyotrophic lateral sclerosis was referred to physical therapy for electrical stimulation of the intrinsic muscles of the right hand.

1. Could this patient benefit from electrical stimulation of the intrinsic muscles of the right hand?

This patient would not benefit from electrical stimulation on the denervated intrinsic hand muscles. Amyotrophic lateral sclerosis is a progressive, degenerative disease affecting both upper and lower motor neurons. Although it is possible to electrically stimulate the denervated muscle and elicit a contraction, stimulation would be futile since the involved lower motor neurons will not regenerate, and reinnervation will not occur.

SUMMARY

While techniques used by the clinician in the electrical stimulation of denervated muscle may vary, the ultimate goal remains the same. The therapist attempts to mini-mize the extent of denervation atrophy by electrical stimulation. Another consideration alluded to earlier in this chapter is the possibility that electrical stimulation following denervation may have a positive trophic influence on axonal regeneration leading to more rapid and more functional recovery.

Although electrical stimulation may be indicated, the therapist and patient must consider the potential financial and time cost associated with a long-term (up to 2 years) electrical stimulation program. Such a program requires commitment of the patient to a comprehensive home program with periodic (i.e., weekly or once every 2 weeks) reevaluation by the therapist. A home program involves the long-term commitment and compliance of the patient and the patient's family. This is an important consideration especially in view of the difficulty in predicting the outcome of the electrical stimulation program.

The future use of electrical stimulation in the treatment of denervated muscle appears warranted. Although a number of basic science and clinical observations strongly suggest that electrical stimulation may benefit denervated muscle, we must depend upon future research to determine ideal stimulation protocols.

REFERENCES

1. Bordier, H: La galvanofaradisation rhythmic. Arch Electr Med 10:331, 1902.
2. Sunderland, S: Nerves and Nerve Injuries. Churchill Livingston, Edinburgh, 1969.
3. Brooke, M and Kaiser, K: Muscle fiber types: How many and what kind? Arch Neurol 23:369, 1970.
4. Engel, WK and Stonnington, HH: Morphological effects of denervation of muscle: Quantitative ultrastructural study. Ann NY Acad Sci 228:68, 1974.
5. Pullam, DL and April, EW: Degenerative changes at neuromuscular junctions of red, white and intermediate muscle fibers. J Neurol Sci 43:205, 1979.
6. Lomo, T: Role of activity in control of membrane and contractile properties of skeletal muscle. In Tjesleff, S (ed): Motor Innervation of Muscle. Academic Press, New York, 1976, p 289.
7. Guth, L and Albuquerque, EX: Neurotrophic regulation of resting membrane potential and extrajunctional acetylcholine sensitivity in mammalian skeletal muscle. In Mauro, A (ed): Muscle Regeneration. Raven Press, New York, 1979, p 405.
8. Shafiq, SA, Milhorat, AT, and Gorycki, MA: Fine structure of human muscle in neurogenic atrophy. Neurology 17:934, 1967.
9. Guth, L: "Trophic" influence of nerve on muscle. Physiol Rev 48:645, 1968.
10. Herbison, GJ, Jaweed, MM, and Ditunno, JF: Effect of activity and inactivity on reinnervating rat skeletal muscle contractility. Exp Neurol 70:498, 1980.
11. Eccles, J, Eccles, R, and Lundenberg, A: The action potential of the alpha motoneurons supplying fast and slow muscle. J Physiol (London) 142:275, 1958.
12. Herbison, G, et al: Effect of electrical stimulation on denervated muscle of rat. Arch Phys Med Rehabil 52:516, 1971.
13. Knowlton, GC and Hines, HM: Kinetics of muscle atrophy in different species. Proc Soc Exp Biol Med 35:394, 1936.
14. Engel, WK, Brooke, MH, and Nelson, PG: Histochemical studies of denervated or tenotomized rat muscle: Illustrating difficulties in relating experimental animal conditions to human neuromuscular diseases. Ann NY Acad Sci 138:160, 1966.
15. Pachter, B, Eberstein, A, and Goodgold, J: Electrical stimulation effect on denervated skeletal muscle myofibers in rats: A light and electron microscopic study. Arch Phys Med Rehabil 63:427, 1982.
16. Jaweed, MM, Herbison, GJ, and Ditunno, JF: Denervation and reinnervation of fast and slow muscles. A histochemical study in rats. J Histochem Cytochem 23:808, 1975.
17. Hoffman, H: Acceleration and retardation of the process of axon-sprouting in partially denervated muscles. Aust J Exp Biol Med Sci 30:541, 1952.
18. Deshpane, S, Albuquerque, E, and Guth, L: Neurotrophic regulation of prejunctional and postjunctional membrane at the mammalian motor endplate. Exp Neurol 53:151, 1976.
19. Axelsson, J and Thesleff, S: A study of supersensitivity in denervated mammalian skeletal muscle. J Physiol 147:178, 1959.
20. Miledi, R: The acetylcholine sensitivity of frog muscle fibers after complete or partial denervation. J Physiol 151:1, 1960.
21. Katz, B and Miledi, R: The development of acetylcholine sensitivity in nerve free segments of skeletal muscle. J Physiol 170:389, 1964.
22. Muchnik, S and Kotsias, B: Characteristics of reinnervation of skeletal muscle in rat. Acta Physiol Lat Am 16:481, 1976.
23. Lomo, T and Slater, CR: Control of acetylicholine sensitivity and synapse formation by muscle activity. J Physiol 275:391, 1978.

24. Guth, L: Regeneration in the mammalian peripheral nervous system. Physiol Nev 36:441, 1956.
25. Aguayo, A, et al: Axonal elongation in peripheral and central nervous system transplants. Adv Cell Neurobiol 3:215, 1982.
26. Cajal, R: Degeneration and regeneration of the nervous system (translated and edited by May, Raoul M.) Hafner Press/Macmillan, New York, 1959.
27. Varon, SS and Bunge, RP: Trophic mechanisms in the peripheral nervous system. Ann Rev Neurosci 1:327, 1978.
28. Brown, MC, Holland, RL, and Hopkins, WG: Motor nerve sprouting. Ann Rev Neurosci 4:17, 1981.
29. Lundborg, G, et al: Nerve regeneration in silicone chambers: Influence of gap length and of distal stump components. Exp Neurol 76:361, 1982.
30. Williams, LR: Exogenous fibrin matrix precursors stimulate the temporal progress of nerve regeneration within a silicone chamber. Neurochem Res 12:851, 1987.
31. Williams, LR: Rat aorta isografts possess nerve regeneration-promoting properties in silicone Y chambers. Exp Neurol 97:555, 1987.
32. Salmons, S and Vrbova, G: The infuence of activity on some contractile characteristics of mammalian fast and slow muscles. J Physiol (London) 201:535, 1969.
33. Pette, D, et al: Effects of long-term electrical stimulation on some contractile and metabolic characteristics of fast rabbit muscles. Pflugers Arch 338:257, 1973.
34. Heilig, A and Pette, D: Changes induced in the enzyme activity pattern by electrical stimulation of fast-twitch muscle. In Pette, D (ed): Plasticity of Muscle. Walter deGruyter, New York, 1980, p 409.
35. Nix, WA, Reichman, H, and Schroder, MJ: Influence of direct low frequency stimulation on contractile properties of denervated fast-twitch rabbit muscle. Pflugers Arch 405:141, 1985.
36. Reichman, H and Nix, WA: Changes of energy metabolism, myosin light chain composition, lactate dehydrogenase isozyme pattern and fiber type distribution of denervated fast-twitch muscle from rabbit after low frequency stimulation. Pflugers Arch 405:244, 1985.
37. Rosselle, N, et al: Electromyographic evaluation of therapeutic methods in complete peripheral paralysis. Electromyogr Clin Neurophysiol 17:179, 1977.
38. Valencic, V, et al: Improved motor response due to chronic electrical stimulation of denervated tibialis anterior muscle in humans. Muscle Nerve 9:612, 1986.
39. Reid, J: On the relation between muscular contractibility and the nervous system. Lond Edin Mon J Med Sci 1:320, 1841.
40. Brown-Sequard, E: Experimental Researches Applied to Physiology and Pathology. H Bailliere, New York, 1853.
41. Langley, JN and Kato, T: The rate of loss of weight in skeletal muscle after nerve section with some observations on the effect of stimulation and other treatment. J Physiol 49:432, 1915.
42. Langley, JN: Observations on denervated muscle. J Physiol 50:335, 1916.
43. Fischer, E: The effect of faradic and galvanic stimulation upon the course of atrophy in denervated skeletal muscles. Am J Physiol 17:605, 1939.
44. Gutmann, E and Guttmann, L: Effect of electro therapy on denervated and reinnervated muscles in rabbit. Lancet 1:169, 1942.
45. Gutmann, E and Guttmann, L: Effect of galvanic exercise on denervated and re-innervated muscles in rabbit. J Neurol Neurosurg Psychiatry 7–17, 1944.
46. Pollack, LJ, et al: Electrotherapy in experimentally produced lesions of peripheral nerves. Arch Phys Med Rehabil 37:377, 1951.
47. Schimrigk, KJ, McLaughlen, J, and Gruniger, W: The effect of electrical stimulation on the experimentally denervated rat muscle. Scand J Rehabil Med 9:55, 1977.
48. Jackson, E and Seddon, H: Influence of galvanic stimulation on muscle atrophy resulting from denervation. Br Med J 2:485, 1945.
49. Liu, C and Lewey, F: Effect of surging currents of low frequency in man on atrophy of denervated muscle. J Nerv Ment Dis 105:571, 1947.
50. Osborne, S: The retardation of atrophy in man by electrical stimulation of muscles. Arch Phys Med Rehabil 32:523, 1951.
51. Guth, L, et al: The roles of disease and loss of neurotrophic function in denervation atrophy of skeletal muscle. Exp Neurol 73:20, 1981.
52. Nix, W: The effect of low-frequency electrical stimulation on the denervated extensor digitorum longus muscle of the rabbit. Acta Neurol Scand 66:521, 1982.
53. Girlanda, PR, et al: Effect of electrotherapy on denervated muscles in rabbits: An electrophysiological and morphological study. Exp Neurol 77:483, 1982.
54. Cole, BG and Gardiner, PF: Does electrical stimulation of denervated muscle, continued after reinnervation, influence recovery of contractile function? Exp Neurol 85:52, 1984.
55. Solandt, D, DeLury, D, and Hunter, J: Effect of electrical stimulation on atrophy of denervated skeletal muscle. Arch Neurol Psychiatry 49:802, 1943.
56. Morris, H: Medical Electricity for Massage Students. Churchill, Ltd, London, 1934, 1940, 1943, 1946, 1953.
57. Thom, H: Treatment of paralysis with exponentially progressive currents. Br J Phys Med 20:49, 1957.

58. Herbison, G, Jaweed, M, and Ditunno, J: Acetylcholine sensitivity and fibrillation potentials in electrically stimulated crush-denervated rat skeletal muscle. Arch Phys Med Rehabil 64:217, 1983.
59. Lomo, T, Westgaard, R, and Dahl, H: Contractile properties of muscle: Control by pattern of muscle activity in the rat. Proc R Soc Lond [Biol] 187:99, 1974.
60. Lomo, T and Rosenthal, J: Control of ACh sensitivity by muscle activity in the rat. J Physiol (Lond) 221:493, 1972.
61. Lomo, T, Westgaard, R, and Engebretsen, L: Differential stimulation patterns affect contractile properties of denervated rat soleus. In Pette, D (ed): Plasticity of Muscle. Gruyter, New York, 1980.
62. Jaweed, M, Herbison, G, and Ditunno, J: Prostaglandins in denervated skeletal muscle of rat: Effect of direct electrical stimulation. Neurosci 6:787, 1982.
63. Sebille, A and Boudoux-Jahan, M: Effects of electrical stimulation and previous nerve injury on motor function in rats. Brain Res 193:562, 1980.
64. Rosselle, N, et al: Electromyographic evaluation of therapeutic methods in complete peripheral paralysis. Electromyogr Clin Neurophysiol 14:549, 1974.
65. Pinelli, P, Arrigo, A, and Moglia, A: In Tibialis Anterior Reinnervation by Collateral Branching With or Without Electrotherapy. Proc Fourth Congr Int Soc Electromyogr Kinesiol, Boston, 1979, p 106.
66. Chor, H, et al: Atrophy and regeneration of the gastrocnemius-soleus muscles. JAMA 113:1029, 1939.
67. Kosman, AJ, Osborne, SL, and Ivey, AC: Comparative effectiveness of various electrical currents in preventing muscle atrophy in rat. Arch Phys Med Rehabil 28:7, 1947a.
68. Kosman, AJ, Osborne, SL, and Ivey, AC: The influence of duration and frequency of treatment in electrical stimulation of paralyzed muscle. Arch Phys Med Rehabil 28:12, 1947b.
69. Kosman, AJ, Osborne, SL, and Ivey, AC: Importance of current form and frequency in electrical stimulation of muscles. Arch Phys Med 29:559, 1948.
70. Wehrmacher, WH, Thompson, JD, and Hines, HM: Effect of electrical stimulation on denervated skeletal muscle. Arch Phys Med 26:261, 1945.
71. Elliott, DR and Thomson, JD: Dynamic properties of denervated rat muscle treated with electrotherapy. Am J Physiol 205:173, 1963.
72. Pockett, S and Gavin, RM: Acceleration of peripheral nerve regeneration after crush injury in rat. Neurosci Lett 59:221, 1985.
73. Slack, JR, Hopkins, WG, and Pockett, S: Evidence for a motor nerve growth factor. Muscle Nerve 6:243, 1983.
74. Slack, JR and Pockett, S: Terminal sprouting of motoneurons is a local response to a local stimulus. Brain Res 217:368, 1981.
75. Thomas, PK: Nerve injury. In Belairs, R and Gray, EJ (eds): Essays on the Nervous System. Festschrift for Prof JZ Young. Clarendon Press, Oxford, 1974, p 44.
76. Pockett, S and Phillip, B: Acceleration of peripheral nerve regeneration. In Gordon, T, Stein, RB, and Smith, PA (eds): The Current Status of Peripheral Nerve Regeneration, Vol. 38, Neurology and Neurobiology. Alan R. Liss, New York, 1988, p 195.
77. Kowarschik, J: Exponential currents. Br J Phys Med 15:249, 1952.
78. Thom, H: Possibilities and limits of electrotherapy of paralysis. Arch Phys Ther 7:3, 1955.

CHAPTER 9

Electromyographic Biofeedback(EMGBF) for Neuromuscular Relaxation and Re-education

Deborah E. LeCraw, M.M.Sc., P.T.
Steven L. Wolf, Ph.D., P.T., F.A.P.T.A.

As early as 1830 electromyographic (EMG) recordings were made from animal preparations; however, it wasn't until 1929 that the single motor unit action potential was recorded and described,[1] following advances in technology and the understanding of anatomy and physiology. In 1938, Jacobsen[2] reported the use of EMG to train subjects to reach deeply relaxed states. In 1948, Price, Clare, and Everhardt[3] examined EMG activity in patients associated with persistent muscle spasm with low backache, and by the late 1950s and early 1960s Andrews,[4] Mims,[5] and Marinacci and Horande[6] addressed the potential use of EMG with the hemiplegic patient.

In 1969, a group of investigators gathered to discuss biologic feedback mechanisms; they coined the term *biofeedback* from *biologic feedback* and also formed the Biofeedback Research Society.[7] This organization, later renamed the Biofeedback Society of America, has grown along with the field of biofeedback applications. Biofeedback applications have developed for many types of physiologic factors including skin temperature,[8] heart rate,[9] blood pressure,[10] skin conductance,[9] as well as for force,[11,12] motion,[13] and position monitoring.[14,15] Whereas these applications are varied and useful in rehabilitation,[7] their discussion is beyond the scope of this chapter.

The purpose of this chapter is to introduce electromyographic feedback (EMGBF) to those clinicians new to or recently acquainted with the topic, and serve as a reference to the EMGBF-experienced clinicians as they make use of this instrumentation and the recent advances in its technology.

To fully understand and interpret the raw EMG signal or a processed, visual representation of the EMG signal, the clinician should understand how the muscle action potential is generated, detected, and processed.

BIOPHYSICAL PRINCIPLES

The Electromyographic Signal

When the anterior horn cell is depolarized by peripheral or supraspinal influences, its axon conducts an action potential to the neuromuscular junction where acetylcholine is released, diffuses across the synaptic cleft, and attaches to receptor sites of the sarcolemma. Depolarization of the postsynaptic muscle membrane continues in both directions of the muscle fiber and is accompanied by movement of ions, which generates an electrochemical gradient in the vicinity of the muscle fibers. An electrode located in this field will detect change in the potential difference or voltage (with respect to ground) associated with depolarization. Such characteristic changes are labeled action potentials.[15]

Krebs[16] emphasized the difference between the electrical and mechanical events occurring during muscle activation and contraction. The electrical event, depolarization of the sarcolemma, is recorded by an EMG instrument. The mechanical event, muscle contraction, occurs only after the depolarization of the sarcolemma results in release of calcium ions from the sarcoplasmic reticulum. The increase in calcium ions within the sarcoplasm promotes physical interactions between actin and myosin filaments, leading to the development of muscle tension.

The number of muscle fibers contracting depends upon the size and number of the motor units activated.[17] Both large and small motor units are found in most skeletal muscles. The development of increased tension of a muscle contraction occurs by increasing the number of motor units firing (recruitment) and by increasing a motor unit's discharge frequency (rate coding). Most participating motor units discharge at about the same rate during weak-to-moderate tonic voluntary contractions. Changes in net discharge frequency are usually seen only during phasic contractions or with strong, sustained muscle contractions.[18]

Signal Detection and Amplification

As muscle membranes in the vicinity of the detecting electrode depolarize, reverse polarity, and then repolarize as a result of changes in ion flow, a triphasic signal is generated reflecting these stages of membrane activity.[15,19] Once the signal is detected by the electrode, the signal is amplified. Equipment usually requiring two active electrodes and a single ground (or reference) electrode necessitates the use of a bipolar arrangement in the detection and filtering of the EMG signal (Fig. 9–1). Each active electrode picks up EMG activity with respect to the reference electrode. Each of the two signals is fed to the differential amplifier, which amplifies the difference between the two signals. Consequently, any components of the two signals having a "common mode" are eliminated, including those signals with a similar amplitude at both detection surfaces. The ability of a differential amplifier to eliminate signals with a common mode is referred to as the common-mode rejection ratio (CMRR).[15] As can be seen in Figure 9–1, the EMG signal undergoes some filtering by the bipolar electrodes as well as by the

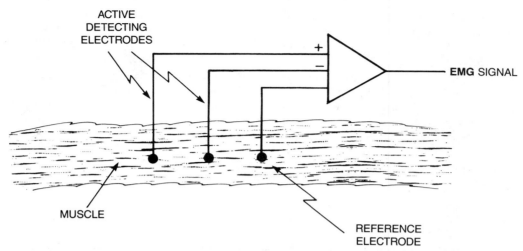

FIGURE 9–1. Bipolar detection of EMG activity. The signals detected at electrodes 1 and 2 are M1 + N and M2 + N, respectively. The EMG activity at each electrode is considered different while the noise at each electrode is considered to be similar. (Adapted from Deluca.[20])

tissues prior to being amplified.[1] Signal detection and amplification are described in detail in Chapter 3.

Because the amplifier will amplify both desired (EMG) and undesired (noise) signals, it is helpful to understand the origins of noise and those measures that can be taken to reduce or eliminate it. According to Basmajian,[20] noise arises from static electricity located on the surface of the subject, for example, clothing; electromagnetic fields from line current, radio signals, and so forth; "thermal" noise from the electrodes; noise generated by the first stage of the amplifiers; and motion artifacts from movement at the electrode-tissue interface and the wire leads connecting the electrodes to the amplifier.

Abrasion of the skin during preparation for electrode placement will reduce artifacts from the electrode-tissue interface by reducing electrical impedance.[20] Motion artifact may be reduced by carefully securing leads to the skin with tape. A variety of measures may be used to reduce static electricity in a patient's hair or clothing: commercially available antistatic sprays are one example. The remainder of the noise present in the environment is dealt with by the differential amplifier. As the muscle activity and noise are detected by each electrode, noise is minimized by the subtraction of the common inputs, as represented in the equation:

$$\text{EMG signal} = (M1 + N) - (M2 + N)$$

where M1 and M2 are EMG seen by the first and second electrodes, respectively, and N is noise. Each electrode picks up the EMG signal as well as other electrical activity generated within its area of pickup (M1 + N and M2 + N). As the signal plus noise are transmitted to the differential amplifier, the *difference* between what is received from the electrodes is amplified and transmitted further.

$$\text{Amplified EMG signal} = \text{gain} \left[(M1 + N) - (M2 + N) \right]$$

In this context gain refers to the amount by which the signal has been amplified. The differential amplifier cancels out the like signals (N) from each electrode. However, perfect cancellation of noise does not occur because (1) subtraction by the amplifier is imperfect and (2) the noise reaching the active electrodes is probably not exactly alike in all aspects, that is, the signals are not all of "common mode." If the signals are sufficiently different in amplitude, phase, or frequency, cancellation will not occur. The actual CMRR is determined by the ratio of the voltage common to both input stages (Ecm) and the voltage common to both input stages that is *not* canceled out, that is, the error voltage, (Ee). This ratio is illustrated as

$$CMRR : \frac{Ecm}{Ee}$$

As the CMRR increases, the cancellation of unwanted currents (noise) appearing at both input stages improves.

Once the EMG signal is detected and differentially amplified, further processing is done to generate a representation of the EMG signal. The signal is visualized by a line moving across a screen or a screen of lights activated in sequence to represent the magnitude of a muscle response. A level detection device is also incorporated within the equipment to determine when a "target" level has been achieved and when the quality of the audio signal has changed (see the section, "Visual Representation of the EMG Signal").

Rectification and Integration of the EMG Signal

Recall that the EMG signal usually has a triphasic pattern which has peaks above and below the zero point (Fig. 3–11, Chapter 3). These positive and negative deflections are a reflection of the changes in ion movement across the sarcolemma. With signal rectification, negative deflections may either be eliminated (half-wave rectification) or inverted (full-wave rectification). The latter is preferred, as all of the signal is retained for further processing. The process of rectification is detailed in Chapter 3. Next, the rectified signal is often smoothed to prepare for integration. Smoothing occurs as high-frequency fluctuations from a signal are suppressed.[21] The degree of smoothing depends upon the filter used. For further information on this topic, refer to Basmajian and Deluca.[15] After the signal has been rectified and smoothed, the EMG voltage of the area under the signal curve may be obtained for a specified time period. This is known as signal integration; integration is the fundamental basis for quantifying EMG activity.

Visual Representation of the EMG Signal

After signal processing, the electromyographic activity may be presented to the patient in a variety of ways. EMG activity may be displayed visually as a line traveling across a monitor, as bars that change levels are integrated value changes, as an array of lights, or as a component of a video game.

Furthermore, as the integrated value of EMG changes, various forms of audio signals can be used. A tone, click, or beep may occur in response to changes in integrated EMG activity with respect to the threshold level set by the clinician. For example, in relaxation training, the audio signal may be silent below a preset threshold level and audible once the integrated EMG activity exceeds the threshold. In facilitatory training, the audio signal may be a faint tone or infrequent clicks at low levels of EMG activity, and may increase in volume and/or frequency of repetition as threshold is approached or surpassed.

Obviously, multiple factors can influence how active surface or indwelling electrodes detect muscle potentials. While EMG provides an opportunity to quantify analog biological activity, it is far from a perfect science. Indeed, later in the chapter we will examine the many factors influencing the EMG signal seen by the patient.

Depending upon the visual and auditory displays available, the clinician may integrate this information into the therapeutic process. Clinical applications are broad and varied. Some examples illustrating the use of EMGBF for adult clients with orthopedic or neurological deficits and for children are provided in the section on clinical applications that follows.

CLINICAL CONSIDERATIONS FOR ADMINISTERING EMGBF

Considerations for Application

Implementing EMGBF training can be fairly simple, largely because training becomes very specific and straightforward. To begin with, there are only two goals that can be used when training a patient to alter EMG activity — either to reduce or enhance muscle activity. The clinician selects the functional activity desired and the muscle groups involved. The presence of paresis or spasticity is identified along with the available joint motion and sensation (e.g., crude and light touch, proprioception). The progression of training (e.g., proximal-to-distal training within a limb segment), type of muscle contraction (isometric, isotonic, or eccentric), and joint-segment training (reciprocal or simultaneous action of muscles about the joint) are identified. Also, the position of the patient during retraining, as well as how that position may change, is considered. The actual evaluation and treatment approaches used are no different from those normally used in the clinic. The primary difference between evaluative and treatment methods that employ EMGBF lies in the use of the information acquired during treatment.

PATIENT SELECTION

Before addressing patient selection, the clinician should consider whether the goal of the treatment is *EMGBF training* or therapeutic exercise in which muscle activity will be monitored primarily by the clinician through EMGBF. If the latter approach is to be adopted, the patient's receptive abilities, motor-planning skills, degree of neglect, or degree of aphasia are of little concern. However, during EMGBF training, these characteristics must be addressed in order to gain the optimal outcome. Bach-y-Rita and coworkers,[21] and Wolf, Baker, and Kelly[22] reported successful progress in retraining hemiplegic patients with mild expressive aphasia. Bach-y-Rita and coworkers also reported progress with patients expressing mild receptive aphasia. Balliet, Levy, and Blood[23] discussed methods by which five hemiplegic patients who had completed 6 to 60 months of rehabilitation and who exhibited neglect, aphasia, and varying degrees of apraxia were treated to improve functional use of their right upper extremity. Two of the patients were considered flaccid whereas three displayed a chronic spastic-flexion posture without contracture. Those with spasticity were able to achieve a gross-assist level of function characterized by limited isolated voluntary movement through a partial range of motion; the ability to perform some tasks requiring proximal stability but with distal synergy present; the ability to hold a door open with some synergy; and the ability to demonstrate elbow extension to assist with rising from a chair.

To participate in EMGBF training, the patient must have sufficient vision to see the visual display, audition and reception to hear and comprehend simple directions, and expressive abilities and motor planning skills to respond to basic instructions. Patients with visual field limitation, hearing difficulties, mild receptive or expressive aphasia, or mild apraxia may still be able to participate and benefit from training. Patients without these deficits may perform quite well and progress in their ability to assume a greater participative role in treatment. For example, in some training sessions the author has had patients *request* time to work independently after the basic training strategy was clear to them.

The final consideration of patient selection is the realistic appraisal of the patient's rehabilitation potential. Obviously, a patient with a known complete spinal cord transection is not an appropriate candidate for EMGBF training. Also, presence of a severe sensory deficit such as a dense loss of proprioception will adversely affect outcome. However, there are few *specific* guidelines for this aspect of patient selection. For example, Wolf, Baker, and Kelly[22] noted that the hemiplegic patients most likely to make functional gains with upper extremity EMGBF training were those with a minimal degree of wrist and/or finger extension and thumb abduction. The final decision regarding use of EMGBF training is, frequently, subjective and may be made on a trial basis.

GENERAL EVALUATION

Before EMGBF training can be effectively incorporated into a treatment plan, a thorough evaluation of the particular disability must be completed. Once known, factors affecting a patient's rehabilitation progress, for example, spasticity, paresis, or joint-movement limitations, can be addressed while EMGBF is being incorporated into the treatment plan. Because EMGBF provides very specific and immediate information concerning muscle activity, it is imperative that the clinician define exactly each goal that is being pursued in the treatment session, how that particular goal relates to the patient's primary goal, and the stage of progression toward functional recovery.

TREATMENT GOALS

Recall that there are only two general goals of training with EMGBF—either enhancement or reduction of EMG activity. *How* these two options are built into a treatment plan will affect how a patient may progress. After the evaluation is complete and functional goals have been established, identify a functional goal toward which to work. Examine the factors affecting the goal (e.g., spasticity, dominance of synergy, weakness, or joint limitations) and begin at this point to consider how these factors will affect the application of EMGBF. For example, if a patient exhibits a significant amount of spasticity, closely spaced electrodes will probably be used during initial relaxation training. Next divide the functional goal into subtasks, and analyze each subtask in terms of muscle activity changes that are required to complete the subtask. Apply electrodes to skin overlying those muscles involved in the subtask. Consideration should be given to appropriate spacing, the potential for volume-conducted activity, the available muscle mass, and other factors affecting the EMG signal. Initiate training with the patient performing the simplest and easiest change in muscle activity, progressing toward increasing the complexity of the training within the confines of the patient's physical and mental abilities. To ensure maximum carryover into functional skills, incorporate functional goals as a part of the training as early as can be done with success and consistency, preferably in the first or second session.

SKIN PREPARATION

When surface electrodes are used, impedance leading to signal attenuation can be attributed to adipose tissue, oils or dirt on the skin, or increased keratinization of the skin, for example, from scarring, callous formation, darker skin color, or greater skin maturity. Proper skin preparation will remove oils, dead skin cells, and excess hair from the epidermis, thereby reducing potentially high impedance sources during recording sessions. If not removed, these elements will attenuate the EMG signals and will likely lead to increased noise levels. Techniques to reduce skin impedance vary and depend on the degree of reduction desired. Techniques include (1) alcohol rub, (2) rub with slightly abrasive electrolytic paste, and (3) dry-skin shaving parallel to the direction of hair growth.

Most frequently, the hair may be clipped or the skin shaved, and, if necessary, rubbed with alcohol, and then the electrodes are applied. If further reduction in impedance is required, rubbing the skin with a slightly abrasive high-salt electrode paste after shaving will sufficiently reduce the skin impedance. If electrical stimulation is to be used along with the biofeedback, care should be taken to keep the area of stimulation free from high-salt electrode paste. The presence of paste residue beneath the stimulating electrodes may result in relatively minor, but uncomfortable, chemical irritation.

To ascertain whether skin preparation is sufficient, the impedance, or total opposition to AC current flow due to resistive, inductive, and capacitive factors, is measured (see Chapter 3). A simple, indirect way to test impedance is to use a DC ohmmeter.[1] During impedance tests, in addition to measuring interelectrode impedance of active electrodes, it is sometimes also useful to measure active-to-ground resistances. For a particular bipolar electrode pair, if there is a marked difference in the active-to-ground resistance, 60 Hz and other electrostatic noise may more likely contaminate the EMG signal.[1]

Subcutaneous fat, scarring, or callous formation over muscle locations cannot be readily modified. The best approach is to prepare the skin appropriately, place the electrodes over the muscle in the proper orientation, and manipulate the sensitivity (gain) of the EMG unit to detect as much EMG activity as possible.

ELECTRODE TYPES AND SIZES

Selection of the electrode size is determined primarily by the size of the muscle from which EMG signals will be monitored. The goal is to gain a reasonable sample of the muscle's activity while avoiding undesired volume-conducted activity from neighboring or underlying muscles, that is, "cross talk." Miniature surface electrodes with recording surfaces of 0.2 cm in diameter have been effectively used during retraining of small muscles located in the face, distal forearm, and hand. Larger electrodes with 1.0 cm recording surface have been successfully used for retraining larger muscle groups. Today most electrode recording surfaces are coated with a silver-silver chloride base.

Increasing electrode size usually will not result in an increase in signal amplitude. Even though more fibers contribute to generating the EMG signal, their individual voltages have proportionately less of an influence on a larger electrode. Debacher examined the EMG activity from pairs of large and miniature surface electrodes over biceps and kept spacing and location constant. He observed that although the area of the large versus the small electrodes differed by a factor of 5, there was no difference in the EMG integral for constant force contractions.[1] Consequently, the electrode size is primarily considered a factor affecting appropriate sampling of muscle activity while avoiding undesired volume-conducted activity.

ELECTRODE PLACEMENT, ORIENTATION, AND SPACING

Those muscle fibers nearest the electrode will have the greatest effect on the signal that is detected. The closer the fibers are to the electrode, the greater the selectivity the electrode will have for those fibers, as the signal-to-noise ratio of the relevant-to-extraneous EMG is increased.[1] Those signals generated by muscle fibers distant from the electrode will be attenuated both by the distance and the impedance of the intervening tissues.[1]

To achieve the most accurate placement over the target muscle, the electrodes should be secured to the body part in the position in which it will be placed during the session. This consideration is particularly important when monitoring EMG activity of the forearm and other areas where the skin movement over the underlying musculature during activities can cause muscles other than those desired to be monitored. Prolonged muscle atrophy and the subsequent increased skin pliability, such as after spinal cord injury, makes this concern especially relevant to treatment.

Orientation of electrode pair with respect to muscle fibers will have an effect on the degree of signal cancellation that occurs as well as the degree of coverage of the muscle from which the EMG sample is taken. Electrodes aligned *perpendicular* to muscle fibers will have potentials affect them simultaneously, and some signal cancellation will occur, resulting in active electrodes monitoring the same motor units. If the electrodes are oriented parallel to muscle-fiber direction, different motor units representing a better sample of the muscle activity will be monitored and extraneous, volume-conducted activity picked up by both electrodes will be reduced.

When determining electrode orientation, first consider the degree of paresis present. For patients with marked paresis, a placement ensuring the least-signal cancellation (parallel) would be selected. If extreme paresis is not a problem, then either a parallel or perpendicular orientation may be used.

Electrode spacing will affect the degree of signal cancellation by the differential amplifier, the signal amplitude, the volume of the muscle examined, and the degree of volume-conducted activity from muscles extraneous to those being directly sampled. Local current flow in a whole muscle will spread throughout the tissue and will follow the volume-conducting properties of the surrounding electrolytic solution.[20] The volume conductor is that conducting medium through which current will spread from a potential source. As a rule, electrodes will detect measurable signals from a distance equal to that of the interelectrode spacing.[15] Consequently, as the distance between electrodes increases, the EMG signal will include input from the muscles immediately beneath the electrodes but also other nearby muscles. EMG activity present from these secondary muscle groups is known as *cross talk*[15] or *volume-conducted activity*[19] and, unless desired, is regarded as an EMG signal contaminant. Understanding this concept is vital in critically interpreting the EMG signal.

Clinical interpretation of the EMG signal in light of volume-conducted activity will vary depending on the goals of the EMGBF session. For example, during relaxation training of a highly spastic lower-extremity adductor mass, the goal is to have the patient learn to induce and maintain a relaxed state. The interelectrode distance early in training is narrow, thus the EMG signal reflects the relaxation of a relatively small portion of the muscle mass. Gradually the patient is trained to control the muscle activity produced as the interelectrode distance is progressively increased. In some cases, the patient is asked to control the EMG activity from an electrode placement in which one active electrode is on the right thigh adductor mass and the other active electrode is on the left thigh adductor mass. Clearly, the EMG signal reflects volume-conducted activity. However, since the goal is to relax such a large muscle mass, the massive volume of activity is not regarded as a signal contaminant.

Similarly, volume-conducted activity is not considered undesirable during the early stages of EMGBF retraining of significantly paretic muscles. The initial goal is to detect *any* measurable EMG activity. Thus relatively large interelectrode distances are selected. As muscle activity becomes apparent with this use of wide electrode placement, the clinician must recognize the probability that volume-conducted activity is present and identify the primary muscle groups contributing to the EMG signal, particularly if spasticity is present or expected to develop. As the patient generates more muscle activity during training sessions, interelectrode distance is gradually reduced. EMGBF training becomes progressively more specific to the point that efforts are made to coordinate muscle groups within a limb segment.

Volume-conducted activity is regarded as a signal contaminant when it leads to misinterpretation of the EMG signal. As EMGBF training focuses on coordination of muscle groups within the limb segment, it is critical to understand the muscle activity represented at each EMGBF channel. For example, if dorsiflexion with eversion during gait is identified as the desired functional goal, the therapist may place an electrode pair over the anterior tibialis to monitor dorsiflexor activity and over the peroneus longus to monitor evertor activity. During dorsiflexion with eversion at heelstrike, the peroneal EMG activity will appropriately rise (Figure 9–2). During the stance phase as the foot is placed flat during the gait cycle and as the patient's weight is transferred to the ball of the foot just prior to and during push off, peroneal EMG activity will again increase quite strongly. This second rise in the EMG activity coming from the electrode pair overlying the peroneus longus reflects peroneal activity as well as volume-conducted activity from the adjacent gastrocnemius muscles (Fig. 9–3).

To avoid confusion during gait training, the clinician may begin training with the swing phase of gait, excluding the production of plantarflexor activity. As training progresses, the patient may be prepared to expect two peaks of muscle activity from the peroneal muscles, one during the swing phase followed by a peak from midstance through the push-off phase in the gait cycle. With proper preparation of the patient, training may progress without hindrance from confusion concerning the EMG signal.

As active electrodes are spaced more closely together, their signal input becomes more similar. Consequently, there is a greater degree of signal cancellation by the differential amplifier,[1] and signal amplitude will diminish. If a narrow electrode placement is used to improve the specificity of the EMG signal, the potential exists that the

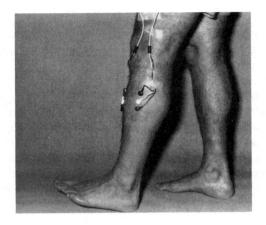

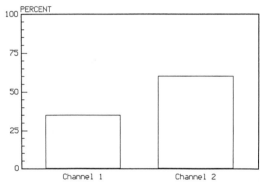

FIGURE 9–2. Relative EMG output from peroneus longus and lateral gastrocnemius during heelstrike. Channel 1 is placed on the plantarflexor muscles; channel 2 on the evertors. Channel 2 detects increases or decreases in evertor muscle activity with dorsiflexion and eversion of the ankle.

EMG signal amplitude may become reduced to levels difficult to read in spite of the most sensitive setting used. If such a situation occurs, the electrode spacing may be widened or the sensitivity increased.

In addition, when monitoring large muscle groups, the signal from narrowly spaced electrodes will usually reflect only a portion of the EMG activity. Particularly if monitoring a two-joint muscle, the EMG activity will reflect the primary action of the muscle where the electrodes are placed. If a paretic muscle is being monitored, the electrode spacing and location may have to be adjusted to display the most appropriate EMG signal.

Some methods used to achieve such electrode-placement consistency from session to session include (1) leaving the electrodes in place between sessions that are only a few hours to a day apart (electrode type will also determine if this is a feasible option), (2) marking the skin around the electrode with nonwashable felt-tip pen, or (3) measuring electrode placement from nearby landmarks and using these measures to determine consistent electrode placement. Even with the most diligent approach to achieve consistent electrode placement from session to session, it is important to keep in mind the limitations of using EMG activity as a measure of quantifying progress. Last, clinicians should never forget the importance of maintaining consistent electrode placements until such time as the treatment strategy (and hence loci of electrode positioning) changes.

FEEDBACK MODES

Depending on the equipment available to the clinician, different modes of EMGBF may be used. A few of the modes available in instrumentation are briefly described. A

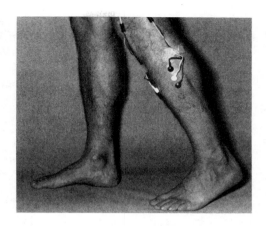

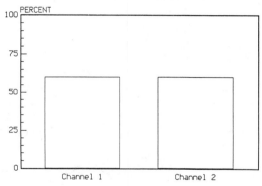

FIGURE 9–3. Relative EMG output from peroneus longus and adjacent muscles during early push-off phase of gait. Channel 1 is placed on the plantarflexors; channel 2 on the evertors. Channel 2 detects the peroneal-muscle activity associated with plantarflexion, as well as volume-conducted activity from the lateral head of the gastrocnemius muscle.

continuous mode displays a running integral of EMG in a visual form, usually as an array of lights, as the needle deflection of a gauge, or as a running graph on a monitor screen. A *work-rest* or *on-off* mode displays a cue to the patient to initiate a muscle contraction or to relax. Usually this mode is a part of a continuous mode and also may be used when neuromuscular stimulation (NMS) is incorporated with EMGBF. A *copy* mode displays a pattern, usually on a monitor, for the patient to trace with the visual display representing muscle-activity output. The trace may be generated from the patient's own EMG output (usually from an intact contralateral homologous muscle group) or manually. The difficulty of the task may be altered by inducing the EMGBF sensitivity (gain) so that the patient has to generate more activity to reach the trace or by slowing the sweep speed, that is, to challenge the patient to recruit muscle activity for a longer duration. Although the best form of *audio* feedback has never been ascertained from objective criteria, we often find *clicks* to be more offensive than tonal changes. Inclusion of "raw" EMG sounds often allows the clinician to *hear* noise or artifact.

SIGNAL SENSITIVITY OR AMPLIFICATION

Gain is the extent to which EMG signals are multiplied by the amplifier. Recall that as the EMG signal is processed by the differential amplifier, the difference in the muscle activity detected at each of the active electrodes with respect to ground is amplified.

When examining muscle activity, the greater the gain, the greater the signal will be amplified. Signal sensitivity has been used as a synonymous term for signal gain. Consequently, at a high gain, the EMGBF instrument will have a high sensitivity for the muscle-activity signal.

Signal gain (or sensitivity) is usually depicted on a "scale" of options. For example, an EMGBF instrument may have scales of 1, 10, and 100 μV of EMG activity. The scale with the *greatest* sensitivities is that of 1 μV because that is the scale sensitive enough to detect the smallest amounts of activity. Conversely, the scale with the *least* gain is the 100-μV scale. The scales used for treatment should be recorded.

SIGNAL TIME CONSTANT

Some EMGBF units will present an option frequently referred to as the EMGBF time constant. Not to be confused with the "time constant" which reflects the frequency components of a signal such as an action potential, EMGBF time constant refers to the sampling frequency of the EMG signal and how frequently that EMG information is relayed to the viewer in the form of an EMGBF signal. Hence, the shorter the EMGBF signal time constant, the more frequently EMGBF information will be updated.

When training in fairly static postures and receiving a rapid update of EMGBF information, the patient may become frustrated as he or she attempts to respond to the EMGBF signal changes as quickly as they occur. On the other hand, when engaged in dynamic movement or fine-motor-control retraining, a longer EMGBF time constant may lead to some confusion if the information relayed to patients is at a slower sampling rate and some information is consequently lost. Select a short time constant (0.1 s) for training dynamic movement, so that minimal delay occurs between the last EMG change and its feedback presentation. Select a longer time constant (0.5 to 1.0 s) for training static activities or postural changes.

DATA ACQUISITION AND MANAGEMENT

When documentation of clinical progress is desired, three primary approaches toward data management are available, depending on the EMGBF instrument being used. If the EMG activity is integrated for a given time segment, then this integral may be measured for any specific task over a specified time period. Task complexities range from simple active movements to complex functional activities. Another approach is to examine changes in patterns of muscle activity. For example, knowing that lumbosacral paraspinal muscle activity is usually symmetrical during forward bending, one can allow progressive training of a patient with asymmetrical EMG activity toward recruiting activity symmetrically. The clinician can describe the progress in terms of peak EMG of each channel or the duration of symmetrical EMG activity. Finally, one may discuss treatment progression in terms of changes in the sensitivity or gain of the instrument during various training efforts. All of these approaches describing changes of EMG activity require inter-session electrode-placement consistency. Under the best of conditions, reliability or consistency of EMG activity cannot be assured. Without such consistency, it is impossible to draw conclusions from changes in EMG activity throughout several sessions.

RELATING EMG TO FUNCTION

An appropriate change in EMG is not necessarily equivalent to a change in function. Similarly, an increase in EMG does not assure an increase in range of motion (ROM) or strength grade or development of isolated movement. Consequently, as a patient's progress is recorded, it is critical to record changes in EMG *along with* changes in ROM, function, strength grade, isolated movement, pain, perception, and level of activity. At the very least, EMG measures provide evidence of whether or not the patient is progressing toward appropriate changes in functional areas.

TREATMENT SCHEDULE, FREQUENCY, AND DURATION

The number of EMGBF sessions required to produce observable changes varies with the number and degree of problems exhibited. The presence of spasticity, severe weakness, or perceptual deficits presents unique obstacles to be dealt with in the course of treatment. The number of treatment sessions for hemiplegic patients needed to measure changes in muscle strength or joint motion range from a few to 30 sessions.[4,6,24-28]

Frequency of treatment sessions is determined subjectively. Baker, Regenos, and Basmajian[29] suggested scheduling patients two to three times per week with treatment durations ranging from 30 to 60 minutes, based on the patient's tolerance. The primary factors affecting the frequency and length of sessions will be the ability of the patient to assimilate the motor skills learned in the biofeedback (BF) sessions and the patient's distractibility and mental and physical fatigue.

FEASIBILITY OF HOME TREATMENT

Feedback training at home is limited only by portability of equipment and, in the case of independent treatment programs, the patient's reliability. Home EMGBF is ideal for those patients with specific motor-control retraining requirements but who are medically stable and functioning independently. For example, a patient with a brachial plexus injury with focal motor weakness but with independency in all activities of daily living is a good candidate. Either the patient or a responsible family member can apply the electrodes and set up the EMGBF unit for the independent training session. As a result, specific, independent motor control retraining can occur during the patient's independent exercise program.

Assessing patient appliances is important when deciding whether to foster a home program. Many patients are motivated and *desire* to improve, but whether they have the *discipline* as well as the cognitive skills to carry out the home program independently must be known. Frequently, this knowledge can only be gained through trial and error.

EVALUATION OF TREATMENT OUTCOMES

In the midst of a treatment in which EMGBF is used to monitor muscle activity, evaluation of treatment outcome may be determined a number of ways. Changes in EMGBF parameters that can be monitored include (1) changes in integrated EMG output for a given time period, (2) changes in frequency of achieving EMG target goals or settings, (3) changes in the length of time the EMG activity is sustained above or below the threshold, (4) changes in the time required to reach threshold. Furthermore, it is appropriate to include in the evaluation of treatment outcome a measure of ROM, mobility, ability to perform functional tasks, or changes in gait (distance and/or time required to ambulate a given distance).

Consideration should be given to several additional factors. First, when training to increase specific muscle activities, *more* does not necessarily mean *better*. Consider the patient with hypertonic muscle groups that are active in synergistic patterns. When being trained to recruit those muscle groups in an isolated manner, the therapist must be cognizant not only of the changes in EMG activity but of the patient's clinical performance as well. Second, a change in EMG activity does not guarantee a change in functional capabilities. Just as the clinician has to relate changes in ROM, strength, and motor control to the overall ability of the patient's functional status, EMG data must also be interpreted with care. The therapist is responsible for relating the outcome of muscle-activity changes to the functional status of the patient.

DISCHARGE CRITERIA

In general, the decision to discharge a patient from receiving physical therapy is based upon the patient's ability to continue to make measurable functional gains. Thus, a patient is usually discharged from EMGBF training when EMG changes associated with functional tasks no longer occur within treatment sessions over the course of several sessions. Patients with chronic neurologic deficits usually make changes in functional abilities slowly; some show increased fine-motor function after 2 to 4 months of EMGBF training. Consequently, the therapist must be prepared to plan each training session with a specific functional goal in mind and clearly document changes that occur toward the goal. At times, the decision to discontinue training is forced by limits imposed by third-party payers, in which case successful EMGBF training may be limited.

PATIENT EDUCATION

The need for patient education about EMGBF depends on how much the patient must attend to the EMGBF signal and her or his ability to do so. If the therapist is primarily using EMGBF as an assessment tool, patient education may be limited to explaining the purpose of the instrument. If the patient is to participate in EMGBF training, the purpose of using EMGBF may be communicated and the amount of detail provided to the patient will depend upon her or his ability to comprehend it. Those patients with receptive aphasia or other cognitive dysfunctions may function quite well during EMGBF training with limited instructions. Very simple instructions with repeated reinforcement may be all that is required to conduct a successful training session. For example, "Mr. Smith, when you straighten your knee correctly, these electrodes (pointing to electrodes over the knee extensors) show how well the muscle beneath is working. When you tighten the muscle, the line on the monitor will rise (pointing to the visual representation of knee extensor EMG activity). When you relax the muscle, the line on the monitor will fall. Let's practice and show you how all this works."

Other details included in a patient's education are (1) orientation of the patient to the auditory and visual displays and differentiation of signals for each channel, (2) information concerning the recruitment and relaxation goals of the EMGBF, (3) description of differences or changes in the sensitivity of different channels, and (4) the relationship between the session's EMGBF goals and functional goals.

CLINICAL APPLICATION FOR MUSCULOSKELETAL PATIENTS

Consideration for Treatment of Low-Back-Pain (LBP) Patients

The most specific description of *electrode placement* for evaluating the EMG activity of lumbar paraspinal muscles also related the placement to findings from cadaveric dissection. This electrode placement is illustrated in Figure 9–4 and is described as:

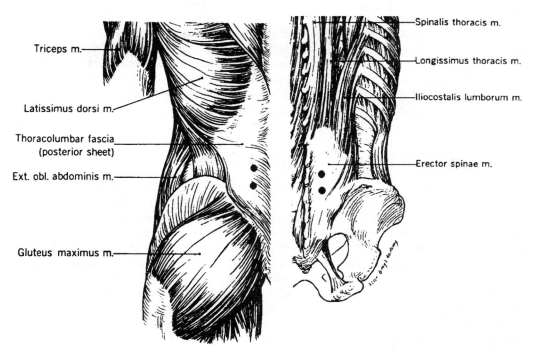

Triceps m.

Latissimus dorsi m.

Thoracolumbar fascia
(posterior sheet)

Ext. obl. abdominis m.

Gluteus maximus m.

Spinalis thoracis m.

Longissimus thoracis m.

Iliocostalis lumborum m.

Erector spinae m.

FIGURE 9–4. Lumbar paraspinal electrode placement. (Adapted from Blumenthal and Basmajian.[53])

> One pair was placed symmetrically at a distance of 3 cm from the midline spinous processes between lumbar vertebrae three and four while a second pair was placed symmetrically from midline between lumbar vertebrae four and five. Numerous dissections from cadaver material indicate that the lower electrode pair is placed over the fascial cleft between the multifidus and longissimus erector spinae muscles while the upper electrode pair is situated over the longissimus muscle bilaterally.[30]

Few reports describe electrode placements in specific detail. In one study in which the placement was described, the distance from the midline was 3 inches,[31] clearly indicating that paraspinal muscle activity was not the predominant activity reflected by the EMG signal. Furthermore, examination of the placement described by Wolf, Nacht, and Kelly[30] revealed that *this placement* overlies the fascia extending from the latissimus dorsi to its origin. This muscle originates from the fascial origin at the lower six thoracic vertebra, the thoracolumbar fascia (which is attached to the lumbar and sacral spinous processes), from the iliac crest and lower three or four ribs. Insertion occurs at the anterior aspect of the humerus, medial to the insertion of the pectoralis major.[32] Consequently, arm movement during the evaluation or treatment of the LBP patient with EMG biofeedback could produce extraneous EMG activity from the latissimus dorsi. In the literature, only one study acknowledged but incompletely controlled for the effects of extraneous arm movement.[33]

EMG ACTIVITY AT REST

Nouwen and Bush[34] recognized several studies testing the hypothesis that LBP patients demonstrate higher resting paraspinal EMG activity than pain-free controls.

Clinicians examining patients with LBP, should consider this hypothesis with caution. Several factors render comparisons of EMG activity *between* patients invalid. Differences in body type will result in differences in signal attenuation. The presence of muscle denervation (a particular concern for clinicians providing target feedback at muscle sites previously subjected to surgery) will alter the EMG activity produced. Wolf and associates[35] also recognized that paraspinal EMG activity levels can vary widely, even among patients who have diagnoses stemming from similar pathological processes.

EMG ACTIVITY DURING ACTIVE MOVEMENT

Using criteria established by Wolf and associates,[35] clinicians can begin evaluating a patient with LBP. EMG activity may be examined (1) at rest, (2) during forward flexion, (3) during trunk flexion to 70° and beyond, (4) during trunk extension from full flexion, and (5) during right and left rotation while the patient is standing with the pelvis stabilized. Clinicians should also perform a thorough evaluation of all signs and symptoms the patient exhibits, including distribution of pain and related pain behavior.

By understanding the basic EMG analysis noted above, appropriate feedback training during dynamic movement can begin. At first, the clinician cannot distinguish between evaluation and treatment activities because the patient appears to undergo training throughout the session. Following patient preparation and electrode placement, the patient is oriented to the EMGBF unit and instructed in the meaning of the visual display, threshold detection, auditory signals, and to activities that could contaminate the EMG signal. The clinician then may elect to have the patient perform movements, postures, or actions that reflect those assumed in work or home activities that may elicit pain. As the patient performs the tasks, the clinician observes the patient's body mechanics and the related EMG activity, and attempts to ascertain relationships between the two. The patient may be instructed to perform a unilateral task on one side followed by the same activity on the other side, with the clinician examining the relative differences in EMG. As the clinician interacts with the patient and instructs him or her in the difference between normal EMG activity and his or her performance, they work together to determine how the patient can alter postures and movements approximating normal EMG activity.

EMGBF INCORPORATED IN THE TREATMENT

Price, Clare, and Everhardt[3] reported in 1948 how patterns of paraspinal EMG changed during movement and how these EMG patterns were related to low-back pain. They observed that areas of pain or tenderness can "migrate" from one muscle group to another or to another region of the same muscle group. It was suggested that the shift of pain was associated with abnormal patterns of muscle activity, either in an attempt to avoid or to relieve pain. Deviations from normal EMG patterns included (1) asymmetry where bilateral symmetry was expected, (2) hyperactivity, and (3) hypoactivity. The authors proposed that hyperactivity occurred by substitution of a less appropriate or effective muscle group to avoid a painful contraction or stretch and that hypoactivity arose from reflex inhibition from pain or from the threat of pain. Consequently, asymmetry of muscle activity was hypothesized to result from an interplay of the described hyperactivity and hypoactivity. Wolf and associates[35] examined lumbosacral EMG activity during trunk flexion-extension, lateral rotation while standing, stooping, and lateral rotation while sitting. Some of the patterns of EMG reported are reviewed in Table 9–1.

TABLE 9-1 EMB Biofeedback Training Strategies during Dynamic
Low-Back Movements

Trunk flexion-extension activity during movement in standing position	1. Symmetrical patterns of the sagittal plane. 2. EMG silence occurred when 70° of trunk flexion was exceeded. 3. EMG activity usually resumed after approximately 20° of trunk extension from full trunk flexion. 4. Extension EMG activity always exceeded flexion activity during trunk movement.
Lateral rotation (standing)	1. During rotation to the *left,* right paraspinal EMG activity exceeded that of the left paraspinal EMG activity. 2. During rotation to the *right,* left paraspinal EMG activity exceeded that of the right paraspinal EMG activity.
Stooping	1. A symmetrical pattern of EMG activity was observed.

In their review of the literature of the relationship between paraspinal EMG and chronic LBP, Nouwen and Bush[34] observed a striking lack of consensus in the relationship between paraspinal EMG and chronic low-back pain. Close examination of the literature suggests that many researchers have overlooked a number of factors influencing the outcome of studies of paraspinal EMG activity. These factors include (1) the differences in the limits of interpretation of unilateral versus combined (right and left) comparisons of EMG activity, (2) the influence of the complex biomechanics of the spine, (3) EMG changes associated with movement, (4) the effect of surgical intervention on EMG activity, (5) the influence of patient position, (6) the effect of arm movements, and (7) the necessity for precise electrode placement.

REDUCTION OF MUSCLE SPASM (RELAXATION TRAINING)

Among patients with either musculoskeletal or neuromuscular problems impeding mobility, one of the earliest treatment goals sought with EMGBF is reduction of hyperactive EMG activity through relaxation training (RT). Musculoskeletal (or orthopedic) problems frequently demonstrate muscle spasm as a protective response to pain or fear of movement. On the other hand, neuromuscular problems arising from central nervous system (CNS) deficits may demonstrate an altogether different kind of muscle reactivity (spasticity) and require a different therapeutic intervention plan and treatment progression. In spite of these different etiologies of muscle spasm and different overall progression of treatment, the basic principles of RT are virtually the same.

The goal of relaxation training is reduction of EMG activity. This goal may be applied toward a single muscle or to a series of muscles in a limb or larger segment of the body. Within each session, experiences with the EMGBF are planned to ensure consistent success by the patient for each task. Tasks are planned to progressively increase in difficulty and complexity. As relaxation improves, the progression of interelectrode spacing is changed from narrow to wide and the sensitivity of the EMGBF unit is from low-to-high levels. Consequently, the patient is required to relax larger muscle masses and achieve even greater relaxation.

During relaxation training, several cues may be offered to the patient to encourage progress. The cues given will reflect the specificity of the RT desired. For example, in RT of large or several muscle groups, the patient may be cued to use mental imagery or deep breathing techniques. For RT of specific muscle groups, cues that might be helpful include instructions to (1) contract and relax a particular muscle group, (2) imagine a "heaviness" or "warmth" within a specific muscle group or limb, (3) practice deep-breathing techniques, or (4) alter body position (e.g., alignment of the trunk).

As the patient achieves successful RT in the clinical setting, the degree of difficulty may be increased by requiring the patient to apply the techniques in a different position or environment. For example, the patient successful at relaxing the biceps in a sitting position might progress to doing so while standing or ambulating. An example of an environmental change is to move from the clinical setting to the patient's workplace. In the latter case, the patient might be called upon to perform the RT techniques performed in the clinical setting while engaging in work activities. Thus, the training learned in the clinic may be practiced during daily activities.

Muscle Re-education in Patients Undergoing Tendon Transfer

In the examples that follow, EMGBF is used as a tool to re-educate muscles, often following surgical intervention. In each case, the patient is evaluated thoroughly, the problems are clearly defined, and a specific treatment is initiated to address the problem at the root of the dysfunction.

Cannon and Strickland[36] reported effective use of EMGBF for patients with difficulty recovering digital flexion following surgical repair of wrist and/or finger flexors. They observed that the protective contraction of the antagonist extensor-muscle groups impeded some patients in their efforts to recover digital flexion. EMGBF was reported to enable patients to visualize and reduce the contradictory extensor-muscle activity and maximally recruit flexor muscles. The authors also used EMGBF to reduce patients' preoccupation with pain while enhancing motivation so they could most fully participate in the therapy program following flexor-tendon surgery.

Hirasawa, Uchiza, and Kusswetter[37] used EMGBF therapy with patients following either tenorrhaphy or tendon transfer after rupture of the extensor pollicis longus tendon. Five patients were treated with EMGBF, all of whom had demonstrated functional deficits "despite intensive postoperative rehabilitation." In their treatment plan, training was initiated on the unaffected side until the patient sufficiently understood the muscle contraction desired and the visual information of the EMGBF instrument. Treatment progressed to the affected side with the patient performing the muscle contraction both actively and with resistance to movement offered by the therapist. Muscle contraction was sustained for 5 minutes followed by 5 minutes of complete rest. Training progressed toward greater active recruitment of muscle activity and less resistance to movement offered by the therapist. The authors report improvement of extension from a manual muscle test grade of poor to that of good or normal in all five cases. Two of the cases demonstrating an interphalangeal (IP) extension lag of the thumb of 10° and 15° progressed to an IP extension lag of 0°. One case with an IP extension lag of 40° progressed to an IP extension lag of 15°.

Treatment of Patients with Joint Instability

Beal, Diefenbach, and Allen[38] reported the use of EMGBF to reduce posterior instability of the shoulder by re-educating patients with "abnormal muscle contraction-relaxation patterns which produced this instability." The basic premise of the EMGBF protocol was to increase posterior deltoid activity—first during humeral flexion with external rotation and then during complex combinations of motions with and without weights. The authors report recovery of their patients where they could resume active sports and were able to avoid surgical intervention.

CLINICAL APPLICATIONS FOR NEUROLOGIC PATIENTS

Those clients with neurologic deficits are among the most difficult to treat because of the complex nature of their multiple symptoms. The presence of weakness, flaccidity, spasticity, or a combination of these three conditions, as well as dysphasia, cognitive impairment, or neglect syndromes challenges the therapist to develop a creative means to efficiently and effectively rehabilitate the client. Through the years, a variety of treatment approaches have been advocated including those by Rood.[39] Also advocated were proprioceptive neuromuscular facilitation (PNF),[40] neurodevelopmental treatment (NDT),[41] and so forth, yet limited documentation exists to substantiate their use. With the increasing availability and improved technology of EMG biofeedback devices, clinicians have the opportunity and responsibility to examine changes in muscle activity as interventions are applied. The client, once having to rely upon the clinician's gross assessment of muscle activity through palpation or observation while awaiting verbal relay of that information, now may also have access to immediate and accurate information regarding the status of the patient's muscle activity.

The medical literature offering insight into the potential clinical use of EMG biofeedback is relatively sparse. For those studies that include some form of neuromuscular re-education, efforts are made to compare EMG biofeedback training with other neuromuscular re-education techniques, rather than combine the use of EMGBF *with* other treatment approaches.[42] There are few investigations devoted to the incorporation of EMGBF into *any* treatment plan.

However, where EMGBF has been incorporated into a treatment plan, the results have favored its use. Inglis and associates[43] conducted a study in which there was a crossover of control subjects into the experimental treatment condition. Two groups of stroke patients had no significant pretreatment differences in motor function. In Part I of the study, the experimental group received 20 treatment sessions of physical therapy plus EMGBF which consisted of audio and visual EMG biofeedback "used to supplement and monitor progressive PT exercises that involved a graduated program of neuromuscular facilitation techniques," while the control group (before the crossover) received the PT exercise without the EMGBF. After both groups completed 20 sessions, the control group received 20 further sessions of PT plus EMGBF to ascertain what benefit might be gained from additional PT plus EMGBF. Although both the experimental and the control groups improved in active ROM and strength, the experimental groups (from Part I and the crossover group from Part II) showed greater improvement.

Burnside, Tobias, and Bursill[44] conducted a controlled trial in which stroke patients were given gait training (to improve dorsiflexion) with or without EMGBF. Immediately after completion of the treatment phase, the EMGBF group showed significantly greater strength of dorsiflexion over the control group, although there were no differences between the groups at that time for ROM and gait ratings. At the 6-week follow-up evaluation, however, the EMGBF group showed significant improvement over the control group in strength of dorsiflexion, ROM, and gait ratings. The authors noted that several of the patients had previously been told to expect no further improvement because they had reached a plateau of neurologic recovery. The authors observed that when they were able to demonstrate the presence of muscle activity through EMGBF, the patients in the experimental group were more apt to try to improve whereas the control-group subjects were difficult to persuade to carry out their exercises without biofeedback.

Wolf and Binder-Macleod[45,46] employed an experimental group procedure with a targeted-training (TT) protocol that proceeded from relaxation of hyperactive muscles to recruitment of weakened antagonist muscles in a proximal-to-distal manner in chronic stroke patients for both the upper (UE)[45] and the lower extremities (LE).[46] For the UE interventions, the EMGBF groups showed significant improvements in integrated EMG activity and ROM, but not for functional tasks. The authors identified those acquiring functional abilities as having, in summary, "(1) demonstrable active ROM for the shoulder, elbow, wrist and fingers; (2) ability to generate substantial biceps EMG but also to reduce biceps activity rapidly following passive stretch or shortening contraction; and (3) ability to relax thenar and finger flexor musculature during passive stretch." They observed that these characteristics might help to predict those patients most likely to benefit from EMGBF. For the LE interventions, the experimental group showed significant improvements in active range of motion (AROM) of the knee and ankle and required significantly fewer or less complex assistive devices for walking.

Another approach developed by Wolf, LeCraw, and Barton[25] involved the process of monitoring homologous bilateral muscle groups and instructing stroke and head-injured patients to match the activity of the involved side with that of the uninvolved side. This motor copy (MC) procedure was based upon the theory of utilizing bilateral descending motor systems to augment therapeutic outcome. The experimental group that received the MC procedure was compared to a control group receiving the TT.[45]

For the MC procedure, bilateral homologous muscle groups were monitored simultaneously for each treatment session. The patients were initially trained to superimpose homologous muscle outputs at rest and during active or passive lengthening of the hyperactive synergistic muscle groups. This was followed by active shortening of the agonist muscles while maintaining reduced levels of EMG of the hyperactive, synergistic muscles. The synergistic muscles were actively shortened in a controlled manner. By varying the gain of each amplifier, patients were provided with the potential to match the EMG outputs from each homologous muscle pair. As each patient achieved this ability to "match" EMG outputs, the difficulty of the task was increased by altering the gains until they became more similar. Consequently, as the gain for the EMG output of the involved muscle group became closer to that of the uninvolved muscle group, the closer to "normal" was the patient's performance. Matching occurred by having the patient superimpose the outputs of both channels of muscle activity during the task performance with or without a template produced on the monitor to serve as a guide for matching. Both the TT and the MC procedures were found to produce improvements in ROM, EMG, and functional performance measure; the TT group improved during the treatment phase and the MC group improved in the follow-up phase.

CLINICAL APPLICATIONS FOR PEDIATRIC PATIENTS

Biofeedback strategies have been used in the pediatric population for management of a variety of pathologies including childhood migraine,[47] urinary incontinence,[48] and fecal incontinence.[49] The majority of studies examining the application of EMGBF in children have focused on those with cerebral palsy (CP).

Various treatment approaches with EMGBF for pediatric patients were evaluated at Emory University Rehabilitation Research and Training Center. Changes in thoracic paraspinal muscle activity were evaluated using EMGBF in a 2-year-old child with spastic quadriplegia secondary to CP.[50] Muscle activity was monitored during (1) crawling versus locomotion using a prone scooter board (Fig. 9–5), (2) ambulation by holding onto the child's hands in the "traditional" assist position versus offering pelvic stabilization with the child's hands secured at the hips by the therapist (Fig. 9–6), and (3) during alternative carrying positions by the mother (Fig. 9–7). The electrode pairs were placed over the posterior midthoracic region bilaterally equidistant from the spinous processes after the skin had been cleansed with an alcohol rub. During the therapeutic sessions, changes in *patterns* of muscle activity were evaluated, with a particular interest in pain involving (1) the difference in the output from one side compared to the other during a specified activity and (2) the overall output of both channels comparing two similar, but different, activities. Before and after the therapeutic sessions, the EMG activity was quantified in an effort to objectively compare these apparent differences in EMG output.

The results were fairly straightforward. The output of the bilateral paraspinal muscle activity was greater when the child was crawling on the floor than when using a prone scooter (Fig. 9–5). It was theorized that the requirement for the child to raise her head up higher to look ahead before crawling contributed to the increased EMG output. During ambulation, the EMG activity produced was more symmetrical and greater when the pelvis was supported and the child was forced to extend her trunk in order to look forward prior to attempting to step forward (Fig. 9–6) than when hand support was given. The final evaluation of the client's paraspinal muscle activity examined changes associated with various carrying positions demonstrated by the mother. Figure 9–7 illustrates a comparison of two carrying positions. Of the three situations, it was most interesting to note the mother and clinician concurrently screening EMG representations as each carrying position was tested. As they examined the output together and discussed the pros and cons of each position, they arrived at a mutually agreed upon decision for the optimal carrying position to facilitate active thoracic extension by the child.

The application of EMGBF in the pediatric population may enable clinicians to accurately assess patient characteristics and treatment outcomes, as well as enhance the care provider's understanding of, and participation in, home therapeutic programs.

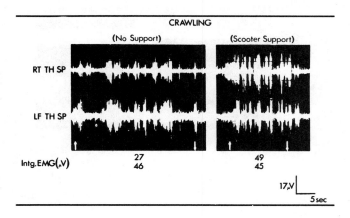

FIGURE 9–5. Raw EMG activity recorded from right and left thoracic paraspinal regions (RT TH SP, LF TH SP) during floor and scooter crawling. Numbers refer to integrated EMG values of upper and lower traces, respectively. (From Wolf, et al.[50] Reprinted from PHYSICAL THERAPY with permission of the American Physical Therapy Association.)

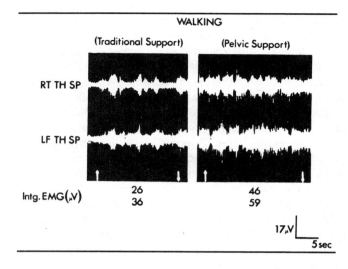

FIGURE 9–6. The EMG activity from right and left thoracic paraspinal regions (RT TH SP, LF TH SP) during ambulation holding patient's hands (left diagram), or pelvis supported (right diagram). Numbers refer to integrated EMG values of upper and lower traces, respectively. (From Wolf, et al.[50] Reprinted from PHYSICAL THERAPY with permission of the American Physical Therapy Association.)

Integration of EMGBF into a comprehensive rehabilitation program is limited only by the clinician's access to, and familiarity with, the equipment, knowledge of anatomy, ability to relate muscle group deficits to functional disabilities, and capability of critically interpreting EMG data.

CLINICAL APPLICATIONS FOR PATIENTS WITH GAIT DEFICITS

Much of the EMGBF literature has been directed toward using this modality to improve gait by correcting footdrop in the hemiplegic patient.[51,52] Varying degrees of success have been reported. In some studies muscle re-education with EMGBF was shown to be an effective tool, enabling clients to eliminate the use of an ankle-foot orthosis (AFO) or to use less cumbersome assistive devices.[52] Moving beyond this

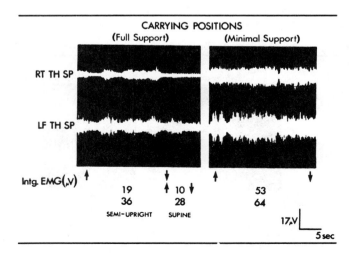

FIGURE 9–7. The EMG activity recorded from the same child as in Figures 9–5 and 9–6, while mother attempts different carrying positions. Arrows define duration of different activities and numbers are integrated values from raw EMG data of right thoracic (*upper trace*) and left thoracic (*lower trace*) paraspinal muscles. (From Wolf, et al.[50] Reprinted from PHYSICAL THERAPY with permission of the American Physical Therapy Association.)

application, clinicians may effectively incorporate EMGBF into neuromuscular re-education of affected hip and knee musculature.

Hip stability is required for a safe level of independent ambulation. Gluteus medius, which provides stability during the stance phase of gait, is often targeted for intensive rehabilitation using EMGBF. Efforts by the client to recruit and strengthen the gluteus medius during mat activities are frequently confounded by the substitution of activity in the tensor fascia latae. Consequently, valuable time may be wasted as the clinician must repeatedly monitor the patient's recruitment efforts and relay back the successes and failures. When the patient attempts to incorporate hip stability into gait training, the learning process is confounded further as the clinician attempts to reinforce for the patient the appropriate sequential activation of these hip stabilizers.

If EMGBF electrodes are applied to the gluteus medius prior to re-education efforts, the clinician can accurately assess and facilitate hip abductor activity during mat exercises as well as during gait training. The patient would also have access to accurate and immediate information regarding his or her voluntary efforts and may be better able to cooperate with the neuromuscular re-education task. Although the electrode application for the gluteus medius is relatively straightforward, the presence of excessive subcutaneous fat in the placement area could significantly attenuate the signal. The only sure way to know whether the appropriate signal can be detected is to proceed with accurate electrode placement and attempt to recruit the muscle activity. First, palpate the peak of the iliac crest and move inferior to the crest. As palpation proceeds over the soft tissue inferior to the crest, the gluteus medius can be detected most easily if the patient is able to initiate abduction. Palpation of gluteus medius promotes accurate placement of the electrodes parallel to the direction of pull of the muscle fibers, with the proximal electrode just inferior to the iliac crest (Fig. 9–8). Narrow spacing is essential to reduce volume-conducted activity from gluteus maximus. Keep in mind that even with the most conscientious attempts to avoid volume-conducted activity, gluteus maximus activity is difficult to avoid and should be considered a potential contaminant to this signal during training.

Another problem encountered in gait training is recruitment of hip flexion with knee extension during the gait cycle. The muscle primarily involved in hip flexion (iliopsoas) is too deep to be effectively monitored through surface electrodes. However, the proximal aspect of sartorius, near its attachment to the anterior superior iliac spine is sufficiently superficial to allow access by surface electrodes (Fig. 9–9). Because the sartorius contributes to hip flexion, its EMG activity (at least partially) affects hip-flexor activity. Again, the electrodes must be narrowly spaced and must be aligned parallel to the direction of the muscle fibers to reduce volume-conducted EMG activity.

Knee-extension muscle activity is most easily isolated from nearby muscle groups by monitoring the rectus femoris muscle with narrowly spaced electrodes placed parallel to the direction of the muscle fibers. Other components of the quadriceps femoris muscle group are accessible for EMGBF, and the potential for volume-conducted activity occurring from the adductor muscle mass or hamstrings muscle group may potentially contaminate the EMG signal.

POSTURAL CONTROL RETRAINING

The acquisition of proximal stability before gaining distal mobility has long been a premise on which rehabilitation interventions have been based — largely for the neurologic population but also for the orthopedic population of patients. The interplay

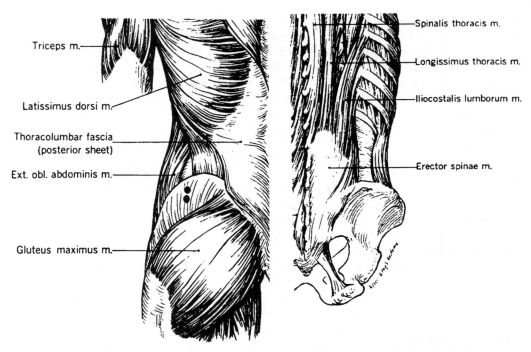

FIGURE 9–8. Electrode placement for monitoring EMG activity in gluteus medius muscle during stance phase of gait. (Adapted from Blumenthal and Basmajian.[53])

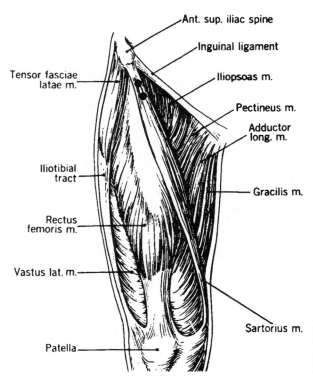

FIGURE 9–9. Electrode placement for monitoring EMG activity in sartorius muscle during swing phase of gait. (Adapted from Blumenthal and Basmajian.[53])

between anterior and posterior muscles of the trunk is of significant importance during attempts to maintain sitting or standing balance, particularly in the patient in the early stages of recovery from CNS dysfunction. Furthermore, correction of trunk alignment has been advocated in patients with CNS dysfunction to reduce hypertonicity in more distal muscle groups of the upper and lower limbs.

The posterior-electrode placement described by Wolf, Nacht, and Kelly[30] may be used to assess patterns of paraspinal muscle responses to perturbations of posture during sitting, transitions between sitting and standing, and postural changes during standing. These placements are illustrated in Figure 9–4. From the assessment, the clinician may compare the patient's response to the activity published by Wolf and associates[35] and establish treatment goals accordingly. The EMGBF may then be used as a tool during the treatment intervention to provide immediate and accurate information to the clinician and patient regarding the client's paraspinal muscle activity, as well as the appropriateness of the therapist's instructions or therapeutic intervention.

The anterior-trunk electrode placement least likely to demonstrate signal attenuation from adipose tissue is directly over the origin of the rectus abdominis muscle just distal to the xiphoid process.[53] Narrow electrode spacing parallel to the direction of the muscle fibers and lateral to the midline of the muscle (Fig. 9–10) will provide information on unilateral changes of the rectus abdominis muscle activity during sitting and standing, similar to those noted for the lumbar paraspinal muscle groups. The potential exists for volume-conducted activity to be present from the heart or respiratory muscles. As the EMG activity is monitored, volume-conducted cardiac or respiratory muscle activity can be discerned by the regular pattern of its signal. In addition, the clinician may wish to monitor muscle groups in the upper or lower extremity if spasticity is present in an effort to discern how changes in posture affect muscle tone.

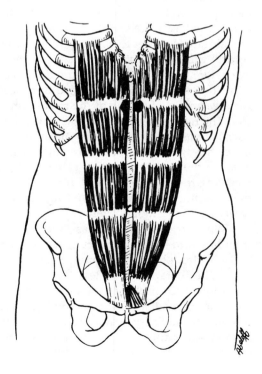

FIGURE 9–10. Electrode placement for rectus abdominis muscle. (Adapted from Basmajian, JV: Primary Anatomy. Williams & Wilkins, Baltimore, 1982, p 136.)

FORCE AND POSITION FEEDBACK

Two forms of feedback which complement that of EMGBF are force and positional feedback. Force feedback relays information concerning the force generated through a limb segment such as the lower limb (12) or through an external device such as a cane.[11] The signal representing forces is transduced through strain gauges, or pressure sensors, into a voltage, the magnitude of which is proportional to the force. Positional feedback provides information concerning position of a joint (e.g., knee, ankle, or finger) or of a body segment, (e.g., head position relative to the trunk.) These signals are transduced through changes in an array of resistors through which a constant current is passed, thus producing a change in voltage (Ohm's law). The potentiometer(s) through which these electronic events are passed is placed in a fixed position in relation to the movement being trained.

COMBINING EMGBF AND NEUROMUSCULAR ELECTRICAL STIMULATION

Two studies have reported incorporating *positional* feedback and NMS. Bowman, Baker, and Waters examined the effects of NMS with joint position feedback of the wrist in hemiplegic patients.[54] Over a 4-week period, the control group received conventional, individualized therapy 5 days per week. The conventional therapy consisted of "passive range of motion, active resisted exercise, classic neuromuscular facilitation and training in activities of daily living." The experimental group received additional positional-feedback stimulation training (PFST) into wrist extension for 30 minutes, twice daily, 5 days per week for 4 weeks. The threshold at which stimulation began was set at approximately 5° below the maximum voluntary ability of the patient. The amplitude of the stimulus was set to a level at which the wrist was fully extended. There was no true control group. The study focused on the outcome of three methods to examine wrist extension. Those methods included (1) *average maximum isometric wrist extension torque* with the wrist initially positioned in *both* 30° of flexion and of extension; (2) *voluntary patterned range of motion* of the maximum angle in which the patient extended the wrist from the normal posturing angle while allowing motion in other joints, and (3) *voluntary selective range of motion* of the maximum angle in which the patient was able to extend his or her wrist before the activation of any muscles of the upper extremity other than wrist and finger extensors. Table 9–2 summarizes the improvement of the group receiving the additional PFST for each of the three outcome variables. As can be seen, the experimental group showed significant improvement over that of the control group receiving conventional therapy.

Winchester and associates[55] incorporated positional feedback with cyclical electrical stimulation to knee extensors of hemiparetic patients. The experimental group received PFST in the following manner. Each day, the patient's minimum threshold angle was set by the therapist at 5° less than the patient's position of maximum volitional knee extension. The amplitude for stimulation was set so that maximal knee extension within the patient's available range of motion was achieved. If the patient could not tolerate the stimulation intensity required to achieve the maximum available range of motion, the stimulation amplitude for quadriceps was reduced to the highest tolerable level. As experimental patients extended their knees beyond the minimum threshold angle,

TABLE 9-2 Significant and Nonsignificant Changes in Tests of Wrist Extension over a 4-week Treatment Period

Method of Examining Wrist Extension	Week 1	Week 2	Week 3	Week 4
Average isometric extension torque				
a. From 30° extension	NS*	S†	S	S
b. From 30° flexion	NS	NS	S	S
Patterned wrist extension	NS	S	S	S
Selective wrist extension	NS	NS	NS	S

*NS = nonsignificant
†S = significant

stimulation was initiated to achieve maximum available range of motion. The number of repetitions ranged between 20 and 50, depending upon each patient's endurance.

In addition to PFST, cyclical stimulation to the involved quadriceps femoris muscle was included in the experimental group to initially acclimate the patient to the sensation of stimulation and to increase quadriceps femoris muscle endurance to allow longer stimulation sessions. Cyclical stimulation consisted of four daily 30-minute sessions of neuromuscular stimulation to the quadriceps femoris muscle with the amplitude of the stimulation set at a level sufficient to obtain a maximum comfortable quadriceps femoris muscle contraction. The amplitude of stimulation and treatment time were increased daily. The goal was to have the stimulation extend the leg against gravity through the full available range for 1 hour, twice daily. Statistically significant increases for the average change in knee extensor torque and for the average change in patterned ROM (the active movement produced during movement in a lower-extremity extensor synergy) were seen in experimental subjects. No statistically significant differences were noted between groups for isolated knee extension.

Individuals who receive joint-position feedback with NMS seem to show improvements in torque production about the treated joint in patterned ROM and selective ROM. Because joint-position feedback trains *motion*, those patients lacking active motion about an involved joint are unable to take advantage of this approach. For the latter population, NMS should be incorporated with *EMG* biofeedback, rather than positional feedback, thereby rendering immediate reinforcement to changes in muscle activity that are insufficient to initiate joint motion. Actual motion at the joint may then be produced by the NMS.

The combination of EMG biofeedback and NMS usually occurs by having the patient attempt to contract the target muscle to a given threshold level of EMG activity. Once the threshold is reached, the NMS is activated and joint motion occurs, thereby providing the patient with visual and auditory reinforcement (through EMG feedback) and proprioceptive input (from joint and soft-tissue receptors as the NMS induces muscle contractions capable of joint movement). If dual-channel capabilities are present in the EMG unit, the antagonist muscle activity may be monitored, controlled, or facilitated, as appropriate, depending on the goals of the treatment session.

This dual-channel approach with a comprehensive treatment program could improve the efficiency of the treatment sessions. Patient treatment for functional-muscle re-education could be initiated earlier in the course of recovery, before motion is seen but when motor activity is likely to be present.

CONCURRENT ASSESSMENT OF MUSCLE ACTIVITY (CAMA)

As clinicians seek to quantify the changes and document the effectiveness of their treatment interventions, more sophisticated, objective, and easily used instruments can assist them in their endeavors. Questions are raised such as, "How can I tell if I am actually recruiting a specific muscle group with this technique?" "How can I document small changes in performance over time and objectively demonstrate that what I see is actually happening?" "I have *two* treatment techniques that are appropriate for this patient. How can I ascertain the more effective of the two so I use limited treatment time most effectively?" Such questions are timely as demands are made upon clinicians to improve the efficiency of their therapeutic programs, as well as objectively document changes in the patient's status as they occur.

Although use of EMGBF may be an effective vehicle in treatment for numerous neuromuscular and musculoskeletal disorders,[56,57] only the patient is required to incorporate the information gained from monitoring the muscle activity into functional use. Wolf, Edwards, and Shutter[50] proposed the use of CAMA, which operates on the principle that muscle biofeedback can be used to inform clinicians about ongoing muscle activity even as the patient responds to the therapeutic interventions. By implementing CAMA, the physical therapist is able to receive quantified documentation about muscle behavior during treatment and can modify a treatment approach to achieve the desired response immediately and continuously. In this manner, the clinician receives more precise information than is available traditionally through palpation of muscle activity and observation of movement exclusively.

Present clinical applications of EMG biofeedback and CAMA are similar in that they both employ ongoing examination of changes in muscle activity during a treatment session. However, there are several characteristics that distinguish between traditional EMG biofeedback training and CAMA. The primary difference between the two methods is that when using traditional training, the patient must be able to understand the EMGBF signal and respond in an appropriate manner. Consequently, those patients with cognitive impairments, receptive aphasia, or visual and/or auditory impairments are not included as potential candidates for using this instrumentation. With the CAMA approach these clients need no longer be excluded because the *clinician* primarily uses the EMGBF information to ascertain how a given treatment approach is affecting the outcome. The client is no longer required to undergo the training, although he or she is not necessarily excluded from the information gained from monitoring the target muscles. Furthermore, the CAMA approach differs from the traditional EMGBF training by allowing direct data acquisition of EMG activity for the clinician, a feature that has only recently been afforded the clinician through advances in EMG biofeedback instrumentation.

Wolf, Edwards, and Shutter[50] examined changes in muscle response during treatment of a right-hemiplegic patient with and without CAMA. The patient was in the Brunnstrom Stage 2 of recovery, with some components of the flexor and extensor synergy patterns as he used his involved upper extremity. Joint approximation was examined in an effort to facilitate elbow extension. Two treatment sessions separated by approximately 30 minutes were conducted, the first was without CAMA (no knowledge of triceps brachii activity was available) and the second was with CAMA (the therapist monitored and watched as the representative of biceps and triceps brachii used the information to adjust his joint-approximation efforts). The treatment phase consisted of maintained joint approximation (2 to 5 repetitions) and passive elbow extension. With the patient lying supine, his elbow was fully flexed and his upper arm was stabilized with the shoulder at approximately 90° of flexion. The therapist asked the patient to "reach up toward the ceiling" twice, with the elbow repositioned into flexion between efforts.

A comparison of the integrated triceps EMG activity with and without CAMA revealed that (1) baseline EMG activity for the biceps and triceps were essentially the same, (2) post-treatment EMG activity of the triceps was also essentially the same, and (3) there was a decrease in biceps activity following the session with CAMA as compared to the session without CAMA. Furthermore, there was an increase in active elbow-extension active range of motion of 15°. This increase in AROM was probably due to reduced resistance to elbow extension as measured through a reduction in biceps muscle activity (Figs. 9–11 and 9–12). The therapist's perception of how she incorporated CAMA into the treatment session is described as follows:

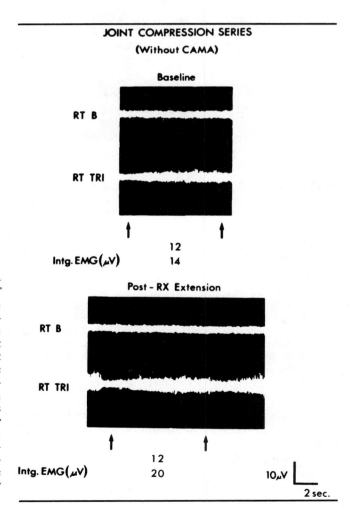

FIGURE 9–11. The EMG recordings from right biceps (*RT B*) and triceps brachii (*RT TRI*) muscles during active elbow extension before (*upper diagram*) and after (*lower diagram*) joint compression exercises without the use of CAMA. Arrows define duration of each activity. Numbers are integrated values from the raw EMG data of biceps (*upper trace*) and triceps (*lower trace*) muscles, respectively. (From Wolf, et al,[50] p 219. Reprinted from PHYSICAL THERAPY with permission of the American Physical Therapy Association.)

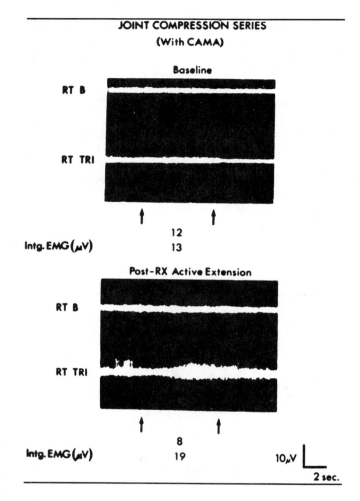

JOINT COMPRESSION SERIES
(With CAMA)

Baseline

RT B

RT TRI

12
13

Intg. EMG (μV)

Post-RX Active Extension

RT B

RT TRI

8
19

Intg. EMG (μV)

10μV

2 sec.

FIGURE 9–12. The EMG recordings from right biceps (*RT B*) and triceps brachii (*RT TRI*) muscles during active elbow extension before (*upper diagram*) and after (*lower diagram*) joint compression exercises with use of CAMA. Arrows define duration of each activity. Numbers are integrated values from the raw EMG data of biceps (*upper trace*) and triceps (*lower trace*) muscles, respectively. (From Wolf, et al,[50] p 220. Reprinted from PHYSICAL THERAPY with permission of the American Physical Therapy Association.)

By using the monitor to see the muscles . . . I was able to more closely gauge when approximation gave me an increase in baseline activity in the triceps so that I could switch to a more forceful quick stretch and elicit a stronger voluntary motion. I also noticed by watching the oscilloscope that after a number of repetitions of volitional resisted elbow extension, I could see when the volitional movement started and biceps EMG decreased. At that point, I would switch back into using my approximation, repeat that several times until I noted that the baseline again began to increase, and then I switched back into my resisted volitional elbow extension. By switching back and forth between those two, I felt that I was able to get a more effective improvement in the terminal extension at the elbow. I believe that this was demonstrated through an actual increase in ROM that was seen.

Having this immediate and accurate information of the muscle activity in the agonist and antagonist, the therapist offered a more effective treatment approach. The changes in the treatment were based on an objective measure (the changes in muscle activity) rather than upon palpation, the force exerted by the patient and subjectively evaluated by the clinician, or on a visual assessment of changes in AROM (also required to be a subjective assessment during the treatment procedure).

Decisions that are made in this manner may occur throughout a treatment session and can be based upon specific, objective information. Using such objective information enables the clinician to rapidly determine a patient's response to a therapeutic intervention, make alterations in the treatment approach, and continue to evaluate the response. The speed at which such decisions may be made is within milliseconds. The rapidity with which patients progress may likely lead to more efficient therapeutic interventions and a more rapid advance toward functional recovery within the limits of their recovery potential.

CASE STUDY

JG, a 33-year-old attorney, underwent surgical removal of a hemispheric astrocytoma from the right tempoparietal lobe. He has left hemiparesis with greater involvement of the left upper limb than the left lower limb. His gait is virtually normal. His occupational therapist referred him for further rehabilitative therapy with EMGBF.

INITIAL EVALUATION OF LEFT UPPER LIMB

1. No deficits in PROM or sensation.
2. Resistance to passive stretch was moderately increased in elbow flexors and extensors, forearm pronators, and wrist and finger flexors.
3. Results of active ROM tests:
a. 160° shoulder flexion (with shoulder elevation and scapular retraction).
b. 90° shoulder abduction (with shoulder elevation and scapular retraction).
c. Full elbow flexion and extension.
d. Full forearm pronation.
e. Less than one-third range of forearm supination (with increased elbow flexion during the attempt).
f. Wrist extension to neutral (with forearm pronated and elbow flexed and supported) with concomitant finger flexion.
g. No wrist flexion.
h. Trace finger-extension and thumb-abduction movements.
i. Full finger flexion — usually in a typical "spastic-type" pattern in which the wrist is flexed and fingers are fully flexed. Unable to flex fingers without concommitant wrist extension.

JG was unable to functionally extend his fingers actively or release an object once he had grasped it. The functional goal was to use a fork in his left hand as an assist for cutting with a knife in his right hand. As JG's functional ability increased, training was directed at overcoming those problems impeding his ability to complete the aforementioned functional task. Throughout the sessions, all training was directed toward achieving the ability to use a fork as described earlier. The training strategy is summarized in Table 9–3.

JG first exhibited an inability to sufficiently open his hand to prepare to grasp the fork with a built-up handle. Because his wrist and finger extensors were very weak and opposed by hypertonic wrist and finger flexors, the initial training was directed toward recruitment of extensors and relaxation of flexors of his wrist and hand with EMGBF combined with NMS for the wrist extensors. As JG's ability to

TABLE 9–3 Overview of Treatment Plan for JG

Function Desired	Desired Motor Control	Available Motor Control	Training Strategies	Progression of Function
Adequate finger extension to prepare to grasp with wrist in neutral position	Recruitment of finger and wrist extensors; inhibition of finger and wrist flexors	Wrist extension in synergistic pattern when fully flexing fingers; trace finger extensors; hypertonic wrist and finger flexors	Recruit FE*; reinforce WE† and FE with NMS and EMGBF; inhibit WF‡ and FF§	Grasp and hold fork
A: Adequate FF to grasp and hold fork	A and B: cocontraction of WE and FF while holding fork.	A: FF adequate to grasp but uncontrolled and dominated by hypertonicity	A: recruit WE and FF while holding fork	Reach forward while holding fork
B: Adequate WE to stabilize wrist while holding fork		B: WE usually tends to incorporate mass FF	B: Limit level of FF recruitment while holding fork	
Adequate WE to stabilize wrist while holding fork and reaching to prepare to place fork	Cocontraction of WE and FF with reinforcement of WE without overrecruiting FF	A: sufficient FF to grasp appropriately	A: cocontract WE and FF while holding fork and reaching to place tines	Place tines on object and begin to press
		B: insufficient WE to stabilize wrist in neutral position before placing tines	B: recruit WE sufficiently to stabilize wrist without overrecruiting FF	
Adequate WF to stabilize wrist during placement of tines and place enough pressure to pierce and hold food	Recruitment of WF to stabilize wrist when pressing on fork	A: sufficient FF to grasp appropriately	Cocontract WE, FE, FF, and WF at appropriate levels to stabilize grip and wrist while pressing on fork	Practice skills with fork use in more and more difficult situations
C. Ability to control degree of FF while holding fork	C. Ability to control degree of FF while holding fork	B: insufficient WF to stabilize wrist while pressing on fork		

*FE = finger extension.
†WE = wrist extension.
‡WF = wrist flexion.
§FF = finger flexion.

open his hand increased, he developed the ability to perform thumb abduction with extension of the second and fifth digits. The third and fourth digits consistently would remain flexed, particularly at the proximal interphalangeal joint (45°) and at the metacarpophalangeal joint (25°). Despite limited finger extension, JG progressed to holding a fork with a built-up handle.

The second problem emerged when JG held the fork in his involved hand. The grasp that was used took advantage of the present gains and limitations. By grasping the fork with digits 3 to 5 with his thumb around the handle and extending the second digit (index finger) along the base of the fork tines, JG could hold the fork in his hand fairly well. He tended to extend his wrist and cocontract the wrist and finger muscles to stabilize fork placement. This cocontraction was reinforced with EMGBF. During EMGBF training, it was also possible to identify muscle activity changes as he lost control of the fork from fatigue or from wrist-flexor spasticity. Once understood, this information was used to enable JG to learn to compensate for these dysfunctions before control was actually lost.

The third stage involved reaching forward while holding the fork. At this point, it became apparent that JG did not have sufficient wrist-extensor strength to maintain wrist stability during reaching. As he would reach and wrist extensors would fatigue, he would invariably drop the fork (finger flexors were inhibited secondary to the tenodesis effect) or his hand would move into a mass flexor grasp (due to hyperactive finger flexors).

Once JG was able to open his hand sufficiently to grasp the fork, hold it securely in his hand, and reach forward while maintaining the grasp with a stable wrist, we approached the task of pressing on the tines of the fork to mimic stabilizing an item to prepare to cut it with a knife held in his right hand. As he reached forward and placed the tines and applied pressure, his grip and wrist stability deteriorated. At this point, training was directed toward progressive recruitment of wrist and finger flexors as pressure was gradually applied to the fork tines. He progressed to applying more pressure through the tines, extending his elbow, and shifting the weight slightly into the left side. As he gained greater control, he made attempts to use the skills he had learned, independent of EMGBF.

A LOOK TOWARD THE FUTURE

Changes in Equipment Type and Availability

In the past 20 years, EMGBF equipment has moved from the basic research laboratory to the clinic with particularly rapid advancements occurring since the early 1980s. Presently, the most basic models of EMGBF will provide some sort of visual display, threshold detection, and a variety of auditory signals with respect to the threshold-level detector. Advances in the computer industry have also influenced EMGBF instrumentation. Increased variety and complexity of the visual feedback signal and improvements in memory capabilities, portability, and quantification of EMG have been realized.

Perhaps the greatest improvement is the capacity for quantification of muscle activity over a given time sequence. With this capability, the clinician has an objective means by which to ascertain performance during an evaluative measure or therapeutic procedure.

Visual feedback capabilities range from an array of lights, which are lit as EMG activity increases, to complex interactive video games. The feedback display can be selected depending upon the treatment goal, ease of visibility, attention span, or age of the patient.

EMGBF instrument size has decreased significantly, allowing lightweight, hand-held devices to possess many capabilities present in the larger devices. This development alone will affect where EMGBF training may be conducted (such as work-site evaluation and training, bedside evaluation and training for the acute-care patient confined to bed rest, or in the arena of home health care), the distance over which training may occur (such as in gait training), and the complexity of movement that can be allowed while examining specific EMG changes. Consequently, clinicians can now evaluate, treat, and educate patients using EMGBF in the settings in which their symptoms are exacerbated or where functional abilities are most greatly challenged on a daily basis whether in the workplace or in the clinic.

Memory capabilities have also improved, allowing the therapist to save the EMG output from a given session and obtain a printed copy. For a given session, the clinician may use this "hard copy" of the patient's performance to identify such components of the session as the average duration of muscle contraction, the peak levels of EMG activity achieved and their relative consistency across attempts to move, and the length of time required to recruit or reduce EMG activity with respect to a particular threshold. The availability of a printed record of objective data permits reliable comparison of performance between treatment and often satisfies the third-party payers' requirement of measurable evidence of improvement for reimbursement.

Finally, with the capability to interface with NMS, functional gains in orthopedic and neurologic applications may be realized earlier in treatment efforts or to a greater degree.

Research Considerations

Improvements in instrumentation provide the means by which EMGBF applications may be systematically examined. These applications with NMS, in the pediatric population, in more complex treatment procedures, and in the earlier phases of acute-care rehabilitation, are a few examples of the areas that require further study. Furthermore, as greater numbers of clinicians seek more objective information concerning rehabilitation techniques that are commonly accepted at present, the ability to examine the supportive rationale of different techniques will be available.

Documentation for Third-Party Payers

Some third-party payers are still reluctant to reimburse treatment sessions referred to as *biofeedback training*. The reason may lie in the lack of specificity in the phrase biofeedback training. Consequently, the more specifically we outline the session activities and indicate how they relate to the goals of the session, as well as how the session goals relate to the overall functional goals, the more likely reimbursement is to occur. Earlier in this chapter, data collection and management were discussed. Included were suggestions for information that would enhance a progress note. By following those suggestions and maintaining accurate, objective records, a patient's progress toward functional goals can be specifically documented. Furthermore, because of the objective nature of the information available to the clinician through EMGBF concerning motor performance, third-party reimbursement for clinical services may be more readily justified.

Additional Considerations

For years, health care providers, consumers, and third-party payers have requested means by which to evaluate patients and substantiate the efficacy of treatment interventions. The intent, in part, has been to move away from reliance upon subjective assessments of a patient's physical status. With the capabilities of the present EMGBF instrumentation, as well as its affordability and accessibility, clinicians have a tool with which they can move toward the goal of improving the objectivity of their assessments.

In addition, the capabilities and scope of this instrumentation will continue to expand. Improved memory capabilities, increased availability for home use (such as integration with videocassette recorders), and improved portability are only a few examples of the future improvements that may be realized in this instrumentation.

SUMMARY

This chapter reviews the history, principles, and considerations for EMGBF. Considerations for clinical application, including equipment, patient selection, evaluation, treatment, and outcome measurement, are discussed. A variety of applications of biofeedback for clinical problems associated with musculoskeletal and neuromuscular diseases are presented, and principles are applied to a sample case history. Suggestions for future research and development of this modality are presented.

REFERENCES

1. Debacher, GA: Electromyography. In Hannay, HJ (ed): Experimental Techniques in Human Neuropsychology. Oxford University Press, New York, 1986.
2. Jacobsen, E: Progressive Relaxation, ed. 2. University of Chicago Press, Chicago, 1938.
3. Price, JP, Clare, MH, and Everhardt, FH: Studies in low backache with persistent muscle spasm. Arch Phys Med 29:703, 1948.
4. Andrews, JM: Neuromuscular reeducation of the hemiplegic with the aid of the electromyograph. Arch Phys Med Rehabil 45:530, 1964.
5. Mims, HW: Electromyography in clinical practice. South Med J 49:804, 1956.
6. Marinacci, AA and Horande, M: Electromyogram in neuromuscular reeducation. Bulletin of the Los Angeles Neurological Society 25:57, 1960.
7. Basmajian, JV: Biofeedback in rehabilitation: A review of principles and practices. Arch Phys Med Rehabil 62:469, 1981.
8. Chapman, SL: A review and clinical perspective on the use of EMG and thermal biofeedback for chronic headaches. Pain 27:1, 1986.
9. Collins, GA, et al: Comparative analysis of paraspinal and frontalis EMG, heart rate and skin conductance in chronic low back pain patients and normals for various postures and stress. Scand J Rehab Med 4:39, 1982.
10. Greenstadt, L, Shapiro, D, and Whitehead, R: Blood pressure discrimination. Psychophysiology 23:500, 1986.
11. Baker, MP, Hudson, JE, and Wolf, SL: "Feedback" cane to improve the hemiplegic patient's gait: Suggestion from the field. Phys Ther 59:170, 1979.
12. Wolf, SL and Hudson, JE: Feedback signal based upon force and time delay: Modification of the Krusen limb load monitor: Suggestion from the field. Phys Ther 60:1289, 1980.

13. Debacher, GA: Feedback goniometers for rehabilitation. In Basmajian, JV (ed): Biofeedback: Principles and Practice for Clinicians. Williams & Wilkins, Baltimore, 1983.
14. Wolf, SL: Biofeedback. In Currier, DP and Nelson, RM (eds): Clinical Electrotherapy, ed 2. Appleton & Lange, Norwalk, CT, 1991.
15. Description and analysis of the EMG signal. In Basmajian, JV and Deluca, C (eds): Muscles Alive. Their Functions Revealed by Electromyography. Williams & Wilkins, Baltimore, 1985, p 65.
16. Krebs, DE: Biofeedback in neuromuscular reeducation and gait training. In Schwartz, MS (ed): Biofeedback. A Practitioner's Guide. The Guilford Press, New York, 1987.
17. Burke, RE: Motor unit recruitment: What are the critical factors? In Desmedt, JE (ed): Progress in Clinical Neurophysiology. Vol 9. Karger, Basel, 1981.
18. English, AW and Wolf, SL: The motor unit. Anatomy and physiology. Phys Ther 62:1763, 1982.
19. Goodgold, JE and Eberstein, A: Electrodiagnosis of Neuromuscular Diseases. Wiliams & Wilkins, Baltimore, 1972.
20. Deluca, C: Apparatus, detection, and recording techniques. In Basmajian, JV and Deluca, C (eds): Muscles Alive. Their Functions Revealed by Electromyography. Williams & Wilkins, Baltimore, 1985, p 38.
21. Bach-y-Rita, P, et al: Rehabilitation medicine management in aphasia. Seminars in Speech Language and Hearing 2:259, 1981.
22. Wolf, SL, Baker, MP, and Kelly, JL: EMG biofeedback in stroke: Effect of patient characteristics. Arch Phys Med Rehabil 60:96, 1979.
23. Balliet, R, Levy, B, and Blood, KMT: Upper extremity sensory feedback therapy in chronic cerebrovascular accident patients with impaired expressive aphasia and auditory comprehension. Arch Phys Med Rehabil 67:304, 1986.
24. Wolf, SL: Essential considerations in the use of EMG biofeedback. Phys Ther 58:25, 1978.
25. Wolf, SL, LeCraw, DE, and Barton, LA: A comparison of motor copy and targeted feedback training techniques for restitution of upper extremity function among neurologic patients. Phys Ther 69:719, 1989.
26. Amato, A, Hermomeyer, CA, and Kleinman, KM: Use of electromyographic feedback to increase control of spastic muscles. Phys Ther 53:1063, 1973.
27. Swaan, D, van Wiergen, PCW, and Fokkema, SD: Auditory electromyographic feedback therapy to inhibit undesired motor activity. Arch Phys Med Rehabil 55:251, 1974.
28. Kelly, JL, Baker, MP, and Wolf, SL: Procedures for EMG biofeedback training in involved upper extremities of hemiplegic patients. Phys Ther 59:1500, 1979.
29. Baker, M, et al: Developing strategies for biofeedback: Applications in neurologically handicapped patients. Phys Ther 57:402, 1977.
30. Wolf, SL, Nacht, M and Kelly, JL: EMG feedback training during dynamic movement for low back pain patients. Behav Ther 13:395, 1982.
31. Stuckey, SJ, Jacobs, A, and Goldfarb, J: EMG biofeedback training, relaxation training, and placebo for the relief of chronic back pain. Percept Mot Skills 63:1023, 1986.
32. Moore, KL: Clinically Oriented Anatomy. Williams & Wilkins, Baltimore, 1985.
33. Nouwen, A: EMG biofeedback used to reduce standing levels of paraspinal muscle tension in chronic low back pain. Pain 17:353, 1983.
34. Nouwen, A and Bush, C: The relationship between paraspinal EMG and chronic low back pain. Pain 20:109, 1984.
35. Wolf, SL, et al: Normative data on low back mobility and activity levels. Implications for neuromuscular reeducation. Am J Phys Med 58:217, 1979.
36. Cannon, NM and Strickland, JW: Therapy following flexor tendon surgery. Hand Clinics 1:147, 1985.
37. Hirasawa, Y, Uchiza, Y, and Kusswetter, W: EMG biofeedback therapy for rupture of the extensor pollicis longus tendon. Arch Orthop Trauma Surg 104:342, 1986.
38. Beal, MS, Diefenbach, G, and Allen, A: Electromyographic biofeedback in the treatment of voluntary posterior instability of the shoulder. Am J of Sports Med 15:175, 1987.
39. Rood, MS: Neurophysiological mechanism utilized in the treatment of neuromuscular dysfunction. Am J Occup Ther 10:220, 1956.
40. Knott, M and Voss, DE: Proprioceptive Neuromuscular Facilitation. Patterns and Techniques, ed 2. Paul B Hoeber, New York, 1956, pp. 86, 102.
41. Bobath, B: Adult Hemiplegia: Evaluation and Treatment, ed 2. Heinman Medical Books, London, 1978.
42. Basmajian, JV, et al: Stroke treatment: Comparison of integrated behavioral physical therapy vs traditional physical therapy programs. Arch Phys Med Rehabil 68:267, 1987.
43. Inglis, J, et al: Electromyographic biofeedback and physical therapy of the hemiplegic upper limb. Arch Phys Med Rehabil 65:755, 1984.
44. Burnside, IG, Tobias, HS, and Bursill, D: Electromyographic feedback in the remobilization of stroke patients: A controlled trial. Arch Phys Med Rehabil 63:1393, 1983.
45. Wolf, SL and Binder-Macleod, SA: Electromyographic biofeedback applications to the hemiplegic patient: Changes in upper extremity neuromuscular and functional status. Phys Ther 63:1393, 1983.
46. Wolf, SL and Binder-Macleod, SA: Electromyographic biofeedback applications to the hemiplegic patient: Changes in lower extremity neuromuscular and functional status. Phys Ther 63:1404, 1983.
47. Labbe, EE and Williamson, DA: Temperature feedback in the treatment of children with migraine headaches. J Pediatr Psychol 8:317, 1983.

48. Sugar, EG and Firlit, CF: Urodynamic feedback: A new therapeutic approach for childhood incontinence/infection (vesicle voluntary sphincter dyssynergia). J Urol 128:1253, 1982.

49. Whitehead, WE, et al: Treatment of fecal incontinence in children with spina bifida: Comparison of biofeedback and behavior modification. Arch Phys Med Rehabil 67:218, 1986.

50. Wolf, SL, Edwards, DI, and Shutter, LA: Concurrent assessment of muscle activity (CAMA): A procedural approach to assess treatment goals. Phys Ther 66:218, 1986.

51. Burnside, IG, Tobias, HS, and Bursill, D: Electromyographic feedback in the rehabilitation of stroke patients: A controlled trial. Arch Phys Med Rehabil 63:217, 1982.

52. Basmajian, JV, Regenos, EM, and Baker, MP: Rehabilitating stroke patients with biofeedback. Geriatrics 32:85, 1977.

53. Basmajian, JV and Blumenthal, R: In Basmajian, JV (ed): Biofeedback: Principles and Practice for Clinicians, ed 3. Williams & Wilkins, Baltimore, 1989, p 369. Electroplacement in electromyographic biofeedback.

54. Bowman, BR, Baker, LL, and Waters, RL: Positional feedback and electrical stimulation. An automated treatment for the hemiplegic wrist. Arch Phys Med Rehabil 60:497, 1979.

55. Winchester, P, et al.: Effects of feedback stimulation training and cyclical electrical stimulation on knee extension in hemiparetic patients. Phys Ther 63:1097, 1983.

56. Wolf, SL: EMG biofeedback application in physical rehabilitation: An overview. Physiotherapy Canada 31:65, 1979.

57. Baker, M, et al.: Developing strategies for biofeedback. Applications in neurologically handicapped patients. Phys Ther 57:402, 1977.

CHAPTER 10

Additional Therapeutic Uses of Electricity

John P. Cummings, Ph.D., P.T.

Although electrical stimulation has traditionally been used by physical therapists to stimulate healthy muscle and to modulate pain, electrical stimulation has several additional therapeutic applications. This chapter describes the application of electricity to enhance wound healing, stimulate bone formation, deliver ions through the surface of the body, and reduce edema.

ELECTRICAL STIMULATION FOR WOUND HEALING

The application of various forms of electrical current to augment wound healing has been widely reported.[1-6] As early as 1668, electrically charged gold leaf was applied to smallpox lesions to prevent scar formation.[7] Charged gold leaf has also been used for its hemostatic effect in vascular surgery[8] and to heal decubitis, diabetic, and ischemic skin ulcers.[2,9] Continuous, very low intensity direct current and monophasic, pulsating current applied directly to wounds have enhanced wound healing in animals[1,3,10] and human subjects.[4-6,11-13]

Although the mechanism responsible for the apparent facilitation of the wound-healing process is not readily apparent, Robert Becker[14,15] has suggested the existence within the body of a direct current electrical system that is responsible for controlling tissue healing. Becker theorized that when the body is injured, the inherent electrical balance of the body is disturbed, resulting in a shift in current flow within this system. Becker referred to this shift in current flow as the "current of injury," which he believes is generated by the injured tissue and is responsible for initiating the healing process. Becker suggested that the ability of anodal direct current to facilitate healing is based on the current amplifying the magnitude of the body's current of injury, which acts as a signal to initiate and maintain the healing process.

Continuous low amplitude (less than 1.0 mA intensity) current has been used to facilitate wound healing in animal subjects.[1,3,16] Carey and Lepley reported different histological responses beneath the anode and cathode and an increase in wound tensile strength which was greater under the cathode than under the anode following stimulation with continuous direct current. In contrast to the findings of Carey and Lepley,[1] Wu, Go, and Dennis[16] reported that polarity does not influence tissue tensile strength. However, Assimacopoulos,[3] in a study of facilitating the healing of mechanically induced wounds in rabbits with continuous direct current, supported the findings of Carey and Lepley that wound healing could be accelerated under the cathode.

Similar results using continuous direct current of intensities ranging from 0.2 to 1.0 mA have been reported in studies using human subjects.[4,5,11–13] Wolcott and associates[4] successfully used low intensity direct current (LIDC) to facilitate healing in a wide variety of wounds. They reported that stimulated wounds healed at rates 2 to 3.5 times faster than nonstimulated control wounds. Furthermore, Wolcott's group formulated a protocol for the application of LIDC using currents of intensities ranging from 200 to 800 μA. Their protocol requires the cathode to be initially placed over the wound for either a 3-day period or until the wound is cultured aseptic. Following this initial period the anode was applied to the wound with the cathode placed 25 cm proximal to the wound. A total of 6 hours of stimulation is given in three 2-hour sessions which are separated by two 4-hour periods of no stimulation. Therefore, the electrodes are applied for 14 hours a day with the current flowing 6 hours a day. More recently, in a similar study using LIDC, Carley and Wainapel,[5] reported that indolent ulcers located either below the knee or in the sacral area and treated with electrical stimulation healed 1.5 to 2.5 times faster than nonstimulated ulcers. Additionally, Carley and Wainapel reported that the wounds treated with LIDC required less debridement than the nonstimulated wounds.

Another possible benefit of electrical stimulation of an open wound with a continuous LIDC is the apparent bactericidal effect that has been reported by numerous investigators both in vitro and in vivo.[4,5,11,17,18] Although some investigators have reported that either cathodal or anodal stimulation has a bactericidal effect, most human studies have demonstrated this effect associated specifically with the cathode.[4,5]

A more recent approach for facilitating tissue healing uses high voltage, monophasic, pulsating current instead of continuous direct current.[6,12,13] Thurman and Christian presented a case study in which they treated a purulent abscess on the foot of a 43-year-old diabetic patient with high voltage, monophasic, pulsating current.[12] They applied the electrodes around the abscess and pulsed the current at a "low frequency" and an intensity "great enough to elicit muscular contractions." Thurman and Christian[12] reported that the abscess responded favorably to treatments given twice daily on weekdays and once daily on weekends. Unfortunately the investigators did not provide a detailed description of the stimulation parameters used with this patient.

In another study on the effect of high voltage, monophasic, pulsating current on wound healing, Akers and Gabrielson[13] assigned 14 patients having decubitis ulcers to one of three groups: (1) whirlpool once a day, (2) whirlpool and high voltage, pulsed stimulation twice a day, and (3) high voltage, pulsed stimulation twice a day. Although the investigators reported that the greatest rate of wound healing occurred in the group receiving only high voltage, pulsed stimulation, they failed to include in their report such necessary information as stimulus characteristics and the duration and number of treatments.

Kloth and Feedar[6] have recently reported a well-controlled study of the effect of high voltage, monophasic, pulsed current on the rate of healing dermal ulcers in humans. In their study, 16 patients with Stage IV decubitus ulcers were randomly assigned to either a treatment group or a control group. Patients in the treatment group received daily electrical stimulation from a commercially available high voltage generator. The stimulation variables were set at a frequency of 105 Hz, an interpulse interval of 50 μs, and a voltage just below that producing a visible muscle contraction (i.e., 100 to 175 V). Each patient in the treatment group received daily 45 minutes of stimulation to the ulcer site, 5 days a week. Initially the anode was placed over the wound with the cathode placed 15 cm caudal to the edge of the anode. This configuration was maintained unless the wound healing reached a plateau. If a plateau in healing occurred, the cathode was placed over the wound, and the anode moved 15 cm rostral to the cathode. Therefore, the electrodes were always positioned with the anode rostral and closer to the neuraxis than the cathode. According to the investigators this configuration was maintained to amplify the "injury potential" as previously suggested by Robert Becker.[19] Patients in the control group had electrodes applied to the ulcers daily, but received no stimulation. Necrotic tissue from the wounds of patients in both groups was debrided both manually and with a proteolytic enzyme ointment, Elase,* as needed.

The ulcers of patients in the treatment group healed at a mean rate of 44.8 percent a week and healed 100 percent over a mean period of 7.3 weeks, while the ulcers of patients in the control group increased in area an average of 11.6 percent a week and increased 28.9 percent over a mean period of 7.4 weeks. The authors further pointed out that the average rate of wound healing in this study, 44.8 percent a week, compared favorably to the 13.4 percent a week reported by Wolcott and colleagues[4] using continuous LIDC. Therefore, both animal and human studies have demonstrated that electrical stimulation may facilitate the healing rate of dermal wounds.

ELECTRICAL STIMULATION FOR OSTEOGENESIS

The use of electrical stimulation in facilitating bone growth or osteogenesis began in 1957 when Fukada and Yasuda[20] demonstrated that bone possessed piezoelectric properties. Their work showed that when external forces are applied to bone, the bone responds by generating electrical potentials. Fukada and Yasuda hypothesized that these potentials might be the signals that control osteoblastic activity and, therefore, may play a role in bone growth and in the repair of bone.

In the mid-1960s Shamos, Lavine, and Shamos[21,22] demonstrated that the piezoelectric potentials originated in the collagenous organic matrix of bone. Yet, in 1966, Friedenburg and Brighton[23] described the presence of freestanding bioelectric potentials in bone, which were dependent upon the viability of the bone cells, and ascertained that chemical gradients within bone were the source of energy for the bioelectric potentials. Friedenberg and Brighton also described negative electric potentials at fracture sites. More recently Borgens[24] observed that steady, endogenous ionic currents (approximately 5 μA/cm^2) enter the fracture sites in the phalanges of living mice.

The identification of such electrical potentials led to the investigation of the response of bone to externally applied electrical and electromagnetic fields. The primary goal of the early experimental work on animals was to determine whether these exogenous potentials could stimulate bone growth and the healing of fractures, with the ultimate goal of accelerating bone healing in humans.

---

*Elase, Parke-Davis (Division of Warner-Lambert), Morris Plains, NJ 07950.

The initial animal studies used very low intensity direct current (2 to 20 μA) applied through implanted electrodes directly to the bone.[25,26] Lavine, Lustrin, and Shamos[26] placed platinum electrodes above and below the experimental bone defect while Bassett, Pawlick, and Becker[25] placed platinum iridium electrodes into the experimental osseous defect. More recently, Brighton[27] has implanted stainless steel electrodes into the fracture site. All of these studies resulted in the acceleration of bone growth in response to electrical stimulation which was observed to occur primarily around the cathode, although some bone also formed between the electrodes. Only occasionally was bone growth observed at the anode. These studies also demonstrated that direct current was more effective than alternating current in facilitating bone growth.

The initial attempts to enhance bone healing in humans by electrical stimulation were done in patients who had a nonunion fracture or a congenital pseudarthrosis of the tibia.[28] In 1971 Friedenberg, Harlow, and Brighton[29] reported successfully treating a patient with nonunion of the medial malleolus, using a current of 10 μA with the cathode implanted across the nonunion. They reported that the nonunion healed in approximately 8 weeks.

In 1979 the Food and Drug Administration (FDA) approved three systems for the stimulation of osteogenesis in the treatment of nonunions.[30] These systems were (1) the semi-invasive system using constant direct current which was developed by Brighton and colleagues;[31,32] (2) the totally implantable, constant direct current system developed by Dwyer and Wickham;[33] and (3) the noninvasive, inductive coupling system of Bassett and associates.[34] In the semi-invasive method either both electrodes are implanted, with one electrode above and one below the fracture site, or only the cathode is implanted into the treatment site, while the anode and power source remain external. In the totally invasive method the entire unit, electrodes and power source, are implanted. The noninvasive approach uses time-varying magnetic fields and time-varying electrical fields to produce electric currents at the fracture site.[35]

Although the invasive, semi-invasive, and noninvasive methods of application are reported to have about the same overall success rate for treatment of fractures of the tibia, each method has its advantages as well as disadvantages.[36] The invasive and semi-invasive techniques subject the patient to a greater risk of infection than does the noninvasive method. However, the cooperation of the patient is more critical in the use of the noninvasive technique.

All three methods are used for the stimulation of the sites of nonunion, delayed union, and congenital pseudoarthosis. In all three techniques, 3 to 6 months of treatment are recommended for nonunion fractures. The clinical contraindications for all three techniques are similar: (1) a gap at the nonunion site which is longer than half of the diameter of the bone at the level of the nonunion and (2) the presence of a synovial pseudoarthrosis. Although patients with quiescent osteomyelitis have been treated with electrical stimulation, treatment with the semi-invasive method was terminated if the infection was reactivated.[36]

According to Lavine and Grodzinsky,[36] although the exact mechanisms by which the various electrical stimuli induce an osteogenic response are still unknown, it is likely that different mechanisms are associated with the invasive technique compared with those of the noninvasive methods, because of the presence of implanted electrodes.

Of particular interest to physical therapists are the reports that the noninvasive application of interferential current facilitates bone healing of nonunion fractures and pseudoarthrosis.[37,38] In 1969, Nikolova-Troeva[37] treated 150 patients with clinical nonunion fractures using interferential current. She stimulated the fracture site with a constant frequency of 100 Hz, at an amplitude of between 10 and 20 mA, for 15 to 20 minutes daily. In patients receiving only interferential current stimulation (no medication), 73 percent of the fractures healed completely.

In another study involving humans, Ganne and associates[38] reported that interferential current facilitated the healing of nonunion mandibular fractures. In nine patients with nonunion mandibular fractures, the fracture site was stimulated with interferential current at 20 Hz for 20 minutes every 2 or 3 days. The current amplitude was set to produce very slight contractions of the underlying facial musculature. In this study the number of treatments varied from 3 to 20, with complete healing occurring in all nine patients. However, the investigators did not address the possibility that the healing may have resulted from an increase in the amount of stress of the mandible secondary to electrically induced contractions of the facial muscles.

In a study on the effect of interferential current stimulation on healing mechanically induced transverse osteotomies of the radius and ulna in a 6-month-old black-headed sheep, Laabs and associates[39] concluded that the rate of healing was accelerated by the interferential stimulation. Laabs and colleagues stimulated the fracture site for 10 minutes three times a week. They also reported that measurements of calcium and phosphorous levels in the regenerated bone indicated full mineralization of the new bone had occurred in the stimulated animal earlier than in the nonstimulated control group.

Regardless of the mechanisms involved in the electrical stimulation of osteogensis, experimental evidence gathered to date suggests that the approach is valuable in facilitating the healing of nonunions, delayed unions, and pseudarthrosis.

ELECTRICAL STIMULATION FOR URINARY DYSFUNCTION

The treatment of urinary dysfunction with electrical stimulation was initially reported by Huffman, Osborne, and Sokol in 1952.[40] Subsequently, electrical stimulation has been used in the treatment of the hyperreflexic bladder,[41] the hyporeflexic (areflexic) bladder,[42] and in cases of myogenic incontinence, such as sphincter weakness and surgical damage to the sphincter.[43,44] According to Jacobs and colleagues,[45] patients who can benefit from chronic bladder stimulation include those with postprostatectomy weakness, cortical incontinence, subcortical incontinence, and stress incontinence.

Correction of urinary dysfunction by electrical stimulation has been achieved using various techniques. Urethral closure may be improved by contracting the striated muscle fibers of the external sphincter and pelvic-floor musculature through electrical stimulation of the pelvic nerves. A second technique involves activating a "pudendal to pelvic reflex" to either depress or totally eliminate uninhibited detrusor contractions.[46] A third technique involves the electrical stimulation of acupuncture points traditionally activated by acupuncturists to inhibit bladder activity.[47]

Stimulation of the Pelvic-Floor Musculature

A number of methods have been used to stimulate the striated muscles of the external sphincter and the pelvic floor musculature. These techniques include anal or vaginal electrical stimulation,[45,48,49] stimulation of the sacral nerve roots,[50] and stimulation of the pelvic floor with interferential current.[51,52]

VAGINAL- AND ANAL-PLUG STIMULATION

Typically, the device used for stimulating the pelvic-floor musculature consists of a plastic anal or vaginal plug with two embedded ring electrodes. The power source is a 9-V battery with stimulation parameters of 8.5 V at 20 to 80 Hz, and a pulsewidth of 0.1 to 1 ms.[45] All stimulation is continuous until the patient needs to void, at which time the stimulator is turned off. Although positive results have been reported, the devices are not widely used because the plugs are often not tolerated by the patients.[53] McGuire and associates[47] have also reported that, with anal-plug electrodes, there is a large current dissipation along the rectal mucosa. This current loss inhibits the effective electrical stimulation of the pelvic-floor musculature. Regardless of the apparent problems associated with anal plugs, after a few months of continuous use, some patients may maintain continence even after the chronic stimulation is stopped. This effect may be a combination of muscle strengthening and neuromuscular re-education.[45]

STIMULATION OF THE SACRAL NERVE ROOTS

Electrical stimulation of the sacral nerve roots has been successful in reducing the residual urine volume following micturation in paraplegic patients.[50,54] Although sacral root stimulation involves a sacral laminectomy and surgical implantation of the electrodes, the technique is low risk, minimizes pain, and separates detrusor from sphincter responses.[55,56]

PELVIC-FLOOR STIMULATION WITH INTERFERENTIAL CURRENT

The use of interferential current to stimulate contraction of the pelvic-floor musculature for the management of stress incontinence and detrusor instability has been reported.[51,52,57] Dougall[51] studied the effect of pelvic floor stimulation using interferential current in 55 female patients between 20 and 72 years of age having urinary incontinence. He reported a 30 percent reduction in the incidence of incontinence in the treated patients, with 60 percent of these patients subjectively reporting improvement 1 year after the treatments were terminated. The technique used by Dougall was similar to that used by McQuire.[57] Treatment was given with the patient in a semireclined position with the hips and knees flexed and supported. Four, large vacuum electrodes were used, two placed symmetrically on the abdomen above the inguinal ligament, 3 cm apart, and two placed on the inside of the thighs, below the inferior border of the femoral triangle. An interferential current of between 0 and 100 Hz was passed between the electrodes at an intensity equal to the maximum limit of patient comfort. Treatments were given for 15 minutes, three times per week for 4 weeks. No other treatment was offered or advice given to the patient during the course of interferential therapy. Success has been attributed to stimulation of the pudendal nerve which increases urethral closure by activating the pelvic floor musculature.

More recently, Laycock and Green[52] compared electrode placements in interferential therapy for the treatment of urinary incontinence with the goal of identifying those electrode placements that provided for maximal pelvic floor stimulation. In electrode positioning, the authors considered the following: (1) proximity to the pudendal nerve, (2) route of least resistance to the flow of an electric current, (3) minimum area of spread of current, (4) patient comfort, and (5) ease of application. The muscular contractions elicited by the interferential stimulation using different electrode sites were compared using a vaginally located pressure-sensitive perineometer capable of detecting, measuring, and recording perivaginal pressure changes produced as a result of the electrical stimulation of the pelvic floor musculature. Laycock and Green concluded that for optimal pelvic-floor stimulation and ease of application the bipolar technique was most effective. For female patients, *one* electrode was placed under either ischial tuberosity with the second electrode over the anterior perineum, immediately inferior to the symphysis pubis. Male patients treated with the bipolar technique had one electrode placed on each side of the gluteal cleft, just anterior to the anus.

Laycock and Green[52] also recommended that specific interferential current parameters be used in the treatment of stress incontinence and detrusor instability. For stress incontinence the authors recommended that a sweep frequency of 10 to 50 Hz be used with a gradual rise and fall to ensure that the full range of frequencies is covered. Recommended treatment time is 30 minutes per session. They also stated that a fixed frequency of 50 Hz is equally effective. If surging current is not available, Laycock and Green recommended stimulation for 6 seconds at 10 Hz followed immediately by 6 seconds at 50 Hz for a total of 30 minutes. According to the authors, the intensity of the stimulus should elicit a maximal contraction of the pelvic floor musculature (i.e., 50- to 80-mA intensity). The authors report a decrease in stress incontinence in patients receiving three treatments per week lasting 30 minutes each, for a total of 12 treatments over a 1-month period. They also recommended that a home program of pelvic floor exercises be stressed as an integral part of the overall treatment program.

In the treatment of detrusor instability with interferential electrical stimulation, the goal is to stimulate the pudendal-pelvic reflex to inhibit detrusor activity, and ultimately re-establish normal urinary reflex activity. Electrical stimulation of the pudendal nerve afferents has an inhibiting or relaxing effect on the detrusor muscle.[58] Since Ohlsson and associates[59] have demonstrated that nerve fibers of smaller diameter (i.e., pudendal afferents) respond to lower frequency stimulation, Laycock and Green[52] recommended that detrusor instability be treated with low frequency (i.e., 50 to 10 Hz) interferential stimulation. They also recommend that the current intensity approach the patient's tolerance. They suggest that treatment lasting 30 minutes be given daily when possible, although good clinical results have been obtained with three treatments per week for 4 weeks. Although the stimulation techniques and parameters described in this part of the chapter are specific to electrical stimulation with interferential current, some of the basic principles of stimulation may be beneficial when stimulating with other types of current (i.e., high voltage, monophasic pulsed current).

Stimulation of Traditional Acupuncture Points

McGuire and associates[47] used transcutaneous electrical stimulation of acupuncture points to successfully inhibit detrusor activity. In 22 patients having a variety of neural lesions accompanied by detrusor instability, surface electrodes were positioned bilaterally over both tibial nerves or both common peroneal nerves. The nerves were stimulated at an intensity of 5 to 8 V, a frequency of 2 to 10 Hz, and pulse widths of 5 to 20 ms. McGuire and associates were able to achieve continence in 90 percent of the patients using constant stimulation. It appears that this type of electrical stimulation may also inhibit reflex detrusor activity.

The possibility that transcutaneous electrical nerve stimulation (TENS) of peripheral nerves may facilitate emptying of the hypotonic bladder was suggested by Jones.[60] TENS was applied to the inner thighs of a 19-year-old female patient with a hypotonic bladder secondary to multiple sclerosis in an effort to improve bladder emptying.[61] Flanigan and associates[61] reported that, following 15 to 30 minutes of stimulation, the patient could initiate voiding and could void to near completion. In this case study, the authors used a conventional neurostimulator having a modified square wave pulse. The current was pulsed at a varying rate of 2 to 110 Hz, and a variable pulse width of 40 to 200 μs. Flanigan and colleagues concluded that bladder emptying was dependent upon the electrical stimulation since withdrawal of the stimulation resulted in the bladder returning to its prestimulation areflexive state.

Although the mechanisms responsible for facilitating normal bladder function using electrical stimulation of acupuncture points and peripheral nerves are not fully understood, clinical use of the technique may be considered a viable alternative to more complicated interventions.

ELECTRICAL STIMULATION FOR PERIPHERAL CIRCULATION

The incidence of deep vein thrombosis (DVT) following major general surgery averages 30 percent, while the postoperative mortality associated with thromboembolic complications averages 1 percent. Nearly 50 percent of the thromboses are formed during surgery, and the majority of them are localized in the calves, particularly in the venous sinusoids of the soleus muscle.[62-64]

Factors contributing to the formation of a thrombosis include changes in blood coagulability, blood flow, and changes in the vessel wall. In the case of postoperative DVT, the most important factors are changes in blood coagulability and blood flow.[64]

According to Jonsson and Lindstrom[64] the patients most likely to develop postoperative thromboembolism are those with malignant disease, those with a previous history of thromboembolism, and the elderly. Jonsson and Lindstrom stressed that the risk of developing deep venous thrombosis in connection with surgery increases drastically with age, and therefore patients older than 40 should receive some type of prophylactic therapy during major surgery. They further emphasized that since the formation of postoperative DVT begins during surgery in most cases, the prophylactic measures should be undertaken from the beginning of surgery.

To date, the most common approaches used to prevent postoperative thromboembolic complications are (1) the use of pharmacologic agents such as dextran and heparin sodium to decrease blood coagulability and (2) mechanical measures, including elevation, compression stockings, and electrical stimulation of the calf muscles, to decrease venous pooling in the legs. The main advantage of the mechanical methods over the pharmacologic agents is that the mechanical measures do not increase the risk of bleeding associated with surgery.[64] The mechanical measure of particular interest to physical therapists is electrical stimulation of the calf muscles. The remainder of this part of the chapter will specifically discuss perioperative electrical calf muscle stimulation for the prevention of DVT.

In the 1960s, Doran and associates[65,66] claimed that electrical stimulation of the calf muscles prevented a decrease in the rate of venous blood flow in the legs during surgery and therefore decreased the frequency of deep venous thrombosis. In 1972, Nicolaides and associates[63] measured the effect of varied impulse frequency on the increase in femoral vein blood flow velocity resulting from calf muscle stimulation. They determined an optimal rate of stimulation to be 12 to 15 pulses per minute. They also suggested that the benefits derived from stimulation may result not only from a reduction in venous stasis but possibly also from increased fibrinolytic activity secondary to the muscle contractions.

In 1973, Becker and Schampi[67] used the radioactive fibrinogen scanning technique to show that a statistically significant reduction in the frequency of postoperative venous thrombosis in the legs could be achieved by electrical stimulation of the calf muscles. Using a Siemens Neuroton 621* stimulator, Becker and Schampi began bilateral stimulation of the calf muscles immediately after induction of anesthesia. Rhythmic contractions of the calf muscles were induced by the intermittent faradic current delivered through four electrodes; one electrode was affixed over the tibial nerve in each leg, just above the popliteal fossa, and one electrode was placed over the Achilles tendons in each leg. The electrodes consisted of 10 by 14 cm tin sheets covered with moist rubber foam sponges. Stimuli having a 10 ms pulsewidth were delivered at a frequency of 30 per minute and at an intensity of 30 mA. Stimulation was terminated at the end of the operation when the patient could move spontaneously. Further stimulation was not possible since it caused "an uncomfortable and in some cases painful sensation in the calf." The investigators did not attempt to continue stimulation at a lower intensity.

In 1975, Rosenberg, Evans, and Pollack[68] demonstrated that electrical stimulation of the calf muscles once every 5 seconds throughout surgery was effective in reducing DVT in patients undergoing laparotomies for benign conditions. However, they also reported that the stimulation was not effective in reducing the incidence of DVT in patients undergoing surgery for malignant disease or for prostate-bladder surgery.

Because previous studies on calf muscle stimulation to reduce DVT used "single electrical impulses" to produce "single twitches" in the calf muscles, Lindstrom and associates[69] investigated the effect of "groups" of impulses resulting in brief tetanic contractions on the formation of DVT. Changes in calf volume were recorded by strain-gauge plethysmography. The investigators demonstrated that bursts of 8 impulses per second, deliver eight times (eight contractions) per minute "reduced calf venous volume approximately three times more efficiently" than stimulation with "single electrical impulses." Lindstrom and colleagues also recognized that in patients under complete anesthesia with muscle relaxation, a stimuli with pulse widths of at least 25 ms were necessary. The intensity of the stimuli in the study ranged from 40 to 50 mA, and was similar to that used by Becker and Schampi.[67]

In a follow-up study, Lindstrom and associates[70] compared the effects of perioperative electrical calf-muscle stimulation using "groups of impulses," to administer the drug Dextran 40 given perioperatively and postoperatively on postoperative DVT and pulmonary embolism. The fibrinogen-uptake test and phlebography were used for DVT screening, while chest x-rays and scintigrams were used to screen for pulmonary embolism. The stimulation parameters were similar to those previously described[69] with the exception of the pulse width, which was increased to 50 ms in the current study. From this study the investigators concluded that both prophylactic methods, electrical stimulation of these calf muscles, and the use of Dextran 40 have similar effects on the incidence of postoperative thromboembolism. However, Lindstrom and colleagues stressed that perioperative electrical stimulation is free from side effects, simple to use, and cost effective. Furthermore, electrical stimulation can be safely used with drugs that interfere with coagulation. An alternate method used to increase peripheral circulation

---

*Siemens Neuroton 621, Siemens Corporation, Erlangen, Germany.

involves the electrical stimulation of the autonomic nervous system and is discussed in Chapter 5.

ELECTRICAL STIMULATION FOR EDEMA REDUCTION

Traumatic edema resulting from the disruption of blood vessels often accompanies such musculoskeletal injuries as acute strains or sprains. Voluntary muscle-pump activity or muscle pump facilitation through electrical stimulation may be effective in facilitating lymphatic and venous drainage, and thereby aid in the resolution of post-traumatic edema. A second approach for the reduction of traumatic edema using electrical stimulation uses sensory level stimulation that does not result in muscle contractions.

The rationale for using motor level, muscle pump facilitation to reduce edema is the same as the rationale for facilitating venous return to decrease the probability of the formation of a deep venous thrombosis. This muscle pump mechanism, elicited either voluntarily or electrically, can effectively lead to a reduction in edema by mobilizing the edema to move from the interstitial compartment to the blood vascular system.

Sensory level stimulation uses the polarity of an electrical stimulus to repel similarly charged substances from the edematous area. Because blood cells and plasma proteins carry a negative charge at the normal blood pH of 7.4,[71] it may be postulated that a negative electrode placed over an edematous area may repel these negatively charged substances from the area of stimulation. If these negatively charged substances are repelled from the treatment area, the fluid component of the edema should follow a concentration gradient and accompany the negatively charged blood cells and plasma proteins, therefore decreasing the amount of edema through a fluid shift.

Although the aforementioned theory has been proposed to explain the use of electrical stimulation to reduce edema, two recent studies in the physical therapy literature cast doubts on the purported effectiveness of high voltage pulsed current (HVPC) in reducing edema. Michlovitz, Smith, and Watkins[72] studied the effectiveness of HVPC in the treatment of acute ankle sprains. They reported no significant changes in the edema control when the electrical stimulation was added to the standard protocol which included ice, compression, and elevation. In a recent study on the reduction of edema following flint trauma to the rat hindlimb, Mohr, Akers, and Landry[73] reported no statistically significant decrease in edema when compared with untreated controls.

The lack of success reported from these studies may be due to the fact that this type of current flows for less than 3 to 5 ms every second. Therefore, one would expect that because the "polar" effect of such a current would be minimal, the ability of the current to effectively repel similarly charged ions would also be minimal. Perhaps a more effective current in managing edema would be a low intensity, continuous, unidirectional current which would be expected to have the appropriate "polar" effects dependent upon the specific polarity used for treatment.

IONTOPHORESIS

Iontophoresis or ion transfer is the noninvasive introduction of topically applied free ions into the skin using direct current. Iontophoresis, based on the principle that an electrically charged electrode will repel a similarly charged ion, was described by Le Duc in 1903.[74] Ions having a positive charge can be introduced into the epidermis and

TABLE 10–1 Ions Commonly Used in Iontophoresis

Ion	Source	Polarity	Indications
Acetate	Acetic acid	—	Calcium deposits
Chloride	Sodium chloride	—	Soften scars and adhesions (sclerolytic agent)
Copper	Copper sulfate	+	Fungal infections
Dexamethasone	Decadron	+	Musculoskeletal inflammatory conditions
Hyaluronidase	Wyadase	+	Edema reduction
Lidocaine	Lidocaine	+	Analgesic agent
Magnesium	Magnesium sulfate	+	Muscle relaxation, vasodilation
Salicylate	Sodium salicylate	—	Musculoskeletal inflammatory conditions
Tap water		+/−	Hyperhidrosis
Zinc	Zinc oxide	+	Dermal ulcers, slow-healing wounds

mucous membranes of the body by the positive electrode, and ions having a negative charge are introduced by the negative electrode.

Historically, iontophoresis with various active ions (Table 10–1) has been used in the treatment of edema,[75] ischemic skin ulcers,[76] hyperhidrosis,[77,78] fungus infections,[75-82] gouty arthritis,[80] calcific tendinitis,[81] musculocutaneous inflammatory conditions,[82] and other conditions. The successful use of iontophoresis with topical anesthetics to produce local anesthesia has also been reported.[83,84] The contemporary use of iontophoresis by physical therapists is primarily in the treatment of musculoskeletal inflammatory conditions, edema, and for the production of local, topical anesthesia of the skin.

Successful treatment of several musculoskeletal inflammatory conditions (i.e., bursitis, tendonitis, etc.) using iontophoresis with dexamethasone sodium phosphate with Xylocaine has been reported by Harris.[79] Harris administered a 1-ml solution containing 4 mg of dexamethasone sodium phosphate combined with 2 ml of a 4-percent Xylocaine solution to 50 patients having various musculocutaneous inflammatory conditions. Each patient received a maximum of three treatments within a 1-week period. Using a commercially available iontophoresis unit, Phoresor,* a current of 1 mA was applied, and increased by 1 mA each minute for 5 minutes. The current remained at an intensity of 5 mA for an additional 15 minutes. In this clinical study, Harris reported that 38 of the 50 patients had excellent pain relief while seven reported moderate relief and five reported little or no long-term pain relief. This study indicates that iontophoresis may be an effective means of delivering ionized anti-inflammatory drugs to inflamed superficial tissues.

A second application of iontophoresis is the reduction of edema using hyaluronidase. In a study of 100 patients, Magistro reported that total edema reduction ranged from 0.6 to 1.9 cm following iontophoresis application of hyaluronidase.[83] Although the permanence of the edema reduction in Magistro's study was difficult to maintain, hyaluronidase administered by iontophoresis appears to enhance fluid absorption.

Another contemporary use of iontophoresis is the administration of local anesthetics.[84-86] Russo and associates[84] compared the duration and depth of anesthesia produced by lidocaine and placebo (physiologic saline) when delivered by iontophoresis, topical application, and subcutaneous infiltration. The investigators reported that

---

*Phoresor, Iomed Incorporated, Salt Lake City, UT.

lidocaine iontophoresis produced local anesthesia of longer duration ($p < 0.001$) than topically applied lidocaine or a placebo by any means of application. Although the anesthesia produced by the lidocaine iontophoresis was of significantly shorter duration ($p < 0.001$) than that produced by lidocaine infiltration, the study did show that lidocaine iontophoresis is effective in producing local anesthesia for about 5 minutes.

Although iontophoresis is noninvasive, sterile, and relatively painless, the practitioner must be aware of the clinical methodology and considerations for iontophoresis. Information on the specific clinical procedures, indications, and contraindications of iontophoresis is easily obtained.[87-89] The reader is encouraged to refer to these sources for specific clinical methods of application.

EVALUATION OF NEW CLAIMS FOR ELECTROTHERAPEUTIC INTERVENTIONS

In the last decade a tremendous increase in the popularity and utilization of electrotherapy occurred in physical therapy. Electrical stimulation has become an accepted and proven agent in the treatment of numerous pathologies ranging from nonunion fractures to the management of scoliosis and urinary dysfunction. However, as we enter the 1990s, we find many new, and often unsubstantiated claims for the benefits of electrotherapy. These claims include, but are not limited to, the use of electrical stimulation for weight loss, body toning, and the potential use of electrical stimulation as a replacement for cosmetic facial surgery.

Throughout the 1980s most physical therapists became knowledgeable in the use of various electrotherapeutic devices. This increased knowledge contributed to physical therapists becoming cautious, discerning users of these devices. When new claims were made regarding the effectiveness of devices, physical therapists demanded to see the clinical and/or basic science research results that substantiated the claims. Therapists also became aware of the importance of relating stimulation parameters and expected physiological effects to manufacturers' and distributors' claims. Specification sheets became as important as ease of operation.

As this century ends, physical therapists must remain critical consumers of electrotherapeutic devices. We must continue to demand accountability. New claims must be substantiated by clinical and/or basic science studies. To achieve this accountability, the therapist must be knowledgeable of the basic principles of electrotherapy. Without a basic working knowledge, the accountability that we expect from manufacturers and distributors, and the accountability that our patients expect from us will be distilled, distorted, or worse, lost.

SUMMARY

This chapter reviews additional therapeutic applications of electricity, including facilitation of wound healing and osteogenesis, neuromuscular re-education of autonomic functions, including pelvic floor control and peripheral circulation, resolution of edema, and iontophoresis. In addition, criteria for objective evaluation of innovative applications of therapeutic electricity are presented to facilitate educated consumerism within the reader. As the use of therapeutic electricity grows, with the advance of technology, it is critical that health care professionals carefully analyze innovative applications, and urge demonstration of efficacy of treatment prior to adoption of new technology and application.

REFERENCES

1. Carey, LC and Lepley, D: Effect of continuous direct electrical current on healing wounds. Surgical Forum 13:33, 1962.
2. Kanof, N: Gold leaf in the treatment of cutaneous ulcers. J Invest Dermatol 43:441, 1964.
3. Assimacopoulos, D: Wound healing promotion by the use of negative electric current. Am Surg 34:423, 1968.
4. Wolcott, LE, et al: Accelerated healing of skin ulcers by electrotherapy: Preliminary clinical results. South Med J 62:795, 1969.
5. Carley, P and Wainapel, S: Electrotherapy for acceleration of wound healing: Low intensity direct current. Arch Phys Med Rehabil 66:443, 1985.
6. Kloth, LGC and Feedar, JA: Acceleration of wound healing with high voltage, monophasic, pulsed current. Phys Ther 68:503, 1988.
7. Robertson, WGA: Digby's receipts. Ann Med History 7:216, 1925.
8. Gallagher, J and Geschikter, C: The use of charged gold leaf in surgery. JAMA 189:928, 1964.
9. Wolf, M, Wheeler, PC, and Wolcott, LE: Gold-leaf treatment of ischemic skin ulcers. JAMA 196:693, 1966.
10. Alvarez, OM, et al: The healing of superficial skin wounds is stimulated by external electrical current. J Invest Dermatol 81:144, 1983.
11. Gault, WR and Gatens, PF: Use of low intensity direct current in management of ischemic skin ulcers. Phys Ther 56:265, 1976.
12. Thurman, BF and Christian, EL: Response of a serious circulatory lesion to electrical stimulation: A case report. Phys Ther 51:1107, 1971.
13. Akers, T and Gabrielson, A: The effect of high voltage galvanic stimulation on the rate of healing of decubitis ulcers. Biomed Sci Instrum 20:99, 1984.
14. Becker, RO: Electrical control of growth processes. Med Times 95:657, 1967a.
15. Becker, RO and Murray, DG: Method for producing cellular dedifferentiation by means of very small electrical currents. Trans NY Acad Sci 29:606, 1967b.
16. Wu, KT, Go, N, and Dennis, C: Effects of electric currents and interfacial potentials on wound healing. J Surg Res 7:122,1967.
17. Rowley, B: Electrical currents effects on E. coli growth rates. Proc Soc Exp Biol Med 139:929, 1972.
18. Rowley, B, McKenna, J, and Chase, G: The influence of electrical current on an infecting microorganism in wounds. Ann NY Acad Sci 238:543, 1974.
19. Becker, RO: The direct current control system: A link between environment and organism. NY State J Med, 62:1169, 1962.
20. Fukada, E, and Yasuda, I: On the piezoelectric effect of bone. J Phys Soc Japan 10:1158, 1957.
21. Shamos, MH, Lavine, LS, and Shamos, MI: Piezoelectric effect in bone. Nature 194:81, 1963.
22. Shamos, MH and Lavine, LS: Physical bases for bioelectric effects in mineralized tissues. Clin Orthop 35:177, 1964.
23. Friedenberg, ZB and Brighton, CT: Bioelectric potentials in bone. J Bone and Joint Surg 48-A:915, 1966.
24. Borgens, RB: Endogenous ionic currents traverse intact and damaged bone. Science 225:478, 1984.
25. Bassett, CAL, Pawlick, RJ, and Becker, RO: Effects of electric currents on bone in vivo. Nature 204:652, 1964.
26. Lavine, LS, Lustrin, I and Shamos, MH: Experimental model for studying the effect of electrical current on bone in vivo. Nature 224:1112, 1969.
27. Brighton, CT: The semi-invasive method of treating nonunion with direct current. Orthop Clin North America, 15:33, 1984a.
28. Lavine, LS, et al: Electric enhancement of bone healing. Science, 175:1118–1121, 1972.
29. Friedenberg, ZB, Harlow, MC, and Brighton, CT: Healing of nonunion of the medial malleolus by means of direct current. A case report. J Trauma, 11:883–885, 1971.
30. Brighton, CT: Foreward. Orthop Clin North America 15:1, 1984b.
31. Brighton, CT, et al: Direct-current stimulation of nonunion and congenital pseudoarthrosis. J Bone Joint Surg 57A:368, 1975.
32. Brighton, CT and Pollack, SR: Treatment of recalcitrant nonunion with a capacitively coupled electrical field. A preliminary report. J Bone Joint Surg 67-A:577, 1985.
33. Dwyer, AF and Wickham, CG: Direct current stimulation in spinal fusion. Med J Aust 1:73, 1974.
34. Bassett, CAL, et al: Electromagnetic repairs of nonunions. In Brighton, CT, Black, J, and Pollack, SR (eds): Electrical Properties of Bone and Cartilage. Grune & Stratton, New York, 1979.

35. Bassett, CAL, Mitchell, SN, and Gaston, S: Pulsing electromagnetic field treatment in ununited fractures and failed arthrodeses. JAMA 247:623, 1982.
36. Lavine, LS, and Grodzinsky, AJ: Current concepts review: Electrical stimulation of repair of bone. J Bone Joint Surg 69-A:626, 1987.
37. Nikolova-Troeva, L: Physiotherapeutic rehabilitation in the presence of fracture complications. Med Wochenschi (Munich) 111:592, 1969.
38. Ganne, JM, et al: Interferential therapy to promote union of mandibular fractures. Aust NZ J Surg 49:81, 1979.
39. Laabs, W, et al: Knochenheilung und dynamischer interferenzstrom (DIC): Erste vergleichende tier experimentelle studie an schafen. Teil I: Experimentalles vorgchen and histologische ergebnisse. Teil II: Physikalische und chemische ergebnisse. Langenbecks Arch Chir 356:219, 1982.
40. Huffman, JW, Osborne, SL, and Sokol, JK: Electrical stimulation in the treatment of intractable stress incontinence: A preliminary report. Arch Phys Med Rehabil 33:674, 1952.
41. Torrens, MJ and Griffith, HB: The control of the uninhibited bladder by selective sacral neurectomy. Brit J Urol 46:639, 1974.
42. Abbate, AD, Cook, AW, and Atollah, M: Effect of electrical stimulation of the thoracic spinal cord on the function of the bladder in multiple sclerosis. J Urol 117:285, 1977.
43. Caldwell, KPS: The electrical control of sphincter incompetence. Lancet II:174, 1963.
44. Caldwell, KPS, et al: Treatment of post-prostatectomy incontinence by electronic implant. Br J Urol 40:183, 1968.
45. Jacobs, SR, et al: Electrical stimulation of muscle. In Stillwell, GK (ed): Therapeutic Electricity and Ultraviolet Radiation, ed 3. Williams & Wilkins, Baltimore, 1983.
46. Teague, CT and Merrill, DC: Electric pelvic floor stimulation. Invest Urol 15:65, 1977.
47. McGuire, EJ, et al: Treatment of motor and sensory detrusor instability by electrical stimulation. J Urol 129:78, 1983.
48. Fall, M: Does electrostimulation cure urinary incontinence? J Urol 131:663, 1984.
49. Plevnik, S, et al: Short-term electrical stimulation: Home treatment for urinary incontinence. World J Urol 4:24, 1986.
50. Brindley, GS, Polkey, CE, and Rushton, DD: Social anterior root stimulators for bladder control in paraplegia. Paraplegia 20:365, 1982.
51. Dougall, DS: The effects of interferential therapy on incontinence and frequency of micturation. Physiotherapy 71:135, 1985.
52. Laycock, J and Green, RJ: Interferential therapy in the treatment of incontinence. Physiotherapy 74:161, 1988.
53. Glen, E: Control of incontinence by electrical devices. In Coldwell, KPS (ed): Urinary Incontinence. Grune & Stratton, New York, 1975.
54. Cordozo, L, et al: Urodynamic observations on patients with sacral anterior root stimulators. Paraplegia 22:201, 1984.
55. Schmidt, RA: Advances in genitourinary neurostimulation. Neurosurgery 19:1041, 1986.
56. Habib, HN: Experience and recent contributions in sacral nerve stimulation for voiding in both human and animal. Br J Urol 39:73, 1967.
57. McQuire, WA: Electrotherapy and exercises for stress incontinence and urinary frequency. Physiotherapy 61:305, 1975.
58. Erlandson, BE, Fall, M, and Carlsson, CA: Scand J Urol Nephrol (Suppl):44, 1977.
59. Ohlsson, B, et al: Effects of some different pulse parameters on bladder inhibition and urethral closure during intravaginal electrical stimulation: An experimental study in the cat. Med Biol Eng Comput, vol 24, p 27, 1986.
60. Jones, U: Experimental considerations and clinical application of electrostimulation for bladder evacuation. Acta Urol Belg 47:515, 1979.
61. Flanigan, RC, et al: Cutaneous stimulation of the bladder in multiple sclerosis: A case report. J Urol 129:1047, 1983.
62. Flanc, C, Hakkar, WW, and Clarke, MB: The detection of venous thrombosis of the legs using ^{125}I-labelled fibrinogen. Br J Surg 55:742, 1968.
63. Nicolaides, AN, et al: Optimal electrical stimulus for prevention of deep vein thrombosis. Br Med J 3:756, 1972.
64. Jonsson, O and Lindstrom, B: Perioperative calf-muscle stimulation for the prevention of postoperative thromboembolic complications. Geriatric Medicine Today 2:86, 1983.
65. Doran, FSA, Drury, M, and Sivyer, A: A simple way to combat the venous stasis which occurs in the lower limbs during surgical operations. Br J Surg 51:486, 1964.
66. Doran, FSA and White, HM: A demonstration that the risk of postoperative deep venous thrombosis is reduced by stimulating the calf muscles electrically during the operation. Br J Surg 54:686, 1967.
67. Becker, J and Schampi, B: The incidence of postoperative venous thrombosis of the legs. Acta Chir Scand 139:357, 1973.
68. Rosenberg, IL, Evans, M, and Pollack, AV: Prophylaxis of postoperative leg vein thrombosis by low dose subcutaneous heparin or peroperative calf muscle stimulation: A controlled clinical trial. Br Med J 1:649, 1975.

69. Lindstrom, B, et al: Prediction and prophylaxis of postoperative thromboembolism: A comparison between peroperative calf muscle stimulation with groups of impulses and dextran 40. Br J Surg 69:633, 1982.
70. Lindstrom, B, et al: Electrically induced short-lasting tetanus of the calf muscles for prevention of deep vein thrombosis. Br J Surg 69:203, 1982.
71. Sawyer, P (ed): Biophysical Mechanisms in Vascular Homeostasis and Intravascular Thrombosis. Appleton-Century-Crofts, New York, 1965.
72. Michlovitz, S, Smith, W, and Watkins, M: Ice and high voltage pulsed stimulation in treatment of lateral ankle sprains. Orthop Sports Phy Ther 9:301, 1988.
73. Mohr, T, Akers, TM, and Landry, RL: Effect of high voltage stimulation on edema reduction in the rat hind limb. Phys Ther, 67:1703, 1987.
74. Le Duc, S.: Electric Ions and Their Use in Medicine. Rebman, Liverpool, 1903.
75. Schwartz, MS: The use of hyaluronidase by iontophoresis in the treatment of lymphedema. Arch Intern Med 95:662, 1955.
76. Cornwall, MW: Zinc iontophoresis to treat ischemic skin ulcers. Phys Ther 61:359, 1981.
77. Haggard, HW, Strauss, MJ, and Greenberg, LA: Fungous infections of hand and feet treated by copper iontophoresis. JAMA 112:1229, 1939.
78. Grice, K, Sattar, H, and Baker, K: Treatment of idiopathic hyperhidrosis with iontophoresis of tap water and poldine methosulphate. Br J Dermatol 86:72, 1972.
79. Abdell, E and Morgan, K: Treatment of idiopathic hyperhidrosis by glycopyrronium bromide and tap water iontophoresis. Br J Dermatol 91:87, 1974.
80. Kahn, J: A case report: Lithium iontophoresis for gouty arthritis. J Orthop Sports Phys Ther 4:113, 1982.
81. Psaki, CE, et al: Acetic acid ionization: A study to determine the absorptive effects upon calcific tendonitis of the shoulder. Phys Ther Rev 35:84, 1955.
82. Harris, PR: Iontophoresis: Clinical research in musculoskeletal inflammatory conditions. J Orthop Sports Phys Ther 4:109, 1982.
83. Magistro, CM: Hyaluronidase by iontophoresis in the treatment of edema: A preliminary clinical report. Phys Ther 44:169, 1964.
84. Russo, J, et al: Lidocaine anesthesia: Comparison of iontophoresis, injection and swabbing. Am J Hosp Pharm 37:843, 1980.
85. Brumett, A and Comeau, M: Local anesthesia of the tympanic membrane by iontophoresis. Trans Am Acad Otolaryngol 78:453, 1974.
86. Sisler, HA: Iontophoresis local anesthesia for conjunctival surgery. Ann Opthalmol 10:597, 1978.
87. Kahn, J: Low-Volt Technique. Joseph Kahn, Syosset, NY, 1973.
88. Cummings, J.: Iontophoresis. In Nelson, RM and Currioer, DP (eds): Clinical Electrotherapy. Appleton & Lange, Norwalk, CT, 1987, p 231.
89. Glick, E and Synder-Mackler, L: Iontophoresis. In Snyder-Mackler, L and Robinson, AJ (eds): Clinical Electrophysiology and Electrophysiologic Testing. Williams & Wilkins, Baltimore, 1989, p 247.

SECTION III

Clinical Decision Making

CHAPTER 11

Application of Therapeutic Electrical Currents in the Management of the Orthopedic Patient

Susan W. Stralka, M.S., P.T.

Electrical stimulation (ES) for innervated muscle is used by physical therapists to facilitate muscular contraction inhibited by pain, to re-educate muscles impaired by chronic disease, and to train new muscle action after tendon relocation.[1,2] Although the efficacy of ES in retarding disuse atrophy has not been clearly demonstrated, some authors, such as Haggmark and Eriksson[3,4] and Stanish and associates,[5] have reported ES to be beneficial in retarding the biochemical changes accompanying immobilization. Research has shown that immobilization following ligamentous injury or surgery of the knee causes significant changes in the characteristics of muscle fibers of the vastus lateralis, as well as decreased oxidative capacity as indicated by succinate dehydrogenase activity.[3] Haggmark and Eriksson[3,4] used percutaneous muscle biopsy to study the postoperative changes in the quadriceps femoris muscles after anterior cruciate ligament (ACL) surgery and found that atrophy of fiber Types 1 and 2 was significant within a week.

ELECTRICAL STIMULATION FOR RECOVERY OF MUSCLE FUNCTION

Recovery of muscle function following joint surgery remains a significant problem in rehabilitation. During rehabilitation of patients following ACL reconstruction surgery a main concern is strengthening the hamstring and quadriceps femoris muscles.[6] In the early phases of rehabilitation, active knee extension from 45° of flexion to 0° is believed to be detrimental to intra-articular repairs and reconstruction.[7] Yasuda and associates[8] have reported that simultaneous contraction or cocontraction of the quadriceps femoris and hamstrings can decrease the amount of stress on the ACL relative to isolated quadriceps femoris muscle contraction. Both volitional and electrically elicited contraction have been increasingly used during the last 10 years. Studies of the effects of electrical stimulation provide evidence that electrical stimulation is effective for augmenting torque of healthy muscle[9-14] and for assisting the recovery of muscle function after certain orthopedic injuries.[15-18] According to McMiken, Todd-Smith, and Thompson,[12] electrical stimulation and voluntary isometric exercise have been equally effective in increasing isometric strength. With appropriate parameters, neuromuscular electrical stimulation (NMES) can affect the five physiologic processes identified by Solomonow[19] as primarily involved in the regulation of muscle tension or force. These processes are (1) action potential firing rate in the individual motor units, (2) selective recruitment of the motor-unit population of a muscle, (3) proprioceptive feedback, (4) synergy of agonist-antagonist activity, and (5) kinesthetics and tactile feedback.

According to Arvidsson,[20] important advantages of the early use of NMES in anterior cruciate ligament repair are maintenance of sensory input, maintenance of muscle integrity, and facilitation of muscle firing which is often difficult because of pain. These benefits are described in his study of integrated EMG activity during maximal voluntary contraction of the quadriceps muscle in 10 patients evaluated on the day following anterior cruciate reconstruction. Arvidsson concluded that pain relief plays a significant role in the ability to normally contract the quadriceps muscle after knee surgery. Pain modulation by electrotherapy, such as neuromuscular electrical stimulation, is accomplished by sensory level stimulation or motor level stimulation. Thus, this is one reason that NMES has been effective in pain control.

CLINICAL DECISION MAKING

The decision to use an electromodality as part of a treatment program should be based on several factors, including the patient's diagnosis, medical status, and mentation, as well as the findings of the pretreatment evaluation. The following guidelines adapted from Michlovitz[21] are helpful in clinical decision making and administration of treatment and will be incorporated into the discussion of the case reports that follow.

1. Evaluate/assess the patient.
2. Establish treatment goals.
3. Determine treatment protocol including the electromodality to be used.
4. Select electrical stimulator with appropriate stimulation characteristics. Identify appropriate electrode type and placement.
5. Familiarize patient with the electromodality and commence treatment program.
6. Establish home program.
7. Evaluate responses to treatment and make necessary adjustments.
8. Determine the time necessary to achieve goal.
9. Determine therapeutic value of treatment.

CASE STUDY

1

The first case study involves a young athlete, CB, who was treated with NMES following reconstructive surgery for an acute anterior cruciate ligament injury.

CB was a 17-year-old high school football player who sustained a left-knee injury during a game. According to the player and coach, there had been no previous injury to the left knee. The player was running down the field and attempted to cut to the right when he was tackled from the side. He heard a popping sound and was unable to straighten or bear weight on his left leg. He was helped off the field by his teammates, and an ice pack was immediately applied to the left knee.

EVALUATE/ASSESS THE PATIENT

Examination by an orthopedist 3 hours after injury revealed moderate effusion of the left knee. Roentgenograms showed no fracture. Active range of motion of the knee was from 15° to 105° of flexion. He displayed a 2+ pivot-shift test, positive Lachman, and anterior drawer signs, but no medial or lateral laxity, posterior instability, or joint line tenderness.

Approximately 48 hours after injury a mechanized arthrokinematic evaluation was performed by the physical therapist using the KT 1000.* The KT 1000 (Figs. 11–1 and 11–2) was developed to assist in the measurement and documentation of the Lachman test, or the passive anterior drawer motion of the tibia relative to the femur. The test was conducted at 30° of knee flexion and was performed bilaterally to permit comparisons. The results of this patient's KT 1000 test are as shown in Table 11–1.

Thigh girth measurements were taken as an indicator of cross-sectional muscle area. Although computed tomography (CT) and muscle biopsy are more reliable methods of determining muscle cross-sectional area,[22] these were not used because of cost factors. In this patient, there was a 2-cm difference in the right and left circumferences at the midpatellar level, probably due to effusion in the injured knee, but there was no difference in the circumferences measured 10-cm proximal to the superior pole of the patella (Table 11–2). Anterior cruciate ligament tear was suspected, and arthroscopic examination was deemed appropriate by the orthopedic surgeon.

Two days after injury, orthopedic assessment with the patient anesthesized revealed a 3+ pivot shift and positive Lachman with a 2+ anterior drawer sign. Again there was no medial or lateral laxity at 0° and 30°. Mechanical arthrokinematic measurements taken at this time are shown in Table 11–3.

Arthroscopic examination at this time revealed a midsubstance tear of the ACL. Reconstructive surgery was performed using the semitendinosus and gracilis tendons, augmented with a Kennedy ligament made of polypropylene.† The patient was placed in a posterior splint with the knee in 45° of flexion for 2 days,

---

*Medmetric Corp. 4901 Morena Blvd., San Diego, CA 92117.
†3-M Orthopedic Products Division, St. Paul, MN 55144.

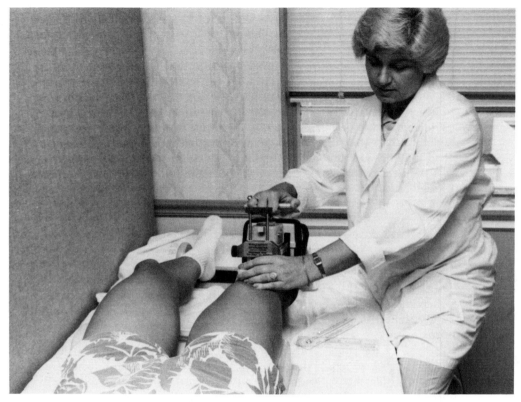

FIGURE 11–1. Assessment of anterior displacement of the tibia using the KT 1000.

then in a controlled-motion brace that permitted movement between 70° and 0°. The motion was increased as joint effusion decreased. The patient was then referred to physical therapy on the first postoperative day. He was evaluated by the physical therapist and goals were established.

ESTABLISHING TREATMENT GOALS

Short-term goals were to maintain normal muscle tone evidenced by patient's ability to generate muscle contraction as compared to the unaffected side to delay significant disuse atrophy and to encourage pain reduction which would not interfere with optimal muscle contraction. Long-term goals were to develop normal muscle strength of the hamstrings and quadriceps as measured by isokinetic comparison and to return patient to a functional activity level as measured by his return to sport activities.

SELECT TREATMENT PLAN, INCLUDING ELECTROMODALITY TO BE USED

NMES was selected to retard the biochemical changes which accompany immobilization following ligamentous surgery, to increase sensory input, and to enhance biofeedback in an attempt to prevent excessive disuse atrophy.

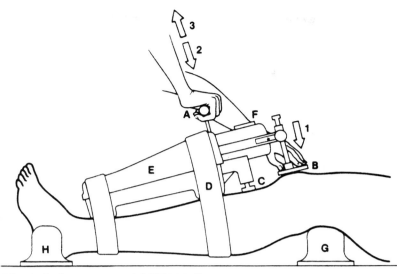

FIGURE 11–2. Arthrometer model KT 1000ᴿ. (*A*) Force handle, (*B*) patellar sensor pad, (*C*) tibial tubercle sensor pad, (*D*) Velcro strap, (*E*) arthrometer case, (*F*) displacement dial indicator, (*G*) thigh support, (*H*) foot support. (1) A constant pressure of 4 to 6 lb applied to the patella sensor pad keeps it in contact with the patella, (2) posterior force is applied, (3) anterior force is applied. (From Malcolm, LL, et al. The measurement of anterior knee laxity after ACL reconstructive surgery. Clin Orthop 196:35, 1985.)

NMES was initiated at this time in the facilitation of a muscular contraction because pain reduced the force of both hamstring and quadriceps contractions. NMES may decrease pain by neurophysiologic means similar to those that operate during transcutaneous electrical nerve stimulation (TENS). Muscle inhibition may subsequently be reduced.

NMES APPLICATION PROCEDURES

Select Stimulator and Stimulator Setting

A dual channel portable neuromuscular stimulator* with an asymmetrical biphasic waveform was selected because it provides adequate stimulus parameters to excite normally innervated muscle as well as a variety of stimulus options.

---

*Medtronic, Inc., Nortech Division, San Diego, CA 92121.

TABLE 11–1 Arthrokinematic Test Results 48 Hours After Injury
(Nonanesthesized Patient)

	Noninvolved	Involved
Anterior displacement:		
15 lb	7 mm	7 mm
20 lb	8 mm	10 mm
Posterior displacement:	4 mm	4 mm
Maximal manual displacement:		
40 lb or greater	10 mm	15 mm
Quadriceps active drawer:	9 mm	13 mm

TABLE 11–2 Thigh-Circumference Measurements

	Noninvolved	Involved
Preoperative		
Midpatella	34.5 cm	36.5 cm
6 cm above patella	41.0 cm	41.0 cm
10 cm above patella	45.0 cm	45.0 cm
Range of motion	0°–135°	15°–105°
At End of Rehabilitation		
Midpatella	34.5 cm	35.0 cm
6 cm above patella	41.0 cm	40.0 cm
10 cm above patella	45.0 cm	44.0 cm
Range of motion	0°–135°	0°–135°

Specific stimulus characteristics are summarized in Table 11–4. The waveform, with a pulse duration of 0.300 ms is preset in the Respond II Stimulator. Pulse frequency was set at 45 pps, which achieved a comfortable tetanic contraction without undue muscle fatigue, which might occur at higher frequencies. Both channels were activated synchronously to produce a co-contraction of the hamstring and quadriceps muscles, thus minimizing loading of the new anterior cruciate ligament reconstruction by excessive anterior displacement of the tibia. Ramp-up (rise) and ramp-down (fall) times were set independently for each channel to allow activation of the hamstrings just prior to activation of the quadriceps muscles in order to further minimize anterior displacement of the tibia.

The duty cycle ratio was initially set at 1 : 2 (10 seconds on, 20 seconds off) to minimize muscle fatigue. For some patients, this ratio will need to be increased to 1 : 3 or 1 : 5 in order to adequately stimulate weak muscles with minimal fatigue. In the case of CB, the duty cycle ratio was decreased to 1 : 1 after the first 30 days of treatment without significant muscle fatigue occurring. The knee was maintained in 45° of flexion in a brace during NMES sessions to avoid injury to the anterior cruciate ligament.

Select Electrode System and Stimulation Site

Two carbon-silicone electrodes with karaya pads (size 4.6 cm by 4.6 cm) from channel 1 were placed on the hamstring muscle group, the proximal electrode 2 cm below the lateral aspect of the gluteal fold overlying the proximal hamstring

TABLE 11–3 Arthrokinematic Test Results with Patient under Anesthesia

	Noninvolved	Involved
Anterior displacement:		
15 lb	8 mm	8 mm
20 lb	9 mm	13 mm
Maximal manual displacement:	10 mm	18 mm
Posterior displacement:	4 mm	4 mm

TABLE 11-4 Stimulation Settings for Simultaneous Excitation of the Quadriceps and Hamstring Muscles

Waveform: asymmetric, biphasic, compensated
Pulse width: 300 μs
Rate: 45 pps

Synchronous stimulation

Rise/fall:
   Channel 1, hamstrings, 2 s ramp-up, 1 s ramp-down
   Channel 2, quadriceps, 4 s ramp-up, 1 s ramp-down
On time: 10 s
Off time: 20 s
Amplitude: to patient's tolerance, fair to fair-plus muscle contraction

musculature and the distal electrode 6 cm above the popliteal fossa medially, in the region of the midhamstring. Care was taken to avoid stimulation of the adductor muscles. Electrodes from channel 2 were applied to the quadriceps muscles. The proximal electrode was placed 4 cm distal and lateral to the femoral triangle; the distal electrode was placed approximately 6 cm proximal and medial to the superior pole of the patella. Electrode configuration is displayed in Figure 11-3.

FAMILIARIZE THE PATIENT WITH THE ELECTROMODALITY AND COMMENCE TREATMENT PROGRAM

To enhance patient compliance, CB was familiarized with the unit preoperatively by applying stimulation to the involved knee to ameliorate postoperative apprehension. Stimulation may also be applied to the uninvolved knee, if not

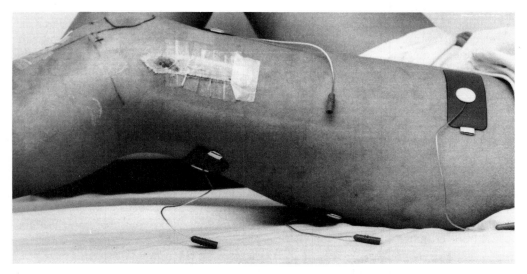

FIGURE 11-3. Electrode placement for hamstring and quadriceps muscle stimulation.

TABLE 11–5 Stimulation Record: Case Study 1

Week 1:   *Starting with First Day of Stimulation*

Day 1: 2–3 muscle contractions; subtetanic contraction four times daily
Day 2: 5 muscle contractions; subtetanic contraction four times daily
Day 3: 10 muscle contractions; gentle tetanic contraction four times daily
Day 4: 10 muscle contractions; fair tetanic contraction four times daily
Day 5: 10 muscle contractions; fair tetanic contraction four times daily
Day 6: 10 muscle contractions; fair plus tetanic contraction two times daily
Day 7–14: start increasing to 45 minutes of stimulation two times daily; fair tetanic contraction achieved at day 14
Day 14–20: increase toward 1 hour of stimulation daily
Day 21–26: 1 hour of stimulation daily adjusting the control as tolerated
Day 27: duty cycle changed to 1:1 ratio, 10 seconds on and 10 seconds off, 10 muscle contractions
Day 28: 12 muscle contractions daily; fair tetanic contractions
Day 29–35: 15 muscle contractions daily; fair tetanic contractions
Day 36–56: 15 muscle contractions daily; fair tetanic contractions
Day 56: home use of NMES discontinued; patient now receiving NMES weekly for cocontraction while at the physical therapy clinic; 10 fair plus cocontractions
Day 112: NMES discontinued in the clinic

initially tolerated on the involved knee. The patient may only tolerate submaximal stimulation on the involved side postoperatively, and it will take time to increase his tolerance to achieve a fair grade contraction. CB tolerated the fair plus cocontraction without difficulty and by the third day was using the unit independently four times daily, to produce 10 muscle contractions during each session. He was encouraged to volitionally cocontract his muscles with the stimulation.

A summary of the stimulation record is presented in Table 11–5. CB was once again instructed to co-contract the quadriceps and hamstring muscles concurrently with the ES. CB slowly progressed up to 1 hour's stimulation time by the 21st day. By the 36th day he was able to accurately execute an appropriate co-contraction assisted by the ES.

NMES alone does not constitute a complete rehabilitation program. For CB, electrical stimulation was integrated into a total rehabilitation program which included isometric, isotonic, and isokinetic exercises, as well as active range-of-motion (ROM) exercises. An isometric exercise program was initiated in the brace on the second or third postoperative day and included quadriceps-, hamstring-, and gluteal-setting exercises, ankle pumping with both lower extremities, and active resistive exercises of the uninvolved lower extremity using proprioceptive neuromuscular facilitation (PNF) patterns and with 5- to 10-lb weights placed on the ankle. Two weeks after surgery, hip adduction, abduction, and extension exercises were added on the involved side. CB periodically received a hot pack prior to knee mobilization and an ice pack following exercise.

CB began ambulation on crutches, touch-down weight bearing, and progressed to full weight bearing on crutches within the first 6 weeks. After receiving the Lennox-Hill brace* 5.5 weeks following surgery, CB was able to ambulate without crutches, since his gait pattern was satisfactory.

---

*Lennox-Hill Brace, Inc., Long Island City, NY 11101.

ESTABLISH A HOME PROGRAM

CB received written and oral instructions detailing his home exercise program. He performed active ROM exercises in the locked knee brace, and active assisted ROM out of the brace, at home after the 10th day postoperative day, when all sutures were removed. During the second week of rehabilitation, progressive resistance exercises (PREs) were begun out of the brace with emphasis on hamstring contraction, while straight-legged PREs for the quadriceps were still done in the brace.

Eight weeks after surgery, the patient was able to begin isokinetic exercises for the hamstrings; isokinetic rehabilitation of the quadriceps was delayed until 12 weeks after surgery to allow sufficient healing of the ACL. Isokinetic quadriceps exercises were performed in the range-limiting brace that prevented knee extension beyond 30°; exercise throughout the full ROM was not allowed until 6 months after surgery.

EVALUATE THE PATIENT'S RESPONSE TO TREATMENT AND MAKE NECESSARY ADJUSTMENTS

If stimulation sites are uncomfortable, if irritation occurs, or if the patient is unable to achieve a tetanic contraction, it may be necessary to adjust the parameters or change the electrode sites. CB did not require modification of electrode placement or stimulus settings.

DETERMINE TIME NECESSARY TO ACHIEVE GOAL

Usually 6 to 8 weeks is the time frame for using NMES for muscle re-education following orthopedic surgery of this type. By this time most patients can cocontract the muscles about the knee without difficulty and will be strong enough to begin isokinetic hamstring rehabilitation. Ideally, the maximal volitional isometric contraction (MVIC) should be objectively measured by torque output with and without the NMES, but this was not possible in CB's case because of the physician's concerns for the maturation stage of the ACL repair. NMES was continued because the patient needed assistance with proximal patellar movement and achievement of the appropriate cocontraction. During outpatient treatment (Table 11–5, day 56) an Electrostim 180* was used to augment volitional contractions. The patient performed co-contraction 10 times per session. The ES 180 was set to deliver 15-second trains with a 5-second ramp-up time; 50 seconds of rest was allowed between contractions. Current intensity was increased according to the patient's tolerance to facilitate a fair-plus contraction. NMES was discontinued as part of CB's home program at this time.

DETERMINE THERAPEUTIC VALUE OF TREATMENT

NMES was discontinued 16 weeks following surgery when the patient was able to consistently perform fair-plus co-contraction and proximal movement of the patella was normal. Rehabilitation continued for a total of 11 months, after

---

*Electrostim Visa, Ltd., 1851 Black Road, Joliet, IL 60435.

TABLE 11-6 Arthrokinematic Test Results at End of Rehabilitation (11 Months)

	Noninvolved	Involved
Anterior displacement:		
15 lb	7 mm	6 mm
20 lb	8 mm	7 mm
Posterior displacement:	4 mm	4 mm
Maximal manual displacement:		
40 lb or greater	10 mm	9 mm
Quadriceps active drawer:	9 mm	8 mm

which the patient was discharged to resume all activities in his brace, including football. Isokinetic dynamometer tests, using a Cybex 11* indicated less than 15-percent torque difference between the involved and uninvolved legs at 60° per second, 180° per second, 240° per second, and 300° per second for both hamstrings and quadriceps. KT 1000 measurements (Table 11-6) were within normal limits when noninvolved and involved limbs were compared. Thigh circumference measurements (Table 11-2) were essentially equal for both legs.

SUMMARY

The benefits of NMES for muscle strengthening have been previously reported. Patients recovering from knee ligament surgery[3] and patients with chondromalacia patellae[15] have shown increases in isometric strength of quadriceps femoris following electrical stimulation training. Currier and Mann's[11] research study of the normal quadriceps femoris musculature in healthy subjects receiving ES showed similar, statistically significant torque improvement as those who performed voluntary exercise regimens, and a greater increase than the nonexercised control group.

Recent research by Delitto and associates[27-28] has shown the importance of NMES for contraction of the thigh musculature with resulting torque increases in both extension and flexion along with increases in thigh circumference. As previously stated, the importance of hamstring contraction to prevent excessive anterior movement of the tibia cannot be overly stressed in the rehabilitation of postsurgical ACL-repair patients.

Other researchers, including Jurist and Otis,[25,26] Paulos and associates,[30] and Malone, Blackburn and Wallace,[7] have repeatedly noted in the literature that forceful end-range knee extension exercises from 0° to 45° in the early phase of rehabilitation cause excessive high-tensile stresses to the ACL and may be detrimental. Many orthopedists and physical therapists suggest ligamentous protection for a full year after surgery until the newly reconstructed ACL reaches biochemical and histochemical maturity.[27] This consideration should be integrated into an electrically facilitated muscle re-education program.

The above case study presents one method of using co-contraction of the

---

*Cybex, Division of Lumex, Inc, Ronkonkoma, NY 11779.

thigh musculature in the early phase of rehabilitation following ACL repair to facilitate strengthening of the quadriceps without jeopardizing the ACL. Presently a three-center study (Washington University, St. Louis; University of Delaware, Newark, Delaware; and Campbell Clinic, Memphis) with a varied patient population is underway to further determine the clinical efficacy of NMES for orthopedic patients. It is our belief that NMES is a useful adjunct to more conventional rehabilitation methods in decreasing the time required for rehabilitation and maximum recovery of muscle function after ACL surgery.

ELECTRICAL STIMULATION FOR RECOVERY OF JOINT MOBILITY

Electrical stimulation may also be a useful adjunct to clinical treatment of musculoskeletal problems, such as rehabilitation following a distal (Colles) fracture of the radius. Regardless of the casting technique, after distal fractures of the radius, regaining normal range of motion is often painful and tedious. Muscle imbalance and wasting, and joint contractures are potential clinical problems associated with immobilization following Colles fracture.[28] NMES may be used to augment voluntary exercises after cast removal.

CASE STUDY

2

MG is a 64-year-old female who fractured her left wrist in a fall on her outstretched hand. She stated that she heard a snap and that any movement of the wrist or fingers was extremely painful.

EVALUATE/ASSESS THE PATIENT

Examination by the orthopedist revealed a moderate effusion of the left wrist. Roentgenograms showed a fracture of the distal radius with slight dorsal angulation. The Frykman classification[29] for this Colles fractures was Grade I, indicating a nondisplaced fracture of the radius only. Clinical findings included tenderness to palpation at the distal radioulnar joint, and pain with movement of the wrist and fingers. After closed reduction, a sugar-tong splint was applied rather than a circular cast because of the edema in the hand and wrist. The arm was immobilized with the wrist in approximately 10° of flexion, and the forearm in neutral position with 8° of ulnar deviation. The elbow joint was permitted 45° to 90° of flexion in the splint. Roentgenograms confirmed the accuracy of reduction and proper sugar-tong positioning of the wrist. Six and one half weeks after injury, roentgenograms showed healing of the fracture site; immobilization was discontinued and MG was referred to physical therapy for evaluation and treatment.

ESTABLISH TREATMENT GOALS

Short-term goals were to decrease pain and edema and increase wrist ROM. Long-term goals were to regain adequate strength and ROM for functional activities.

SELECT TREATMENT PLAN, INCLUDING ELECTROMODALITY TO BE USED

NMES was selected to increase sensory, visual, and proprioceptive input, as well as assist ROM in an attempt to prevent fibrous restrictions and joint contractures. NMES was initiated at this time to facilitate wrist motions of flexion and extension reciprocally. As stated in the previous case report, NMES may also be helpful in decreasing pain and, thus, reflex muscle inhibition.

NMES APPLICATION PROCEDURES

Select Stimulator and Stimulator Setting

A dual channel portable neuromuscular stimulator* was selected because it provides adequate stimulus parameters to excite normally innervated muscle as well as a variety of ES options. These parameters were described in Case Study 1. The pulse frequency was set at 30 pps to ensure a smooth tetanic contraction without undue muscle fatigue. The unit was set on reciprocal stimulation which first stimulated the wrist extensors and then the wrist flexors (Table 11–7). Reciprocal stimulation was chosen to stimulate the extensor and flexor muscle groups, produce ROM, and decrease swelling through muscle-pumping action. Ramp-up (rise) and ramp-down (fall) times were set at 4 seconds and 2 seconds, respectively, for both channels to allow for a gradual buildup of stimulation with less time for ramp-down. The duty cycle was set at a 1:1 ratio; 12 seconds on and 12 seconds off. This ratio may vary from patient to patient depending on individual muscle fatigue.

Select Electrode System and Stimulation Sites

Two carbon-silicone electrodes (4.6 cm by 4.6 cm) from channel 1 were placed on the skin overlying the forearm extensors. One electrode was placed on the proximal third of the forearm overlying the extensor muscle bellies (Fig. 11–4). Placement of the electrodes was determined by locating the site over the extensor

---

*Medtronic, Inc, Nortech Division, San Diego, CA 92121.

TABLE 11–7 Stimulation Settings for Reciprocal Stimulation of the Wrist Extensors and Flexors

Waveform: Asymmetric biphasic, compensated
Pulse width: 300 μs
Rate: 30 pps

Reciprocal stimulation

Rise/fall: 4 s ramp-up, 2 s ramp-down
On time: 12 s
Off time: 12 s
Amplitude: patient's tolerance, fair to fair-plus muscle contraction

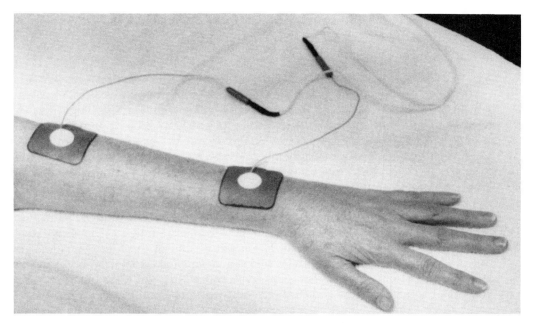

FIGURE 11–4. Electrode placement for wrist extension.

muscles from which stimulation produced the desired movement. The second electrode from channel 1 was placed on her distal forearm 5 cm proximal to the wrist crease. Electrodes from channel 2 were placed on the flexor surface of the forearm: the proximal electrode on the upper third of the forearm and the distal electrode centrally over the flexor tendons approximately 7.6 cm proximal to the wrist crease (Fig. 11–5).

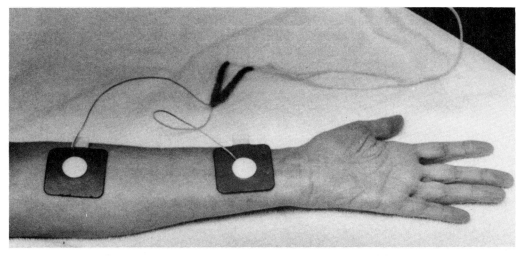

FIGURE 11–5. Electrode placement for wrist flexion.

FAMILIARIZE THE PATIENT WITH THE ELECTROMODALITY AND APPLY TREATMENT PROCEDURES

One of the most important factors to ensure patient compliance with the NMES program following cast removal for a Colles fracture is prestimulation education. The patient should be familiarized with the unit, and the unit may be applied to the uninvolved wrist to ameliorate prestimulation apprehension. Although MG tolerated sufficient stimulation to produce a fair contraction initially, it is not unusual for the patient to take a week to build up tolerance to a fair contraction. Once the desired muscle contraction was achieved and the patient was comfortable with adjusting the unit's parameters,[5] she was instructed to use the unit three to four times daily to produce 10 to 15 muscle contractions during each treatment. Again, it is important to observe the quality of muscle contraction and decrease repetitions as needed to minimize muscle fatigue. The stimulation record of MG is presented in Table 11–8. By the end of the fifth week, MG no longer used the NMES because ROM had significantly increased (see Table 11–9), strength had improved to a good plus level, and the patient was able to perform functional activities, such as daily household activities, without difficulty.

MG also received soft tissue massage, active and active-assisted ROM exercises to wrist, elbow, and digits, putty and weight exercises, joint mobilization, and functional training using a BTE work simulator program* (Fig. 11–6). The first time using the BTE, MG used each attachment 60 seconds to establish a comfortable exercise level. Distance was also a factor as the total of all the degrees of rotation were accumulated during exercise. The goal of the BTE was to increase the exercise level (force/resistance) and distance from day 1 to discharge from therapy. The goal was achieved. As in Case Study 1, MG also received hot pack treatment before exercise and ice packs following exercise as needed to diminish muscle guarding and pain. She was observed to make sure that the hot pack did not increase the edema. At the third week of rehabilitation, ultrasound was applied distal to the fracture to reduce joint stiffness prior to mobilization and ROM. Then Grade 1 and Grade 2 mobilization and ROM exercises were under-

---

*Baltimore Therapeutic Exercise, Hanover, MD 21076.

TABLE 11–8 Stimulation Record: Colles Fracture

Second Case Study: MG

Starting with First Day of Stimulation
Day 1: 5 muscle contractions; fair level, twice daily
Day 2: 5 muscle contractions; fair level, twice daily
Day 3: 7 muscle contractions; fair level, three times daily
Day 4: 8 muscle contractions; fair level, three times daily
Day 5: 8 muscle contractions; fair level, three times daily
Day 6: 10 muscle contractions; fair-plus level, three times daily
Day 7: 10 muscle contractions; fair-plus level, three times daily
Day 8–14: 10 muscle contractions; fair-plus level, three times daily
Day 15–34: 10–15 muscle contractions; fair-plus level, four times daily
Day 35: NMES discontinued following BTE testing

TABLE 11–9 Range of Motion

| | Day 1 | | Day 35 | |
	Active	Passive	Active	Passive
Wrist flexion	10°	15°	75°	78°
Wrist extension	25°	32°	70°	70°
Radial deviation	12°	15°	25°	25°
Ulnar deviation	18°	24°	32°	34°
Supination	45°	50°	80°	85°
Pronation	30°	35°	75°	82°
Shoulder/fingers	WNL*		WNL	

*WNL = within normal limits.

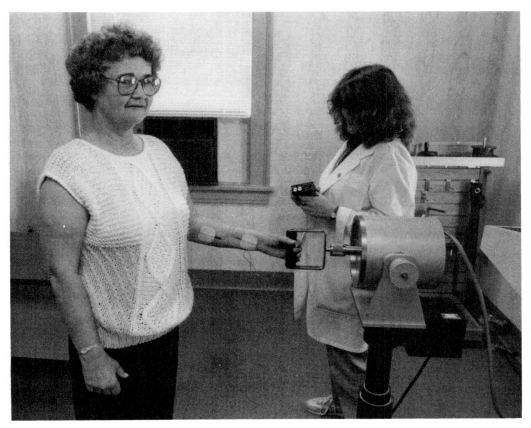

FIGURE 11–6. Patient undergoes functional training using a Baltimore Therapeutic Exercise (BTE) work simulator.

taken to improve wrist mobility. Additional forms of electrotherapy such as TENS for pain control or high voltage pulsed current for edema reduction or prevention may also be incorporated into the treatment regimen as needed. These applications are reviewed in Chapters 5 and 10, respectively.

ESTABLISH A HOME PROGRAM

Both oral and written instructions were reviewed with MG to prepare her to apply the NMES at home. MG was started on a home program following her second visit to physical therapy. Since MG was being seen twice weekly for physical therapy, we were able to check her ability to use the NMES. Once the cast was removed 6 weeks after fracture, MG used the NMES twice daily for five to six contractions for the first week. Along with the NMES, MG was instructed in hand exercises using putty and active and active-assisted hand exercises. As the rehabilitation program progressed, the NMES treatment duration was increased (Table 11–8).

EVALUATE THE PATIENT'S RESPONSE TO TREATMENT AND MAKE NECESSARY ADJUSTMENTS

MG required an electrode placement change because her skin became erythematous during the fourth week of stimulation. The proximal electrode on channel 1 was moved approximately 2.54 cm distally and the desired motion was still achieved. Channel 2 did not require movement of electrodes.

DETERMINE THE TIME NECESSARY TO ACHIEVE GOALS

In MG's case, the clinical effectiveness of NMES was determined by comparing BTE measurements as well as functional improvement.

DETERMINE THE THERAPEUTIC VALUE OF TREATMENT

NMES was discontinued after 5 weeks of treatment, when MG was able to consistently perform good muscle contractions and had 90 percent of normal ROM of the wrist and fingers compared with her uneffected wrist and hand (Table 11–9). BTE measurements were also significantly improved over pretreatment values, as were pinch test and dynamometer measurements.

SUMMARY

Although the value of NMES in regaining ROM after Colles fractures has not been well documented, in the case of MG, NMES appeared to facilitate a faster, less painful, and less tedious return to function for this patient after her Colles fracture. Advances in NMES application and treatment protocols are occurring rapidly. A therapist should keep up with these new developments. Further studies of the efficacy of NMES for regaining ROM and strengthening are needed to identify maximally effective treatment protocols and the parameters for these protocols. Well-designed clinical studies comparing different parameters are necessary for clinical efficacy and reimbursement.

REFERENCES

1. Cummings, G: Physiological basis of electrical stimulation in skeletal muscle. CATAJ 7:7, 1980.
2. Scott, PM: Clayton's Electrotherapy and Actinotherapy, ed 7. Williams & Wilkins, Baltimore, 1975.
3. Haggmark, T and Eriksson, E: Fiber type area and metabolic potential of the thigh muscle in men after knee surgery and immobilization. Int J Sports Med 2:12, 1981.
4. Haggmark, T and Eriksson, E: Cylinder or mobile cast brace after knee ligament surgery. Am J Sports Med 7:48, 1979.
5. Standish, WD, et al: Effects of immobilization and of electrical stimulation on muscle glycogen and myofibrillar ATPase. Can J Appl Sport Sci 7:267, 1982.
6. Paulos, L, et al: Knee rehabilitation after anterior cruciate ligament reconstruction and repair. Am J Sports Med 9:140, 1981.
7. Malone, T, Blackburn, TA, and Wallace, LA: Knee rehabilitation. Phys Ther 60:1602, 1980.
8. Yasuda, K, et al: Muscle exercise after anterior cruciate ligament reconstruction of the knee, Part I, The force given to the anterior cruciate ligament by separate isometric contraction of the quadriceps or the hamstrings. Nippon Seikeigeka Gakkai Zasshi 59:1041, 1985.
9. Romero, JA, et al: The effects of electrical stimulation of normal quadriceps on strength and girth. Med Sci Sports Exerc 14:194, 1982.
10. Laughman, RK, et al: Strength changes in the normal quadriceps femoris muscle as a result of electrical stimulation. Phys Ther 63:494, 1983.
11. Currier, DP and Mann, R: Muscular strength development by electrical stimulation in healthy individuals. Phys Ther 63:915, 1983.
12. McMiken, DF, Todd-Smith, M, and Thompson, C: Strengthening of human quadriceps muscles by cutaneous electrical stimulation. Scand J Rehabil Med 15:24, 1983.
13. Kramer, JF and Semple, JE: Comparison of selected strengthening techniques for normal quadriceps. Physiotherapy Canada 35:300, 1983.
14. Selkowitz, DM: Improvement in isometric strength of the quadriceps femoris muscle after training with electrical stimulation. Phys Ther 65:186, 1985.
15. Johnson, DH, Thurston, P, and Ashcroft, PJ: The Russian technique of faradism in the treatment of chondromalacia patellae. Physiotherapy Canada 29:266, 1977.
16. Eriksson, E and Haggmark, T: Comparison of isometric muscle training and electrical stimulation supplementing isometric muscle training in the recovery after major knee ligament surgery. Am J Sports Med 7:169, 1979.
17. Godfrey, CM, et al: Comparison of electrostimulation and isometric exercise in strengthening the quadriceps muscle. Physiotherapy Canada 31:265, 1979.
18. Lainey, CG, Walmsley, RP, and Andrew, GM: Effectiveness of exercise alone versus exercise plus electrical stimulation in strengthening the quadriceps muscle. Physiotherapy Canada 35:5, 1983.
19. Solomonow, M: Restoration of movement by electrical stimulation: A contemporary view of the basic problems. Orthopedics 7:245, 1984.
20. Arvidsson, I, et al: Reduction of pain inhibition on voluntary muscle activation by epidural analgesia. Orthopedics 9:1415, 1986.
21. Michlovitz, S: Thermal agents in rehabilitation. FA Davis, Philadelphia, ed 2, 1990.
22. Haggmark, T, Jansson, E, and Svane, B: Cross-sectional area of the thigh muscle in man measured by computed tomography. Scand J Clin Lab Invest 38:355, 1978.
23. Delitto, A: Personal communication, 1987.
24. Delitto, A, et al: Electrically elicited co-contraction of thigh musculature after anterior cruciate ligament surgery: A description and single-case experiment. Am Phys Ther J 68:45, 1988.
25. Jurist, KA and Otis, JL: Anteroposterior tibiofemoral displacement during isometric extension efforts: The role of external load and knee flexion angle. Am J Sports Med 13:254, 1985.
26. Paulos, L, et al: Knee rehabilitation after anterior cruciate ligament reconstruction and repair. Am J Sports Med 9:140, 1981.
27. Sisk, TD: Personal communication, 1987.
28. Benton, LA, et al: Functional Electrical Stimulation: A Practical Clinical Guide. Rancho Los Amigos Rehabilitation Engineering Center, Downey, CA, 1981.
29. Frykman, G: Fracture of the distal radius including sequelae-shoulder-hand-finger syndrome, disturbance in the distal radioulnar joint, and impairment of nerve function. Acta Orthop Scand (Suppl): 108, 1967.

CHAPTER 12

Electrotherapeutic Applications for the Neurologically Impaired Patient

Roberta Packman-Braun, M.Ed., P.T.

The decision whether or not to use electrotherapeutic interventions in the physical therapy program should be made in exactly the same way as the decision to use any other physical modality. The first step in any therapeutic treatment course is a complete patient evaluation. This includes a history as well as physical and functional evaluations. Once the evaluation is completed, a problem list can be generated. For each patient problem a treatment goal should be established. In working toward any clinical goal the therapist has a variety of treatment options. Some of these alternatives involve hands-on intervention by the clinician or active participation by the patient, whereas others involve the use of various physical modalities. Electrical stimulation (ES) and electromyographic (EMG) biofeedback should be viewed as two of the many treatment alternatives used by physical therapists. Most often the appropriate course of action entails some combination of the available alternatives. In the process of selecting a treatment mode, several options can usually be eliminated as less appropriate for the specific problem under consideration. For instance, while ice, electrical stimulation, and active muscle pumping are all possible means of managing edema, the first two would be more appropriate than the latter in the presence of acute musculoskeletal trauma. Other alternatives are contraindicated in other specific cases, for example, whereas active exercise and electrical stimulation might both be possible means of strengthening weak muscles, electrical stimulation would be inappropriate for muscle strengthening in the patient with a demand cardiac pacemaker. Once the most effective and safe treatment options have been identified, the therapist can make a final decision based on more practical factors. These might include therapist or patient time constraints, equipment availability, cost, and so forth.

The purposes of this chapter are to review the *clinical decision-making process* associated with the use of ES and EMG biofeedback (EMGBF), and suggest the selection of appropriate electrotherapeutic procedures and equipment for the neurologically impaired patient. Patient selection considerations are reviewed. Two hypothetical case studies involving patients with neurological pathology are presented along with discussion of possible applications of electrotherapeutic modalities in the treatment program. In addition, guidelines for preparation of a stimulation protocol and for selection of appropriate equipment to meet program goals are provided.

SELECTION OF APPROPRIATE CANDIDATES FOR ELECTRICAL STIMULATION

Before a definitive decision is made, it should be determined that there are no contraindications to the use of ES in a given patient. A variety of factors should be weighed when evaluating a potential ES candidate. Age, mentation, and attention span may be limiting factors if the ability to understand and follow directions is required for the treatment application under consideration, for example, when biofeedback is used to achieve relaxation or facilitation. Level of cooperation is also important if active participation is required. These considerations are not as relevant for applications that do not require the patient to actively participate; for instance, ES has been effectively used to increase passive range of motion (PROM) in comatose patients with knee-flexion contractures.[1]

Some patients have a true phobia of electricity and this fear should be respected. However many people who are at first wary of the idea of using ES, are reassured when the treatment is presented in a confident and competent manner. If a motor level of stimulation intensity will be used for treatment, the anxious patient can first be acquainted with a sensory-level stimulus and allowed to become comfortable with the concept and sensation of ES before the intensity is increased.

Several medical conditions may make ES an inappropriate choice. These include the presence of a demand cardiac pacemaker,[2,3] and pregnancy, cancer, and epilepsy.[3] For an ES application other than those utilizing direct current, an intact peripheral nervous system is required. Obesity often limits the effectiveness of an ES treatment program as it is more difficult to reach targeted structures at intensity levels within the sensory tolerance of the patient. Patients with hypersensitive or fragile skin may experience skin irritation or breakdown from electrode gel and tape used along with the ES device. Edema, if it overlies the areas targeted for stimulation, can present a problem by dispersing the current away from targeted structures. Of course edema itself may be treated with ES, and in this case electrode placement over the edematous area may be perfectly appropriate. In the same way, electrode placement over an open wound is inappropriate unless wound healing is the goal of stimulation.

A program of stimulation should be consistent with the overall program goals and restrictions. For instance, if a patient with phlebitis is allowed no active muscle contraction in an extremity, then ES should not be used to elicit a contraction in that extremity; or if some PROM is prohibited following joint surgery, then ES should not be used to elicit the prohibited motion at that joint.

When use of ES as part of a home program is being considered, several additional factors come into play. Patient or attendant reliability is important under these circumstances because of the need to maintain equipment, duplicate electrode placements and stimulation settings, and monitor unusual responses. Even a reliable patient may not be physically capable of duplicating electrode placements or maintaining a unit properly. Ability of the patient or attendant to perform these skills should be evaluated before the decision is made to provide a patient with an electrical stimulator as part of a home program. Financial coverage for unit rental or purchase should be investigated before the idea of ES as a home program alternative is pursued. A patient may be suitable in every other way for treatment with ES but have no means of obtaining a stimulation device for home use.

PROBLEM MANAGEMENT: THE DECISION WHETHER TO USE ES

Once it has been determined that there are no major negative considerations to the use of ES in a given patient, use of ES should be considered for its documented and theoretical effectiveness in the management of the exhibited problems and compared with the other treatment alternatives. If the comparison is favorable and practical considerations allow, electrical stimulation may be selected as the treatment of choice.

Two hypothetical case studies are provided here. Immediately following each case study, patient problems and therapeutic goals are identified. Considerations for the use of ES in the management of each patient problem toward the achievement of each of the treatment goals are then presented.

CASE STUDY 1
HISTORY

The patient is a 76-year-old male with left hemiparesis secondary to a right cerebrovascular accident (CVA) which occurred 4 weeks ago. He was hospitalized at that time and received physical therapy at bedside for about 2 weeks, and therapy in the physical therapy department for 1 week. He is admitted at this time to a rehabilitation hospital for continued treatment. The patient's past medical history is unremarkable except for a history of hypertension.

He is a retired plumber who lives alone in the upper half of a duplex apartment. There are 13 steps up to the second floor of the building with a rail on the right on ascent. The patient is a widower and has one son, age 53 years, living about one-half hour from the patient's home. He hopes to return home and reside alone.

SKELETAL STATUS

Physical examination reveals a left glenohumeral subluxation of about two fingers' breadth. Dependent edema is noted in the left ankle, with the circumference measuring 25 cm at the distal border of the lateral malleolus. The right-ankle circumference is 22 cm at this level. PROM is within normal limits at all joints with the exception of left-ankle dorsiflexion which measure 0° and left-wrist extension which measures 0° to 15°.

NEUROMUSCULAR STATUS

Active Movement

The patient has complete functional use of the right upper and lower extremities. He is able to isolate movement at all joints and is able to sustain a contraction when minimal resistance is applied. The patient has no functional use of the left upper extremity (UE) at this time. He is able to produce minimal volitional activation of shoulder elevation, protraction, and retraction. Any attempt to move the left UE is accompanied by flexion-synergy influence, noted as shoulder abduction and internal rotation, elbow flexion, wrist flexion and pronation, and finger flexion at all joints. No isolated movement is seen at this time. In the left lower extremity (LE), without strict attention to task, attempts at any component movement elicits a pattern of hip flexion, abduction, and external rotation; knee flexion; minimal ankle dorsiflexion and strong inversion. Extension movements at any joint also occur in synergy in a pattern of hip extension, adduction and internal rotation, knee extension, and ankle plantarflexion and inversion. With close attention to the task, the patient shows minimal isolation of knee extension and ankle dorsiflexion.

Sensation

Light touch (LT), pinprick (PP), and proprioception are intact in the right extremities and trunk. The left extremities and trunk have diminished sensation of LT and PP throughout. Proprioception is absent in left upper extremity and in left ankle and foot, and diminished at the hip and knee.

Reflexes

Biceps, triceps, patellar, and achilles: all 3+ on left, 2+ on right.

Tone

No tonal abnormalities are noted in the right upper and lower extremities and trunk musculature. The left trunk musculature has minimally increased tone in lateral trunk flexors. The left upper extremity has moderately increased tone in the pectorals, biceps, and wrist flexors and minimally increased tone in the triceps. In the left lower extremity, tone is moderately increased in the quadriceps femoris and plantarflexor muscles.

FUNCTIONAL STATUS

The patient is independent in wheelchair (WC) propulsion using his right upper and lower extremities. He is also independent in the management of his WC brakes and footrests. Armrest management is not applicable as the patient uses a standing pivot transfer which does not require armrest removal.

Transfers from sit to stand, and from WC to mat table or back, require moderate assistance (mod A) of one to help stabilize the left knee and ankle and extend the patient's trunk to achieve an upright position.

In bed mobility, the patient can independently roll to his right and left sides, and move from sitting to supine, or the reverse when movement is toward his right side. When moving between supine and sitting with movement toward his left

Problem List	Short-Term Treatment Goals (to Be Achieved within a 2-Week Period)
1. Decreased PROM, left wrist and ankle	1. Increased PROM (by 5°) for wrist extension and ankle dorsiflexion
2. Left glenohumeral subluxation	2. Reduced glenohumeral subluxation
3. Dependent edema, left ankle	3. Edema reduction
4. Decreased volitional activation and control of left upper- and lower-extremity muscles	4. Increased volitional and control of left-extremity musculature
5. Decreased strength, right- and left-extremity musculature	5. Increased strength (ability to sustain a contraction during moderate resistance), right- and left-extremity muscles
6. Increased tone, left pectorals; elbow extensors; elbow, wrist, and finger flexors; knee extensors; ankle plantarflexors and invertors	6. Tone reduction, left pectorals; elbow extensors; elbow, wrist, and finger flexors; knee extensors; ankle plantarflexors and invertors
7. Decreased LT and PP sensation, left extremities with absent proprioception of left upper extremity and left ankle and foot	7. Increased awareness of and compensation for sensory deficits to improve function and maintain integrity of skin.

8. Gait deviations:
  a. Retracted pelvis
  b. Insufficient hip flexion
  c. Hip external rotation and adduction used to advance left LE
  d. Decreased hip extension and abduction during stance
  e. Decreased knee flexion (swing)
  f. Occasional knee buckling at midstance
  g. Insufficient dorsiflexion for swing-phase clearance
	8. Improved gait pattern

9. Dependent transfers [moderate assist (mod A)]	9. Transfer with (min A)
10. Dependent moving sit <–> supine toward the left side [minimal assist (min A)]	10. Independent bed mobility
11. Dependent ambulation [(mod A)] in parallel bars and elevations	11. Increased level of ambulatory independence on all surfaces and elevations

side, he requires minimal assistance (min A) to push up from left side-lying to the short-sitting position.

The patient ambulates two lengths of the parallel bars with mod A of one for balance, to stabilize the left knee during the stance phase, and to assist with left-leg clearance during the swing phase. Gait deviations include (1) pelvic retraction on the left side throughout the gait cycle, (2) insufficient left hip flexion during swing with external rotation and adduction used to advance the left LE, (3) decreased knee flexion during swing, (4) decreased ankle dorsiflexion during swing (a "drop foot" gait pattern), (5) left ankle medial/lateral instability (initial contact on stance is the lateral border of the forefoot), and (6) and occasional left knee buckling. Management of stairs, curbs, and ramps is dependent at this time and the degree of assistance required has not yet been assessed.

A problem list of all abnormal findings can be generated and treatment goals can be established once the evaluation is completed. The problem list and list of associated treatment goals for Case Study 1 are provided in the table opposite.

MANAGEMENT CONSIDERATIONS

The treatment plan serves as a bridge between the problem list and the program goals. Treatment alternatives for a given problem should be selected individually or in combination in light of their documented effectiveness in achieving the desired result, and in keeping with limitations imposed by a specific patient's unique characteristics.

Short-Term Goal (STG) 1: Increasing PROM (Left Wrist Extension and Left Ankle Dorsiflexion)

For the problem of decreased PROM the goal of treatment is to increase the available range. The conventional treatment alternatives consist of manual and gravity-assisted stretch of the muscle groups restricting joint motion with or without ultrasound, and application of a three-point pressure system around the joint through splinting or bracing. Electrical muscle stimulation applied to the antagonist of the shortened muscle group at the end of the available joint ROM can also be used to provide stretch.[1,4]

Some joints cannot be effectively moved through full range with the use of ES because of inability of the stimulation to overcome the weight of the limb, as in the case of the hip or shoulder. For motions around these joints manual and gravity-assisted techniques and three-point pressure systems are the most effective treatment modes. Severe spasticity in shortened muscle groups at any joint may override attempts to stimulate antagonistic muscle groups. A long ramp-on time may be used in an attempt to avoid activating the stretch reflex in a spastic antagonist.

For soft tissue tightness around the elbow, wrist, knee, and ankle, manual stretching, bracing, or splinting, and electrical stimulation all have the potential to provide the elongation of the musculotendinous unit necessary to increase joint PROM. There are several advantages to selecting ES for this purpose. With ES there is little time required on the part of the therapist, who needs only to set up the electrodes and stimulator and intermittently supervise the stimulation process, since the patient is not an *active* participant during this treatment. Manual stretch techniques require a greater commitment of therapist time. In the time saved, the therapist can work with this patient or another patient on some activity for which active intervention is necessary. The patient can concurrently work on other activities during the stimulation session, for example, exercise the lower extremity muscles while his or her wrist receives electrically induced PROM. The stimulation session can even take place away from the physical therapy (PT) department, for example while the patient is eating lunch, sitting in his or her room between therapy appointments, or at home. If a dual-channel unit is utilized, more than one joint can receive PROM simultaneously in a way that could not be accomplished manually. These factors help to optimize the use of available treatment time.

An important advantage of electrical stimulation is its ability to serve more than one function at a time. If the patient has some volitional activation of the muscle group being stimulated, strengthening may occur during the ROM program. This is especially important in the hemiparetic patient where weakness often occurs in the overstretched, overpowered antagonists to a shortened spastic muscle group. If the patient is instructed to work with the cycling stimulation, neuromuscular re-education may be enhanced. If edema is present in the area, the electrically induced contractions that provide PROM and stretch may also work to decrease edema in a way that manual PROM and stretch cannot. The opportunity to capitalize on the treatment time utilization efficiency of ES can be very important in the treatment of the hemiparetic patient. This patient population often has a high degree of physical involvement and many areas must be targeted for therapeutic intervention within a single treatment session.

ES does not necessarily have to be chosen in preference to other methods of increasing PROM. It may be used as a supplement to manual stretch and/or the use of splints or braces. These treatments can be scheduled to follow one another with the ES applied within or outside the clinical setting. The stimulation can be even applied while a three-point pressure system, for example, a dynamic splint, is being worn; or manual stretch can be timed to coincide with the stimulated muscle contractions of the antagonist to the shortened muscle group.

If motor return does not occur, provision of PROM to various joints becomes a long-term concern with respect to cleanliness, cosmesis, comfort, and ease of donning clothing. Portable, battery-operated ES units are readily available for rental or purchase, allowing use of this modality after discharge to provide PROM to the same joints treated with ES in the clinic.

STG 2: Glenohumeral Joint Reduction

For the problem of glenohumeral joint subluxation in the hemiparetic patient, the management alternatives include positioning, for example, with lap boards and arm troughs, upper extremity orthotic devices (slings), and electrical stimulation to the supraspinatus and posterior deltoid muscles to provide glenohumeral approximation.[5,6] There are several advantages to the use of electrical stimulation. Many traditional slings, while serving their function of approximation at the shoulder, maintain the upper limb in a synergy-facilitating posture.[7-9] When active movement of the distal extremity is present, it is often restricted by the orthotic device.[8,9] Static positioning of joints may also support the development of soft-tissue shortening in the area. Electrical stimulation serves to reduce the subluxation proximally without interfering with distal limb function. Although the Bobath roll and hemiharness also allow distal function, the effective approximation provided by these devices is often questionable.[9,10] This is especially true when patients apply the orthosis themselves and when they are active with frequent changes of position. Small changes in the positioning of these devices often result in ineffective joint approximation. Electrical stimulation is capable of effectively reducing glenohumeral subluxation, as seen on x-ray (Fig. 12-1). When the electrodes are placed and secured properly, the approximation of the joint is quite reliable for the duration of each train of stimuli.

Wearing a conventional upper extremity orthosis 24 hours a day is impractical and uncomfortable. This is unfortunate, because poor joint positioning during movement in bed can contribute to the severity of the subluxation. Proper positioning of the glenohumeral joint can be provided by using ES for increasingly longer periods as tolerance to the stimulation increases.[11]

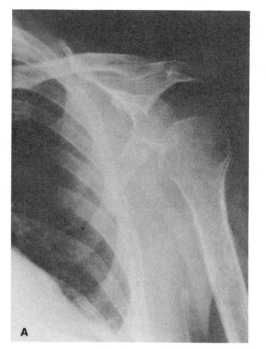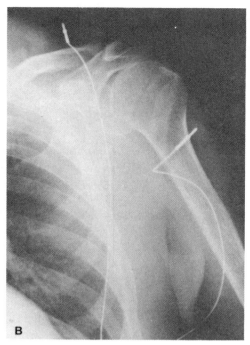

FIGURE 12–1. Approximation of the glenohumeral joint with electrical stimulation. (From Benton, et al[5] with permission.)

The problem of glenohumeral joint subluxation is not usually resolved during the hospital stay. The availability of portable stimulation devices make ES a feasible alternative for management of glenohumeral joint subluxation until such time as spasticity develops and the subluxation is resolved. ES may be continued if subluxation persists.

STG 3: Edema Reduction

Dependent ankle edema may be managed by elevation of the limb, compression, volitionally activated muscle pumping, and electrically stimulated muscle contractions to augment venous return.[12,13] The hemiparetic patient is often incapable of isolated dorsiflexion and/or plantarflexion of the effected ankle. ES can elicit cyclic contraction of the dorsiflexors and/or plantarflexors of hemiparetic patients to augment venous return and reduce dependent edema. The advantage of using ES is obviously the ability to activate appropriate muscles in the absence of volitional activation. In addition, volitionally activated muscle pumping requires the attention of the patient, where electrical stimulation can provide externally activated muscle pumping while patients attend to some other activity or even while they sleep. Numerous extended sessions of repetitive muscle contractions can be provided throughout the day with an ES device. It would be unrealistic to expect patient compliance with a similar program of active muscle pumping around an edematous joint. It is possible to provide PROM, stretch, neuromuscular re-education (with attention to task), and in the presence of some volitional activation, even strengthening while reducing edema with ES. Edema management with ES can also be easily combined with positioning and compression for a more complete treatment program.

STG 4: Increased Volitional Activation and Control of Left Extremities' Musculature by Neuromuscular Re-education

Many techniques are used in the attempt to help the hemiparetic patient regain control of the affected limbs. These include positioning and some form of external facilitation (tapping, patting, or applied resistance) superimposed upon the patients' own attempts to control their body movements.[7,14] Attention to task and an attempt to volitionally control movement must specifically accompany any facilitation technique if neuromuscular re-education is to occur. Motor planning, afferent input about the quality and quantity of movement, and relevant data from motor memory are all prerequisites for neuromuscular re-education.[15,16] In addition to more conventional techniques, ES,[5,17-19] biofeedback[20,21] and ES in combination with biofeedback[22,23] can all be used to enhance neuromuscular re-education.

ES may be used to elicit motor activity of a quality the patients are incapable of voluntarily producing. The afferent volley created by the muscle contractions and associated movement are integrated in the central nervous system and will contribute to the brain's ability to successfully effect motor activity.[5,24] The ES exercise may take the simple form of eliciting a strong contraction of a minimally active muscle. The therapist working with patients on neuromuscular control can use a handheld remote switch to provide the ES synchronized in time with the patients' own attempts to activate the muscle. If the patients are reliable and capable of independent activity, the stimulation device can be set (using an interrupted mode) to provide a series of electrical stimuli, each capable of eliciting a strong contraction. The patients can be instructed to await the onset of the ES and to time their volitional attempts at movement with the electrical stimulus. The patients are instructed to stop voluntary efforts when the stimulation ceases and to relax during the "off cycles" of the stimulation device. In this manner the patients can work on the activity independently, with intermittent therapist supervision. Reliable patients working alone on tabletop exercises can use a heel switch controlled by the unaffected foot to provide the ES synchronized with their own efforts at muscle activation.

Functional electrical stimulation (FES) can also be used to elicit a strong muscle contraction at the time in a functional activity when the affected muscle would normally be active, for example, to facilitate the hip abductors during weight-bearing activities on the affected side. In this case, a remote-control heel switch placed under the heel on the affected side is set to activate stimulation when pressure (i.e., weight bearing) is applied and to terminate stimulation when pressure is removed to synchronize stimulation of the hip abductors with weight bearing on the affected limb. If, due to poor weight shift to the affected side, the stimulus is not reliably triggered using the heel switch in the shoe on the affected leg, the switch (set to provide stimulation when pressure is *removed*) can instead be positioned in the shoe on the unaffected leg, or even in the shoe of the therapist who weight shifts along with the patient as she or he spots the patient from behind. The same activity could be performed in a tall-kneeling position with the heel switch placed under one knee.

This type of ES application may be used to enhance equilibrium reactions. The dorsiflexors may be stimulated while sitting or standing balance is challenged in a posterior direction. During large ball activities with the patient lying prone over the ball, elbow extensors may be stimulated at the time when protective extension would be appropriate.

ES can be used to provide a sensory "reminder" to a strong, but inappropriately inactive, muscle during an activity when that muscle would normally be active, similar to the use of tapping. In this case a stimulus that reaches sensory threshold but is below motor threshold is used, for example, sensory level stimulation to the dorsiflexors during the early swing phase of gait as a reminder that it is time for them to become active. The weight shift and equilibrium reaction activities previously described in this section could also be performed while using a sensory level stimulus applied to the skin overlying strong, but inappropriately inactive, muscle groups.

ES may also be used to facilitate an active movement deviating from synergy which the patient is unable to perform independently. The sensory information relayed as a result of these active movements may enable the brain to be more effective in motor planning of the same movements. An example of this application is the hemiparetic patient who has some active hip flexion and knee extension but cannot combine them to achieve a straight leg raise (SLR). In this case ES can be applied to the quadriceps muscles. The ES supplements the patients' active efforts to maintain knee extension as the hip is flexed. They are thus able to complete an active movement deviating from synergy. The timing of the electrical stimulus with the patients' efforts can be controlled by therapists using handheld remote switches or by an interrupted mode of stimulation. In coordinating the patients' volitional efforts with the ES applied in an interrupted mode, patients are instructed to await the onset of the stimulus and then to perform a SLR. Patients may be instructed to "hold" the SLR at some point in the range for a period of time (for example, for a count of three, if stimulus on time is set at 5 seconds) and then to slowly lower the leg during the ramp-down period. When the stimulation ceases (during each off cycle) the patient is instructed to relax. This sequence can be repeated over and over as long as attention span and muscle endurance allow.

Similarly, patients who can dorsiflex the ankle when the knee is in flexion but cannot do so when the knee is actively extended can be positioned with their knees supported in flexion while stimulation is applied to the dorsiflexors (Fig. 12–2). Patients are instructed to await the onset of the stimulus and then to extend their knees with their ankles dorsiflexed. Again, patients are instructed to *hold*, then slowly lower the leg, and to rest when the stimulus ceases. The dorsiflexors and the knee extensors can be stimulated during the activity if this is necessary to complete the out-of-synergy movement.

Electrically stimulated muscle contractions can be used to position an extremity for activity, in much the same way that a device like an air splint is used. For example, if the patient's affected upper extremities tend to pull up into elbow flexion during lower-extremity exercise, the elbow extensors can be stimulated during that activity to maintain the elbow in an extended position. ES may be applied to the wrist and finger extensors of a patient with increased UE flexor tone to provide positioning and prevent clawing of the wrist and fingers during upper-extremity exercise. In Figure 12–3 the patient is sitting with his arm supported on an elevated table in 90° of shoulder flexion and 90° of elbow flexion. A skateboard

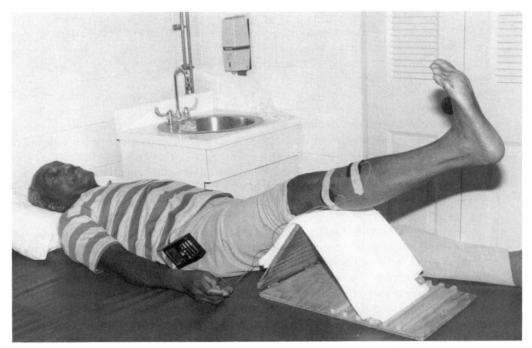

FIGURE 12–2. Electrical stimulation can be used to produce an out-of-synergy movement, for example, knee extension combined with ankle dorsiflexion.

is positioned under the forearm and the patient is instructed to actively extend the elbow. Without ES, as he makes the effort to do so, the wrist flexes and the fingers claw around the end of the skateboard (Fig. 12–3A). In order to control this undesirable motion, electrodes can be placed to activate wrist and finger extensors in a cycling interrupted pattern of stimulation (Fig. 12–3B). The patient is instructed to await the onset of the stimulus which extends his wrist and fingers and then to actively extend his elbow. When the stimulus ceases, the patient relaxes his elbow extensors and passively returns the affected elbow to the flexed position using his unaffected extremity. He then awaits the next stimulus before actively extending again. In this case, proper positioning of the wrist and fingers is provided and a rest interval is built into the motor control activity by virtue of the interrupted stimulation, instead of requiring external monitoring and assistance by the therapist.

EMGBF devices can also be used to assist in programs of neuromuscular re-education. EMG activity of a muscle group can be monitored, the audio and/or visual display made available to the patient and the therapist, and the patient instructed to try to enhance or minimize the activity of that muscle through manipulation of the display. The ". . . patient is given feedback as to how a specific muscle or muscle group is performing with respect to the therapeutic task and may reorient his or her voluntary efforts at recruitment or relaxation accordingly (or in light of suggestions offered by the clinician)."[25] Muscle activity thresholds may be set by the therapist for the patient to use as targets or goals. Recording of activity of muscles on the unaffected side can also be used to provide a target or

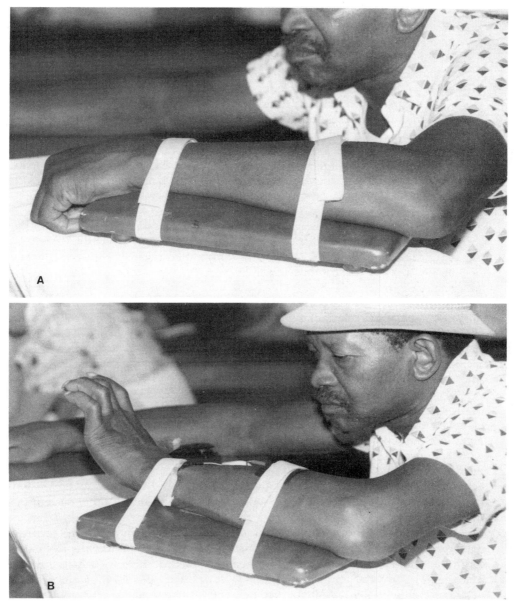

FIGURE 12–3 (A) and (B). Electrical stimulation can be used to position the wrist and fingers during upper-extremity exercise with skateboard.

goal for activity of affected musculature.[26] For example, with bridging activities in the supine position with hips and knees flexed, dual-channel biofeedback may be used to monitor the activity of the gluteus maximus muscle bilaterally and the patient can be instructed to attempt to have the activity on the involved side equal that of the uninvolved side. This technique is called *motor copy* and appears to work best with large, proximally located muscle groups.[27] As is the case with superficially applied ES, EMGBF using surface electrodes is not well suited for re-education of deep-lying muscle groups.

Biofeedback may be used to enhance or diminish isometric, concentric, and eccentric muscle contractions. Muscle activity may be monitored during relatively isolated muscle activity. For example, gluteus medius activity, seen in this patient only with gross flexion of the left lower extremity, may be monitored and displayed as the patient in a supine position attempts to abduct the hip; or the overly active gastrocsoleus muscle may be monitored and displayed as the patient in a sitting position attempts to relax his plantarflexors. Biofeedback can also be used to enhance or diminish muscle activity during more complex activities such as weight shifting or gait. For example, during the stance phase of gait, the patient might attempt to increase the biofeedback signal of his monitored hip abductors as weight is shifted onto the extremity. Patients with hyperactivity of the gastrocsoleus muscle, which interferes with limb clearance, may work to decrease signal activity of the monitored plantarflexors during the early swing phase of gait so that the dorsiflexors can work unchallenged to clear the foot from the floor. The biofeedback signal provides patients with information regarding the effectiveness of their attempts to control muscle activity.

There are instances when biofeedback may be used to provide the therapist with information regarding the efficacy of the treatment approach, for example, positioning, manual manipulations, or facilitation techniques, without drawing any patient attention to the display.[25] In these cases it is often useful for the therapist to monitor not only the activity of the muscle that he or she is trying to facilitate, but also to monitor the activity of the antagonist to that muscle group. The therapist can thereby observe not only the degree to which the patient is producing the desired muscle activity, but also if the effort exerted is causing undesired activity in the antagonist group. For example, if the patient attempted to extend the affected elbow during bilateral resisted rowing activities,[14] the affected elbow flexors and extensors would be monitored with EMG biofeedback (Fig. 12–4). The therapist could thus receive immediate and ongoing feedback as to whether the exercise was actually facilitating more triceps activity or inadvertently activating the biceps. The activity might then be modified with respect to positioning, degree of resistance, number of repetitions, and so on, in order to improve treatment effectiveness.

Devices which combine the use of electrical stimulation and EMG biofeedback can also be used to facilitate neuromuscular re-education. The devices monitor motor activity and in addition have an adjustable threshold for initiation of ES. The therapist sets the ES activation threshold at the upper limit of the patient's active recruitment ability. Patients are instructed to volitionally activate the muscles, and when the present EG threshold is reached, the ES is activated. The ES then elicits a muscle contraction of even greater magnitude (i.e., one which the patient is yet not actively capable of producing). The ES threshold, that is, the level of EMG activity that will trigger the electrical stimulus, can be modified as the patient gains greater volitional muscle control. An advantage of units which utilize an EMG threshold for ES activation over those providing ES alone is that they ensure the presence of volitional effort at the time that facilitation is provided. EMGBF is more sensitive than the therapist's own observational skills, provides more immediate feedback to patients regarding the effects of their physical efforts, provides timely information to the clinician regarding treatment efficacy, and can

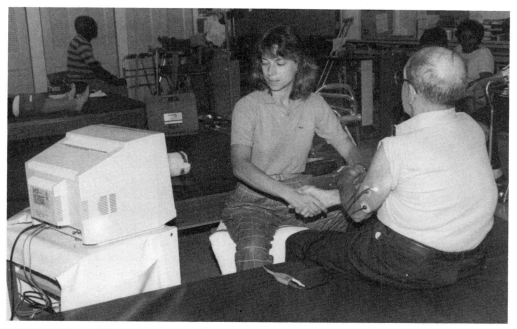

FIGURE 12-4. Therapist observes the effect of bilateral resisted rowing facilitation activity on EMG activity of the biceps and triceps.

provide a quantitative measure of therapeutic outcomes. This is important for the therapist's justification of continuation or termination of the treatment program. Motivation and performance levels of patients tend to be greater when achievable short-term goals are set.[28] Use of EMGBF may allow for successes to be experienced at a time when visible movements and functional gains have plateaued.

Some limitations to the use of EMGBF also exist. EMGBF with surface electrodes is only appropriate for superficial muscle groups. Use of EMGBF can be time consuming because of the one-on-one patient/therapist interaction. The unit and electrodes must be set up and disassembled for each treatment, and patients must receive adequate instruction if they are expected to work independently. Patient ability to work along with the biofeedback device is dependent on attention span, mentation, and level of cooperation.

STG 5: Increasing Strength

In the presence of muscle weakness, conventional treatment regimens consist of active exercise. These may take the form of isometric, concentric, or eccentric muscle contractions. Positioning and the use of external loads can be used to provide assisted or resisted exercise. Biofeedback,[29] ES,[30-32] and the combination of these modalities[22] are other treatment alternatives for strengthening weak muscles.

An isometric contraction can be produced using either a single or synchronous dual-channel ES protocol. Isotonic contractions can also be elicited with single- or dual-channeled ES devices, with varying degrees of resistance provided through the use of positioning or external loads. Weakened quadriceps muscles can be electrically stimulated with the patient sidelying and the lower extremity positioned on a raised powder board in a gravity-reduced position for knee extension. As strength increases occur, the patient can be positioned supine with the leg supported under the knee to work the quadriceps against gravity. Finally ankle cuff weights can be added to provide increased resistance to the electrically induced muscle contraction. Electrical stimulation can be used in conjunction with isokinetic devices in order to provide strength training. Eccentric training may be achieved by combining ES with an isokinetic device like the KINCOM,* which offers an eccentric mode.

Some deep muscle groups, for example, the hip flexors, are more difficult to stimulate by ES delivered through surface electrodes. Stimulation with higher frequency pulses may give better stimulus penetration, and therefore may be more effective for deeper muscle exercise. Active exercise may be the appropriate choice for these groups. For more superficial muscle groups either active exercise, ES, or some combination of these approaches is a reasonable treatment course.

One advantage of ES for muscle strengthening is that attention span is not a limitation as it is with active exercise. This is especially relevant with the neurologically impaired patient. When ES is used to increase strength, the patients need not attend to the treatment. They can work on some other problem simultaneously, eat lunch, or even nap while the stimulation is being applied.

Another advantage is the availability of multichannel stimulators that can be used to simultaneously strengthen more than one muscle group. For example, the wrist extensors and the quadriceps could be exercised at the same time. This would be difficult to accomplish actively even in a patient with fairly normal attention capabilities. Finally, patient compliance may be improved using ES over multiple volitionally activated repetitions. This factor should not be overlooked when unsupervised activity is expected of the patient.

A disadvantage associated with EMS for strengthening, is the rapid onset of muscle fatigue associated with electrically induced contractions, as compared to volitional activation of muscle.[5] Care must be taken to optimize stimulation characteristics and minimize fatigue whenever a program of ES involving repetitive contractions is planned.

Biofeedback devices and devices that combine EMGBF with ES can again be used to help the patient maximize muscle use. Here, as in the case of neuromuscular re-education,[33] thresholds are set to provide goals or targets for active efforts. These devices may be most effective in increasing activity and strength of very weak muscles that cannot yet resist external loads, or when it is difficult for patients to recognize whether they are achieving the desired contraction without some external form of biofeedback.[34] EMG biofeedback with superficial electrodes is ineffective in monitoring activity in deep muscle groups. Adequate mentation, attention span, and cooperation are required for all biofeedback applications.

STG 6: Tone Reduction

Conventional means of dealing with spasticity include icing, gentle stroking, medication, and so forth. ES may be applied to the spastic muscle[34,35] or its

---

*Kincom. Chatler, 4717 Adams R., Hixson, TN 37343.

antagonist[4,18,36] depending upon the stimulation characteristics chosen in an effort to decrease spasticity through fatigue or reciprocal inhibition (see Chapter 7). For example, in the presence of increased tone in the biceps muscle at the elbow, either the biceps or triceps muscle group may be targeted for ES. Biofeedback may also be used to decrease muscle tone.[25,37] The use of electrical modalities to decrease tone in no way precludes the additional use of more conventional tone reduction methods. It is advantageous to use a combination of methods during the treatment course to decrease tone.

Advantages of ES for tone reduction include a small time requirement (for setup) on the part of the physical therapist. Treatment with ES can be delivered while the therapist is with another patient and can even take place outside of the physical therapy department. If tone reduction protocols, which involve antagonist stimulation, are chosen, an additional benefit of increased strength in the antagonist muscle may be realized. This is especially important because weakness is often present in the reciprocally inhibited, overstretched antagonist to the spastic muscle group. Some volitional activation of the weakened muscle groups must be present in order for strength gains to occur. The serial contractions of the stimulated muscles can simultaneously provide PROM to the joint and may serve to reduce edema. In addition, if the patient with some volitional activation is instructed to work with the stimulus to achieve muscle activity, neuromuscular re-education is possible.

EMGBF can also be used to normalize muscle tone. The activity of the spastic muscle is monitored and displayed auditorally and/or visually to the patient. It may be most effective to set the device so that muscle activity produces noise or visual display and relaxation reduces this feedback. The patient thus works to quiet the visual or auditory display by reducing motor activity in the muscle group(s) being monitored. Just as stability should first be achieved before mobility is superimposed, control of spastic muscle activity should first be worked on at rest and then in conjunction with movement of the involved extremity.[25] For example, patients should first practice relaxation of their spastic biceps muscles in a supine position or sitting with their arms at rest, before attempting to maintain that relaxation during some arm movement such as shoulder flexion with elbow extension. Intact cognition and patient cooperation, accessible muscle groups, and cost and availability of equipment are concerns consistent with those previously mentioned for other EMGBF applications.

STG 7: Management and Enhancement of Sensory Awareness

Any patient with extensive sensory deficits should be instructed in pressure-relief methods, skin inspection, and proper skin-care techniques. The problem of decreased sensation is an important one in the rehabilitation of the hemiparetic patient, as it appears that patients who exhibit sensory deficits along with their paresis have a poorer prognosis for functional recovery.[7,38] In the treatment of the hemiparetic patient with decreased sensation, the clinician is constantly attempting to increase sensory input to the central nervous system through facilitation techniques like tapping, patting, and so on, and also to facilitate the patient's use of intact sensory pathways which are intact in order to compensate for areas of deficit. Both ES and EMG biofeedback are useful adjuncts to these treatment goals.

ES, whether applied at sensory- or motor-threshold intensity, provides a barrage of afferent messages to the CNS. It is thought that the added afferent input will enhance the redevelopment of effective sensory pathways from the area of stimulation.[39] Biofeedback devices can help to compensate for the sensory deficit by augmenting intact senses. A limb-load monitor consisting of a pressure-sensitive heelplate and auditory signal can help the patient with an insensitive lower extremity to recognize weight shift to the insensitive limb. EMG biofeedback can also help the patient to make better use of pathways which may be intact but underused. For example, patients, when instructed to bend their elbows, may not be able to produce the desired movement, yet when biceps brachii activity is monitored electromyographically and they are instructed to manipulate the auditory or visual signal, they may indeed find a means of accomplishing the desired movement. The input they receive from the biofeedback display provides them with afferent information that they use in their motor planning and subsequent activity.

STG 8: Normalizing Gait Patterns

The conventional management of gait deviations takes numerous forms including pregait mat activities, exercise, facilitation, component activities in the upright position, orthotic application, and progressive gait training in the parallel bars and ultimately with assistive devices. ES as an orthotic substitute[17-19,40-42] and EMG biofeedback[21] may also be considered gait training options.

As mentioned in the section on neuromuscular re-education. EMG biofeedback can be used during gait training in order to cue the patient to augment or diminish the activity of the monitored muscle group. For instance a patient with some volitional control of dorsiflexion who does not consistently exhibit dorsiflexion on swing phase can be instructed to increase the biofeedback display associated with the monitored tibialis anterior muscle at the end of stance. Conversely, if the lack of dorsiflexion exhibited following the roll-over and push-off phases of gait is thought to be a result of hyperactivity of the plantarflexors then the patient can be instructed to try to decrease the display associated with tibialis posterior muscle activity during initial swing. EMG biofeedback can be used to facilitate correction of gait deviations involving any muscle group whose activity can be monitored with surface electrodes. Adequate mentation, attention span, and cooperation are requirements for this treatment application as they are for any activity requiring active patient participation.

While ES with remote (heel or hand switch) triggering timed to coincide with the patient's individual gait pattern can be a useful adjunct to many gait training programs, there are gait deviations that cannot be effectively managed through the use of this modality. Deviations like pelvic retraction and decreased hip flexion, with external rotation and adduction used to advance the involved extremity, are not well suited to the use of ES because the affected muscles are too deep to be reached with surface electrodes. It may be noted that these gait deviations also do not lend themselves to more conventional orthotic management as traditional braces do not provide pelvic protraction or hip-flexion assistance. Again in the case of insufficient knee flexion for swing, neither conventional bracing nor ES applied as an orthotic substitute are suitable choices for management. Conventional knee-ankle-foot orthoses (KAFO) are not capable of providing a knee-flexion assist. Knee flexion for limb clearance during swing is for the most part passively provided as a result of momentum generated by hip flexion.[41] Dorsiflexion-assist ankle-foot orthoses (AFOs) and ES applied to the dorsiflexors may be used to enhance a mass-flexion pattern of the lower extremity and increase knee flexion for swing. Most often the problem of insufficient knee flexion is best managed by mat activities, facilitation, exercise, and progressive gait training.

There are gait deviations that are well suited to orthotic management. This can take the form of conventional ankle-foot orthoses made of plastic or metal and leather, ES using a remote control switch, or through some combination of these alternatives. Gait deviations of this patient which may be modified include knee instability (stance), ankle medial/lateral instability (initial foot/floor contact), and insufficient dorsiflexion (swing).

Several considerations help to clarify the management decision with respect to these gait deviations. One dilemma that therapists wrestle with is that of bracing "too early," in the neurologically impaired patient who has the potential for return of neuromuscular function. The therapist must weight the need to ensure safe joint positioning for ambulation versus the tendency for conventional orthoses to discourage active contraction of the muscles whose function is supported by the brace. ES provides effective joint positioning by eliciting activity from the weakened or inactive muscle groups. ES has the potential to strengthen these muscles when volitional activation is present, while serving the orthotic function. The problem of bracing too early is therefore eliminated.

Another problem associated with conventional orthoses is that while they provide desired positioning during one phase of gait, they may interfere with motions essential to the normal completion of other phases of the gait cycle. For example, a double-upright AFO with a 90° posterior stop provides dorsiflexion for limb clearance during swing but prevents a normal push off at end stance and a conventional KAFO provides knee stability for stance but interferes with knee flexion for limb clearance during swing.

When ES is chosen as an orthotic substitute, the timing of the stimulus during ambulation is usually controlled by a pressure-activated heel switch. Because of this, corrective positioning provided during swing phase will be terminated during stance, and corrective positioning for stance will be terminated during swing, producing a more normal gait pattern. If dorsiflexion during swing phase (for limb clearance) were the goal of stimulation, there would be no interference with push off during stance because weight bearing on the heel switch in early stance would inactivate the stimulation to the dorsiflexors. Similarly, were the knee extensors stimulated for stance stability, there would be no interference with knee flexion during swing as non-weight bearing on the heel switch at end stance would inactivate the stimulation to the quadriceps muscle.

Setting the posterior stop of a conventional AFO in a dorsiflexed position to correct a "drop-foot" gait pattern causes an increase in the flexion moment at the knee as the foot-ankle complex moves from heelstrike to foot flat.[42] In a patient with insufficient quadriceps strength to stabilize the knee, this can result in knee buckling. When ES is used to provide dorsiflexion during swing, the electrical stimulus ceases upon weight bearing, thereby allowing the ankle to move freely into plantarflexion from heelstrike to foot flat; no increased flexion moment is created at the knee. This may be quite important for the hemiparetic patient in whom knee instability is a problem. In cases of knee instability, where the addition of an anterior stop would be indicated on a conventional AFO, the electrical orthosis can also be used. The same electrical device that stimulates the dorsiflexors for swing can also be used to stimulate the quadriceps for knee stability during stance, with both functions (working reciprocally) controlled by a single heel switch. Electrical stimulation devices utilized for gait training are lightweight and portable. They do not require use of any special type of shoe, because the heel-switch control, which fits in the shoe, is quite small. Like plastic AFOs, FES devices provide good cosmesis when the patient wears long skirts or slacks, and are less cosmetic when short pants or skirts above the knee are worn. Both plastic AFOs and FES as orthotic substitutes are more cosmetic than are metal and leather AFOs.

ES may facilitate neuromuscular re-education as well. The stimulation positions the limb for function by eliciting active muscle contractions, and in doing so, provides added afferent information to the CNS. With attention to task and attempts at volitional activation, this afferent input may contribute to neuromuscular re-education of the stimulated area. Because the elicited contractions occur at the point in the gait cycle when muscles would normally be active, there may be some training specificity with respect to the stimulated muscles' function during ambulation.

Long-term dependency on an orthosis is, of course, undesirable if avoidable. While conventional orthoses simply promote dependency, the potential strengthening and neuromuscular re-education benefits of ES as an orthotic substitute may allow for eventual weaning from the use of the device.[18,19]

Some limitations to ES do exist. Rapid stimulation of muscles that are antagonists of moderately-to-severely spastic muscle groups may result in quick stretch and undesirable activation of the spastic muscles. This involuntary activity can override the stimulated contraction and result in a loss of orthotic function. For example, rapid stimulation to the tibialis anterior muscle in the presence of excessive gastrocsoleus spasticity can result in facilitated plantarflexion rather than desired dorsiflexion during swing. Increasing stimulus ramp on time provides more gradual achievement of peak stimulus intensity and more gradual movement through the ROM. Unfortunately it is not always possible to prolong the ramp time of the stimulus while providing the desired orthotic function at the point in the gait cycle when it is needed. For this reason ES may not be a viable orthotic alternative for the patient with moderate-to-severe spasticity in the muscle antagonistic to those targeted for stimulation. Often a non-weight bearing trial stimulation session of the muscle group in question can clarify this issue early in the treatment course.

Another problem associated with the use of ES for orthotic substitution stems from the fact that the heel switch control is solely pressure activated or inactivated. Therefore, if the unit is set to provide a swing phase correction, for example, a balance dorsiflexion contraction, then the stimulus will remain on whenever there is no weight bearing on the switch. This is true not only during ambulation (Fig. 12–5A) but also for static standing during which the weight is shifted over the uneffected extremity (as it often is in the hemiparetic patient) and for sitting (Fig. 12–5B). In this case the ankle would continue to dorsiflex with the patient sitting or standing without sufficient weight bearing on the affected lower extremity. Undesirable results include unnecessary muscle fatigue, balance impairment, inappropriately timed afferent input, and cosmetically unacceptable posturing during static standing and sitting.

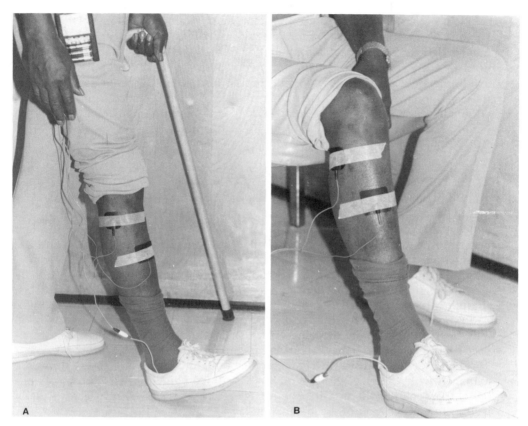

FIGURE 12–5 A and B. The same orthotic heel-switch setup that provides dorsiflexion for the swing phase of gait (*A*) causes the ankle to remain constantly dorsiflexed whenever the patient is non-weight bearing on the switch, as in sitting (*B*).

Relatively small changes in electrode position can dramatically influence effective joint positioning. When ES as an orthosis is used outside the clinic, it is necessary to have a patient or attendant, who can reliably duplicate effective electrode placement at home, note changes in joint position during the wearing period, and correct electrode placement should that be indicated. The patient or attendant must also be responsible for battery replacement or recharging, gel application, skin inspection, and adjustment of intensity controls. Because the ES protocol is more complex than a conventional orthosis, there is of course a greater chance of mechanical breakdown as well as human error. Safety is a primary concern because any human or mechanical error can result in ineffective joint positioning and increase the risk of a fall. Implanted electrodes and more sophisticated control mechanisms may soon solve these problems. These factors are less significant during the supervised use of ES in the clinical setting. ES as an orthotic substitute might most appropriately be chosen for short-term trials in the home for patients with good potential for neuromuscular recovery and for supervised gait training in the clinic. Cost for short-term rental of portable stimulation units is very reasonable and may be justified by the possibility of decreased need for conventional bracing following the ES gait-training period.

It is not always necessary to choose between more conventional orthoses and ES for gait training. In cases where more conservative or more cautious management is deemed appropriate, a combination of methods is quite feasible. ES may be used to elicit contractions of the affected muscles with the heel switch placed inside the shoe of the conventional orthosis. In this way, there is activity of the muscles which may lead to strength gains and/or neuromuscular re-education, while safety is enhanced. It is also possible that a less-supportive brace can be used when applied in conjunction with the ES in this manner.

STG 9, 10, and 11: Dependent Transfers, Bed Mobility, Ambulation

Problems such as dependent transfers and dependent ambulation, which are identified during the functional evaluation, are managed with direct work on the deficient skill itself, for example, through transfer training and also through breaking the activity into its component parts, such as moving forward on the chair, proper foot alignment, leaning forward, pushing up, balancing, pivoting, and so forth, identifying which components are lacking, and working on the accomplishment of each deficient component individually. The completion of each component is dependent on more basic component activities such as PROM, AROM, strength, weight shift, and so on. Various forms of electrical stimulation may be used to facilitate these necessary skills as an adjunct to traditional functional training in the management of functional problems.

Many of the physical therapy problems identified in Case Study 1 can be managed with electrical stimulation alone or in combination with more conventional therapeutic options. Other neurological conditions lend themselves equally well to the application of electrical stimulation.

CASE STUDY 2

The patient is a 21-year-old male with C-6, C-7 quadriplegia following a spinal cord injury sustained in a motor-vehicle accident 10 weeks ago. The patient received acute care at a general hospital where the spinal column was stabilized using a Halo vest. He received physical therapy at bedside for 2 weeks consisting primarily of gradual elevation of the head of the bed to offset orthostatic hypotension—progressing toward use of a recliner wheelchair and PROM to all four extremities. This was followed by 6 weeks of therapy in the physical therapy department. The patient was discharged home for 2 weeks for psychological reasons and is now referred to the rehabilitation hospital for continued therapy. The patient's past medical history is unremarkable. He smokes two packs of cigarettes per day.

The patient, a college junior majoring in liberal arts, was living with a male friend in a second-floor apartment close to the college they were attending at the time of the accident. The patient's parents live in a split-level home in the same city with six steps up or down to levels other than the main floor. The main level contains the living room, dining room, kitchen, and a small powder room. Full bath and bedrooms are on the upper level. Insurance coverage is private insurance.

The patient presently has rented a manual wheelchair, sliding board, and commode for use at home.

PHYSICAL STATUS

Physical examination reveals mild-to-moderate dependent ankle edema bilaterally. The patient reports that antiembolic stockings and lower-extremity elevation were not consistently used at home. A pressure sore is present over left-ischial tuberosity. It is 2.3 cm by 2.3 cm in diameter without significant depth. A cigarette burn is also present on the right proximal thigh. The patient reports that weight shifts were not faithfully carried out at home. Some loss of muscle bulk is noted bilaterally in the LE and trunk musculature.

PROM is within normal limits throughout the extremities except for the following: neck flexion, extension, rotation, and lateral flexion were not assessed due to halo immobilization; shoulder flexion and abduction are 0° to 130° bilaterally with excursion limited by the halo vest; SLR measures 0° to 110° bilaterally; and ankle dorsiflexion is minus 5° on the right, 0° on the left. Tightness of the wrist and finger flexors is present and desirable for tenodesis; the finger joints have full extension range with the wrist positioned in flexion and full wrist extension is available with the fingers positioned in flexion.

NEUROMUSCULAR STATUS

Strength

Strength in the neck muscles was not assessed due to Halo device. Shoulder musculature is 4/5 throughout on right, 4−/5 on the left within the available ROM.[43] Elbow flexion is 4−/5 bilaterally; elbow extension is 2−/5 on left, 1/5 on the right. Wrist extension is 3+/5 bilaterally; wrist flexion is 1/5 bilaterally. Finger extension is 1/5 bilaterally, with 0/5 finger flexion noted at this time. Trunk musculature was not evaluated fully because of Halo vest. No evidence of abdominal muscle function was noted with attempts to cough. Lower extremity muscle strength is 0/5 throughout.

Sensation

Light touch, pinprick, and proprioception are intact to C-6 level, diminished at C-7, and absent below.

Tone

Occasional mild extensor spasms are noted in lower extremities. These spasms do not interfere with functional activities at this time.

Vital Capacity

The patient's vital capacity is 30 percent of normal for his body size.

FUNCTIONAL STATUS

The patient is independent in wheelchair propulsion using plastic-coated hand rims, negotiating distances of about 150 ft before fatiguing. Management of ramps is dependent due to the Halo device and to the patient's subsequent inability to lean forward. Negotiation of curbs was not assessed at this time due to motion limitations caused by the Halo device and restrictions regarding spinal stabilization. The patient is independent in the management of his WC brakes using extensions and requires assistance with management of leg rests and lower extremities secondary to restrictions imposed by the Halo device. The patient is independent in weight-shift activities in the WC. He removes an armrest and uses hooking and sideleaning to clear each buttock.

Transfers from the wheelchair to the mat or commode using a transfer board require mod A of one for balance and to aid in push up due to restrictions of the Halo device. Car transfers using a transfer board require maximum assistance. Transfers to other surfaces were not assessed at this time.

All bed mobility activities are limited by the Halo device. Rolling requires mod A, LE management on and off the mat requires moderate to maximum assistance, sitting to supine requires mod A, and supine to sitting requires max A, that is, the patient himself is capable of accomplishing approximately 25 percent of the work involved in the task. Ambulation assessment is not indicated.

Problem List	Short-Term Treatment Goals*
1. Dependent edema, both ankles	1. Decreased ankle edema
2. Grade 2 decubitus ulcer, left buttock	2. Wound closure
3. Decreased PROM in both shoulders, ankles	3. Increased PROM ankles (by 5°)
4. Decreased sensation in hands, trunk, and lower extremities	4. Increased reliability for weight shifting, skin inspection, and skin-care technique
5. Atrophy of LE musculature	5. Delayed LE atrophy
6. Decreased strength in upper-extremity musculature	6. Increased strength in upper-extremity musculature (by one-half MMT grade)
7. Decreased vital capacity (VC)	7. Increased vital capacity
8. Limited WC propulsion endurance (150 ft)	8. Increased indoor WC propulsion endurance (175 ft)
9. Dependent WC management of leg rests and LEs (mod A)	9. Ability to instruct assistant in management of leg rests and LEs
10. Dependent side transfer with board (mod A)	10., 11., 12. Ability to participate within limitations of the Halo device and to instruct attendant in assistance in the performance of (10) side transfer with board, (11) bed mobility skills, and (12) advanced WC skills
11. Dependent bed mobility (mod-max A)	
12. Dependent advanced wheelchair skills (elevations, uneven surfaces)	

*Short-term goals (especially with respect to function) are greatly affected by limitations imposed by Halo-vest stabilization device.

MANAGEMENT CONSIDERATIONS

STG 1: Edema Reduction (Both Ankles)

Dependent edema in the spinal cord injured patient is managed in much the same way as it is in the hemiparetic patient. Elevation and compression are the conventional methods used to address this problem. Volitional muscle pumping of the dorsiflexors and/or plantarflexors is most often not possible secondary to the deficits left after the spinal cord injury. Here, as in the hemiparetic patient, ES can be used to elicit muscle contraction, or pumping, and so assist in venous return.

Again, in addition to more effective edema reduction, an advantage associated with the use of ES along with more conventional approaches is the ability to simultaneously accomplish more than one goal. There is some evidence that an ES program of this kind may reduce the incidence of deep vein thrombosis.[12-13] The cyclic stimulation of the dorsiflexor musculature around the ankle can also provide PROM to the ankle joint. Muscle re-education and strengthening of dorsiflexors or plantarflexors are not possible in the course of the edema-reduction program in the patient with complete spinal cord transection as they were in the hemiparetic patient. With this patient, the peripheral nerve pathways are intact, but CNS input is lacking. Decreasing atrophy of the stimulated muscles may be a feasible associated goal, although this area requires further investigation with respect to stimulation characteristics and program requirements.

STG 2: Wound Healing (over Left-Ischial Tuberosity)

Conventional management of open wounds includes whirlpool, water-pick debridement, packing, and topical dressings along with positioning, weight shift, cushions, and pressure-reducing mattresses. Treatment with ES is another viable alternative for the clinician working toward wound closure.[44-46] A wide variety of ES units with stimulation characteristics appropriate to this goal are commercially available (see Chapter 10).

There is no need to choose between treatment with ES and more traditional methods of wound management. The use of ES can easily be combined with more conventional wound healing techniques. More rapid and more complete healing has been reported when ES is used in conjunction with conventional techniques to promote healing.[44-46] This is, of course, desirable as it decreases the chances of infection, decreases the length of the hospital stay (and the associated costs), and accelerates the return to normal function. Portable units make this therapy available for professionally administered bedside or home-based treatments.

STG 3: Increasing PROM (Shoulder Flexion and Abduction, Ankle Dorsiflexion)

Shoulder range limitations evidenced at this time are associated with the spinal stabilization device. Should these limitations remain following removal of the device manual and gravity-assisted stretch would be indicated. As stated before, ES is not effective for providing PROM at the shoulder or hip where muscle groups are deep and the weight of the limb is often too great to be overcome by the electrically stimulated contraction. Active ROM exercise of shoulder muscles is preferred for this patient.

Plantarflexor tightness can be managed here, as in the hemiparetic patient, through stimulation to the dorsiflexors at the end of the available dorsiflexion ROM. Should edema be present around the ankle joint, edema reduction may be a concommitant benefit of this program of stretch. Delayed atrophy in the stimulated muscles is another, less well-documented potential benefit (see Chapter 8).[47,48]

STG 4: Improving Skin-Management Techniques

Lack of sensation associated with the complete spinal cord transection is managed by teaching the patients or their attendants to perform regular weight shifts in all positions and also to perform regular visual inspection of the skin in insensitive regions. Because only the peripheral nervous system is intact below the level of the lesion, therapy directed toward increasing afferent messages sent from the periphery to the central nervous system is not appropriate as it is in the hemiparetic patient. For this reason, ES and biofeedback are not effective means of dealing with the sensory deficits seen in this spinal cord injured (SCI) patient.

STG 5: Delaying Muscle Atrophy

Loss of muscle bulk can present problems to the spinal cord injured patient in terms of poor psychological adjustment and loss of cushion between bony prominences and externally applied pressures. There is no conventional means by which the patient can exercise to prevent or decrease the occurrence of muscle atrophy below the level of the spinal cord lesion. Many patients simply learn to deal with the changes associated with the loss of muscle bulk along with their other adjustments to the disability. Electrical muscle stimulation may be used in the attempt to maintain lower extremity muscle bulk in the SCI patient.[47-50] Success is dependent upon patient compliance with long-term treatment.

Programmed electrical stimulation exercise units such as the REGYS I (Fig. 12–6) and the ERGYS I systems* are specifically designed for patients with spinal cord injuries but intact peripheral nerves to lower extremity muscles. Potential benefits associated with programs using these devices include maintenance of or increase in muscle bulk, improved cardiopulmonary status, relaxation of muscle spasms, and increased local circulation.[48-50] However, it should be remembered that the problem of muscle inactivity is a permanent one in this case, and that any treatment initiated toward the management of muscle atrophy must continue indefinitely in order to remain effective. Therefore, it is important to weigh the time (total treatment time including setup and dismantling is 1½ to 2 hours) and cost requirements of maintaining a program of this kind against the potential benefits. Feasibility of a post-discharge home program of ES should be determined before the decision is made to use ES in the clinic for the purpose of atrophy delay.

---

*Therapeutic Technologies, Inc., 2200 West Commercial Blvd., Ft. Lauderdale, FL 33309.

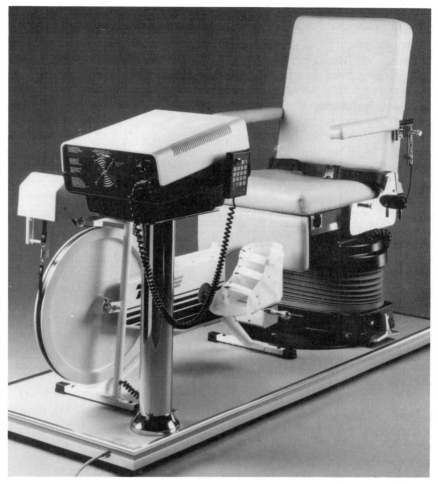

FIGURE 12–6. The REGYS I programmed electrical exercise unit. (Courtesy of Therapeutic Technologies, Inc., Tampa, Florida.)

STG 6: Increasing Strength

In the presence of weak muscles following spinal cord injury the treatment program is much the same as that outlined for the hemiparetic patient. The program may consist of active exercise in the form of isometric, isotonic, or eccentric muscle contractions with assistance or resistance provided as indicated. ES,[30-32] EMG biofeedback,[51] or a combination of these modalities are also treatment alternatives which may be used to achieve strength gains in weak muscles.

There are advantages to the use of ES for strengthening in the SCI patient, as there are in the hemiparetic patient. By using a dual- or multichannel ES unit more than one muscle group can be exercised at a time. The patient need not attend to the ES program and can even work on some other activity while the stimulation is being applied. Once again treatment time is optimized as multiple treatment goals may be simultaneously addressed. Should any edema be present in the stimulated area, the induced muscle contractions associated with the strengthening program may help to reduce it. The cyclic muscle contractions can also be used to simultaneously provide PROM or stretch to a shortened antagonist muscle, while the agonist is being strengthened.

Another advantage of ES is that it can elicit a contraction which is stronger than the one that the patient produces volitionally. The activity and the associated elicited afferent volley may facilitate volitional recruitment of additional motor units that are innervated but essentially inactive.

As previously stated, use of ES is inappropriate for the strengthening of muscles such as the hip flexors which are too deep to be effectively stimulated with a superficially applied stimulus. It should also be remembered that the ES program must be consistent with the program goals. In the present patient problem, a tenodesis grasp has been achieved by allowing selective tightening of the wrist and finger flexors. Although the wrist and finger extensor muscles show weakness, it is important not to stimulate these groups in such a way that both wrist and finger extensors are stimulated simultaneously. ES can still be used to strengthen the wrist extensors as long as finger extension is prevented (e.g., through the use of a glove with velcro closure around the dorsum of the hand, which maintains the flexed position of the finger joints) and to strengthen the finger extensors with the wrist stabilized in a flexed position.

Often the muscles at the level just spared by the spinal cord injury lesion are weak. This may at first be due to edema in the vicinity of the lesion. Regaining the use of all the available musculature is extremely important in the quadriparetic patient. Here every spinal level significantly affects projected functional gains (Table 12–1).

EMG biofeedback devices and devices which combine ES with EMG biofeedback can be used to assist the SCI patient to recruit existing but dormant muscle function. Superficial muscle activity that is barely a trace (1/5) level by manual muscle test evaluation can be effectively monitored by these means. The patient's manipulation of the EMGBF signal and the setting of thresholds for EMG response or for ES activation are performed in the same manner described for the hemiparetic patient. The advantages of having immediate and ongoing feedback for the patient's attempts at muscle function continue to apply here, as do the expense and availability considerations associated with these devices. As with ES, EMGBF with superficial electrodes is not suitable for the rehabilitation of deep-muscle groups.

STG 7: Improving Cardiopulmonary Function by Increasing Vital Capacity

Decreased cardiopulmonary function in the SCI patient is conventionally managed through the use of resisted diaphragmatic breathing exercises, incentive spirometry, and overall conditioning exercises such as isotonic or isokinetic upper-extremity ergometry and wheelchair aerobics. Electrical stimulation can also be used to treat this problem. Programmed electrical exercise units (e.g., REGYS I) using pedal ergometry and applying stimulation to quadriceps, hamstrings, and gluteal muscle groups have been shown to improve cardiopulmonary parameters in SCI patients (Fig. 12–6).[52] This result is desirable for its functional implications and because cardiopulmonary complications have been identified as a major cause of death following SCI.[53] Additional potential benefits to the program include maintained or increased muscle bulk,[48–50] increased circulation,[49] relaxation of muscle spasms, and psychological benefits.

Time and cost requirements for ES programs of this nature are presently quite high. Equipment availability is also somewhat limited, although both clinical and home units are commercially available and in some cases, are covered by third-party insurance coverage. Conditioning activity of this nature must be ongoing in order for benefits to be maintained. Further investigation is required to determine whether these ES programs are of greater ultimate cost benefit than more conventional, less expensive, more readily available treatment alternatives.

STG 8, 9, 10, 11, and 12: Improving Wheelchair Management, Transfers, Bed Mobility, Advanced Wheelchair Skills, and the Ability to Instruct Assistant

Functional deficits are managed for the SCI patient as they were for the hemiparetic patient through work on the deficient skill itself and work on the component parts of that functional skill. The completion of each component is dependent on the presence of more basic-skills blocks, such as adequate PROM, AROM, strength, weight shift, and so on, whose acquisition can be facilitated with ES. The patients should also become competent in instruction of assistants in the performance of skills of which they are incapable due to the limitations of the Halo-vest stabilization device.

SELECTION OF APPROPRIATE ELECTROTHERAPEUTIC PROCEDURES AND EQUIPMENT

The selection of ES as a treatment modality is analogous to the decision to use heat. Just as heat is a broad heading for various modalities such as hot packs, ultrasound, diathermy, and infrared, where heat is generated and/or delivered in different ways, so does the broad heading ES encompass a variety of devices in which the electricity is produced and delivered in many different ways. Just as specific forms of heat are most appropriately chosen for different patient problems, specific forms of electrical stimulation are most appropriately chosen for the management of different types of problems. For example both biphasic and monophasic (pulsatile current) can be used to retard disuse atrophy, but in the presence of denervated muscle only the use of monophasic-pulsed current, with a sufficient pulse duration, would provide a successful form of stimulation. It is very important to understand the electrical characteristics that are required in order to obtain a desired physiologic effect; otherwise while ES may be an appropriate general treatment choice, the device, or stimulation, characteristics selected may prove ineffective. The stimulus characteristics required to produce specific physiologic effects are discussed in Chapters 5 through 10 of this text.

Once the decision has been made to use ES, and the necessary features of stimulation have been identified, an electrical stimulator can be selected. Because manufacturers may choose to package the various features of ES in many combinations, it is not practical to rely on a general category of electrical device as named by the industry (e.g., low voltage stimulators) to provide any given function. There is at present no standardization among the features offered on any category of devices. To achieve the therapeutic goal, the clinician can use any machine that offers the necessary stimulation charac-

TABLE 12-1 Anticipated Functional Levels in Spinal Cord Injury

	Pulmonary Hygiene	AM Care	Feeding	Grooming	Dressing	Bathing	Bowel and Bladder Routine
C-3, C-4	Totally assisted cough.	Total dependence.	Unable to feed self. Drink with long straw after set up.	Total dependence.	Total dependence.	Total dependence.	Total dependence.
C-5	Assisted cough.	Independent with specially adapted devices with set up.	Independent with specially adapted equipment for feeding after set up.	Independent with specially adapted equipment for grooming after set up.	Total dependence.	Total dependence.	Total dependence.
C-6	Some assistance required in supine positions. Independent in sitting position.	Independent with equipment.	Independent with equipment. Drink from glass.	Independent with equipment.	Independent upper dressing. Assistance with lower dressing.	Independent uppers and lowers with equipment.	Independent for bowel routine. Assistance with bladder routine.
C-7	As above.	Independent.	Independent.	Independent with equipment.	Potential for independence in upper and lower dressing.	Independent with equipment.	Independent.
C-8, T-1	As above.	Independent.	Independent.	Independent.	Independent.	Independent.	Independent.
T-2-T-10	T-2-T-6 as above. T-6-T-10, independent.	Independent.	Independent.	Independent.	Independent.	Independent.	Independent.

Bed Mobility	Pressure Relief	Transfers	Wheelchair Propulsion	Ambulations	Orthotic Devices	Transportation	Communications
Total dependence.	Independent in powered recliner wheelchair. Dependent in bed or manual wheelchair.	Total dependence.	Independent in pneumatic or chin-control driven power wheelchair with powered reclining feature.	Not applicable.	Upper-extremity. Outside-powered orthosis. Dorsal cockup splint.	Dependent on others in accessible van with lift.	Read with special adapted equipment. Specially adapted phone. Unable to write. Type with special adaptions.
Assisted by others and equipment.	Most require assistance.	Assistance of one person with or without transfer board.	Independent in powered chair indoors and outdoors. Short distances in manual wheelchair with lugs, indoors.	Not applicable.	As above.	As above.	Same as above.
Independent with equipment.	Independent.	Potentially independent with transfer board.	Independent manual wheelchair with plastic rims or lugs indoors. Assistance outdoors and with elevators.	Not applicable.	Wrist-driven orthosis.	Independent driving with specially adapted van.	Independent phone. Write with equipment. Type with equipment. Independent turning pages.
Independent.	Independent.	Independent with/without transfer board except to/from floor with assistance.	Independent manual wheelchair indoors and outdoors except curbs.	Not applicable.	None.	Independent driving car with hand controls or specially adapted van. Independent wheelchair into car placement.	Independent with equipment for phone, typing, and writing. Independent turning pages.
Independent.	Independent.	Independent including to/from floor.	Independent manual wheelchair indoors and out.	Not applicable.	None.	As above.	Independent.
Independent.	Independent.	Independent.	Independent.	Exercise only (not functional) with orthoses.	Knee-ankle-foot orthoses with forearm crutches or walker.	As above.	Independent.

(Continued)

TABLE 12–1 Anticipated Functional Levels in Spinal Cord Injury (*Continued*)

	Pulmonary Hygiene	AM Care	Feeding	Grooming	Dressing	Bathing	Bowel and Bladder Routine
T-11–L-2	Not applicable.	Independent.	Independent.	Independent.	Independent.	Independent.	Independent.
L-3–S-3	Not applicable.	Independent.	Independent.	Independent.	Independent.	Independent.	Independent.

Source: Developed by the Occupational and Physical Therapy Departments of the Regional Spinal Cord Injury Center of the Delaware Valley. Magee Rehabilitation Hospital, 1513 Race Street, Philadelphia, PA 19102; and Thomas Jefferson University Hospital, 11th and Walnut Streets, Philadelphia, PA 19107.

teristics (parameters). For example, a conventional TENS unit may be used to fatigue a spastic muscle as long as it is programmed for continuous stimulation at motor threshold and high rate.

It is wise to take an organized approach when making decisions about features necessary for achievement of a given therapeutic goal. This can be done by preparing a protocol related to the specific goal in question. Each of the following ten elements should be addressed: waveform, rate or frequency, pulse duration, amplitude (intensity), modulations (including interruptions, ramping, and bursts), special features (including number of channels, remote switch, portability, and control accessibility), electrode type and placement, session length and frequency, and projected time of re-evaluation.

SAMPLE PROTOCOL

To develop an electrical stimulation protocol, the clinician would proceed element by element in a logical and organized fashion, defining the necessary requirements of each component for achievement of the treatment goal. In order to demonstrate this process, the hemiparetic patient problem of *decreased PROM* (Case Study 1) is considered. The goal of stimulation is defined as *increased PROM*, initially by 5°. The sample protocol including each of the above-mentioned elements is summarized in Table 12–2. The rationale for the selection of each component is presented below.

Rationale for Protocol Requirements

1. *Waveform:* Pulsatile with sufficiently rapid rise time to avoid physiologic accommodation.

Bed Mobility	Pressure Relief	Transfers	Wheelchair Propulsion	Ambulations	Orthotic Devices	Transportation	Communications
Independent.	Independent.	Independent.	Independent.	Potential for independent functional ambulation indoors with orthoses. Some have potential for stairs with railing.	Knee-ankle-foot orthoses or ankle-foot orthoses with forearm crutches.	As above.	Independent.
Independent.	Independent.	Independent.	Independent.	Independent indoors and outdoors with orthoses.	Ankle-foot orthoses with forearm crutches or canes.	As above.	Independent.

Rationale: No *net pulse charge* is necessary to achieve this goal. A waveform with or without a net pulse charge can be used. A *sustained muscle contraction* is desired. Therefore, the use of continuous direct current, which produces only a twitch contraction at the closing and opening of the circuit, is inappropriate. The time required for the waveform (be it monophasic, biphasic, or multiphasic) to go from 0 V to its peak amplitude must not be so long as to allow the nerve to accommodate to the stimulus (e.g., greater than 10 ms).

2. *Pulse-repetition rate:* Tetanizing (preferably just-tetanizing, approximately 25 to 50 pps)

   Rationale: A *sustained contraction* is desired and therefore a low rate producing only twitch contractions is inappropriate. A rate closer to just-tetanizing is preferable to avoid unnecessary fatigue, which may occur when higher rates are used.[5]

TABLE 12–2 Protocol for Increasing Passive Range of Motion

1. *Waveform:* Pulsatile (i.e., monophasic, biphasic, multiphasic) with sufficiently rapid rise time to avoid physiologic accommodation.
2. *Pulse-repetition rate:* Tetanizing (preferably just-tetanizing, ~25–50 pps).
3. *Pulse duration:* Any (i.e., long or short) pulse sufficient to produce a strong muscle contraction given the available intensity.
4. *Intensity:* Sufficient to produce a muscle contraction that carries the part through the available joint range of motion, and that receives a MMT grade of fair plus (3+/5) when brake tested at end range (may be low or high, dependent upon the pulse duration).
5. *Modulations:* Interruption; duty-cycle fixed at, or adjustable to, 1:3 or 1:5; adjustable ramp-on time; adjustable ramp-off time (desirable, but not absolutely necessary).
6. *Special features:* Easy access to controls.
7. *Electrode placements:* Over motor points of antagonist(s) to shortened muscle group(s).
8. *Session length:* 30 minutes.
9. *Session frequency:* Three times/day; daily.
10. *Re-evaluation time:* Every 3 to 4 days.

3. *Pulse duration:*   Any (i.e., long or short) pulse sufficient to produce a strong muscle contraction given the available intensity.

    Rationale: Pulse duration (width) requirements are interdependent with stimulus intensity. With the *available intensity* the *duration parameter of the strength-duration (S-D) curve* for the tissue to be stimulated must be met. The *peripheral nerve is intact,* therefore an exceptionally long pulse duration is not necessary to meet the requirement of the strength-duration curve. If high intensity stimulation is available, a relatively short pulse duration can be used to produce a strong muscle contraction. If stimulation intensity is lower, pulse duration must be longer. This rationale is presented in detail in Chapters 4 and 7.

4. *Amplitude:*   Sufficient (with a given pulse duration) to produce a muscle contraction that carries the body part through the available joint range of motion, and which receives a MMT grade of fair plus (3+/5) when break-tested at end range.[5]

    Rationale: Amplitude that produces a 3+/5 strength muscle contraction is used because the aim is to move the joint through the range of motion and to give some *stretch to shortened soft tissue structures at the end of the available range.* Intensity sufficient to produce a stronger muscle contraction is not appropriate because it may cause "jamming" of the joint at end range.[5]

    Amplitude requirements are interdependent with pulse duration in that *at any given pulse duration,* the intensity must be sufficient to meet the requirement of the S-D curve for the tissue to be stimulated. Therefore, in order to produce the desired motor response with a stimulus of relatively short pulse duration, for example, 40 μs, the intensity must be relatively high. If the pulse duration is longer, for example, 300 μs, the intensity requirements decrease. If the pulse duration is exceptionally short, the high intensity required may be too uncomfortable for the patient.

5. *Modulations:*   Interrupted, duty cycle fixed or adjustable to 1:3 or 1:5; adjustable rise time; adjustable fall time.

    Rationale: Interruptions are necessary in order to elicit a series of contractions with rest intervals. Continuous current would produce a single sustained contraction that would more rapidly result in muscle fatigue.

    A *duty cycle* (ratio of stimulus on time-to-off time) of 1:3 (25 percent time on) or 1:5 (17 percent time on) is desirable. The long rest intervals between trains of stimuli help to avoid fatigue and achieve the desired repetitive contractions over a period of time.[5,54] A stimulus peak on time of approximately 5 seconds provides a stretch at the end of the available joint range of motion.

    An *adjustable ramp-on time* is desired. An adjustable ramp time allows for a gradual achievement of peak amplitude and results in a more gradual movement of the limb. This can be important in the presence of increased tone in the antagonists to muscle groups targeted for stimulation in order to avoid quick stretch and undesired activity of these groups. A 2-second ramp-on time is usually sufficient for patient comfort and can be used in this patient for stimulation of muscles of the paretic limbs that do not have moderately to severely spastic antagonists.

    An *adjustable ramp-off time* is useful. An adjustable ramp-off time is desirable in the presence of low or absent tone for a stimulation program involving movement through the range with the part in an antigravity position. The gradual decline in the stimulus intensity and the resultant gradual decrease in the force of the contraction serves to protect joint structures from being suddenly subjected to the force of gravity at the end of the stimulation period. If no ramp-off time is provided on the stimulation unit, positioning may be utilized to minimize these stresses.

6. *Special features:* Easy access to controls.
    Rationale: In this case, the ES unit will be used in the clinic where *accessibility* is a time saver for the therapist. No *remote switch* is necessary as cyclic stimulation will be used. *Portability* is not necessary for this application when used in the clinical setting. The *number of channels* available for stimulation is not a factor, although if more than one muscle group is to be stimulated, a multichannel unit will be a time saver.

7. *Electrode placements:* Over motor points of antagonist to shortened groups.
    Rationale: These electrode placements will produce a strong muscle contraction with the least intensity required.

8. *Session length:* 30 minutes, three times per day.[4]
    Rationale: The length of the treatment program should be based on the literature available with regard to ES and the therapeutic goal. In the absence of objective clinical data, program guidelines should be based on the therapist's clinical experience with other techniques used to achieve the same goal. Results should be carefully monitored and reported with the intent of clarifying similar decisions in the future.
    In patients with hemiplegia, three daily 30-minute sessions of ES have been shown to be effective in increasing PROM.[4] In addition, a study on duty cycle and fatigue revealed a marked drop in the force of muscle contraction after 30 minutes of stimulation at duty cycles of $1:3$ or $1:5$.[54] Longer sessions might therefore not provide sufficient contraction force to cause stretch at the end of the available range of motion.

9. *Session frequency:* 7 days per week.
    Rationale: Frequency of treatment should be established in much the same way as session length. Programs of ES performed daily have been shown to be effective in increasing joint PROM.[4]

10. *Re-evaluation time:* Every three to four days.
    Rationale: PROM can often be increased within even a single session of stretch. Unfortunately these increases are not always maintained from session to session. It is therefore appropriate to allow several days to pass in order to assess the true effectiveness of the treatment program designed to increase PROM.

SELECTION OF AN APPROPRIATE STIMULATION DEVICE

Once a protocol like the one in Table 12–2 has been developed, it can be compared with the features offered on the stimulation devices that are available to the clinician, and an appropriate unit can be selected. For example, assume that the four ES units described in Table 12–3 are available in the PT department. (It may be useful for the clinician to prepare a table such as the one provided here to clarify at a glance the features provided on the ES units available in his or her own department.) The therapist would compare the sample protocol requirements with the features offered on each of the available units. In the example offered, the comparison reveals that devices A, C, and D would all be appropriate choices for use with the protocol for increasing PROM outlined above. Unit B does not offer the necessary modulations identified in the protocol as it has no interrupted mode and no ramp adjustments, and is therefore unsuitable for use in this stimulation program.

TABLE 12-3 Sample ES Devices

ES Device	Waveform	Pulse Duration (μs)	Frequency (pps)	Intensity (mA)	Modulations	Special Features
A	Twin-peak monophasic	80 (fixed)	0-120	0-2500	Continuous interruptions: surge on, 0.5-60 seconds; surge off, 0.5-60 seconds	Single channel (may bifurcate); Easy control access; Minimum portability
B	Symmetrical biphasic	40-200	2-100	0-60	Continuous pulse duration and rate modulation.	Dual channel; portable; easy control access
C	Asymmetrical balanced biphasic	250 (fixed)	0-100	0-100	Interruptions: on time, 2-55 seconds; off time, 2-55 seconds; adjustable ramp on, 0-10 seconds; adjustable ramp off 0-10 seconds	Dual channel; synchronous and reciprocal modes; portable; easy control access
D	Multiphasic 2500 Hz sine-carrier frequency	200 (fixed)	50 (bursts) (fixed)	0-100 0-100	Continuous Interruptions: on, 15 seconds; off, 50 seconds; adjustable ramp on, 1-5 seconds	Single channel (may bifurcate); minimum portability; easy control access

EVALUATION OF TREATMENT EFFECTIVENESS

In any therapeutic program it is important to periodically re-evaluate the patient in order to determine whether or not the current treatment course is an effective one. Although the use of ES is presently considered to be an addition to the more traditional treatment approaches, the means for evaluating its effectiveness in the management of a given problem is quite conventional. The clinician need only look as far as the means by which the problem was originally identified in order to find the method for evaluating the efficacy of the ES program. For example, given the sample problem of decreased PROM, the tool for initial evaluation and for evaluation of program effectiveness would be goniometry. An effective program would result in an increase in PROM as measured in this way. A lack of progress seen over a reasonable period of time would indicate the need to review treatment methodology and/or strategy.

SUMMARY

Electrical stimulation may be used in the management of a great many problems commonly seen in the neurologically impaired patient. Once the patient has been evaluated and problems and goals have been identified, ES should be compared to the other treatment options on the basis of appropriateness to the patient problem and the specific patient in question, documented and theoretical effectiveness, and more practical considerations such as time requirements, equipment availability, and cost. If the comparison is favorable, ES may be selected as the treatment (or one of several treatments) of choice. Once the decision is made to use ES, an organized approach should be taken first to design a stimulation protocol and then to choose an appropriate unit for stimulation, in order to optimize the results of the treatment. ES treatment effectiveness should be periodically re-evaluated and modified as indicated. In all of these respects, use of ES is no different than use of any other treatment modality and should be integrated into a total rehabilitation program.

It must be noted that every ES application mentioned in this chapter requires further investigation with regard to optimal stimulation characteristics. Whereas ES has been shown to be effective in producing a number of positive results, there has been minimal standardization of methods in the investigations performed to date. This statement is not made to discourage the reader from the use of ES but rather to encourage future investigation into and improved documentation of the uses of ES and the stimulation characteristics required to produce desired results. Stimulation characteristics are readily quantifiable and many of the results of stimulation are easily measurable using currently available evaluation methods. Every therapist has a responsibility to help to clarify the application and thereby improve the effectiveness of the many treatments that we as a profession provide.

REFERENCES

1. Munsat, TL, McNeal, D, and Waters, R: Preliminary observations on prolonged stimulation of peripheral nerve in man: Recent advances in myology. Proceedings of the Third International Congress on Muscle Disease, 1974, p 42.
2. Eriksson, M, Schuller, H, and Sjolund, B: Hazard from transcutaneous nerve stimulation in patients with pacemakers. Lancet 1:1319, 1978.

3. Electrical muscle stimulator (EMS) labeling, indications, contraindications, warnings, etc. FDA publication, July 11, 1985.
4. Baker, LL, et al: Electrical stimulation of wrist and fingers for hemiplegic patients. Phys Ther 59:1495, 1979.
5. Benton, LA, et al: Functional electrical stimulation: A practical clinical guide. The Professional Staff Assoc of the Rancho Los Amigos Hospital, Downey, CA. 1981.
6. Baker, LL and Parker, K: Neuromuscular Electrical Stimulation of the Muscles Surrounding the Shoulder. Phys Ther 66:1930, 1986.
7. Bobath, B: Adult Hemiplegia: Evaluation and Treatment. William Heinemann Med Books, London, 1978.
8. Voss, D: Should patients with hemiplegia wear a sling? Physiother 49:1029, 1969.
9. Davies, PM: Steps to Follow: A Guide to the Treatment of Adult Hemiplegia Based on the Concept of K and B Bobath. Springer-Verlag, New York, 1985.
10. Moodie, NB, Brisbin, J, and Morgan, AMG: Subluxation of the glenohumeral joint in hemiplegia: Evaluation of supportive devices. Physiotherapy Canada 38:151, 1986.
11. Eiguren, BE: Respond II shoulder subluxation protocol. Medtronic Neuro Division, 6951 Central Ave NE, PO Box 1250, MN 55440, 1984.
12. Lindstrom, B, et al: Electrically induced short-lasting tetanus of the calf muscles for prevention of deep vein thrombosis. Brit J Surg 69:203, 1982.
13. Doran, FSA, Drury, M, and Sivyer, A: A simple way to combat the venous stasis which occurs in the lower limbs during surgical operations. Brit J Surg 51:486, 1964.
14. Brunnstrom, S: Movement Therapy in Hemiplegia. A Neurophysiological Approach. Harper & Row, Philadelphia, 1970, p 71.
15. Brooks, VB: Motor control. How posture and movements are governed. Phys Ther 63:664, 1983.
16. Luria, AR: Restoration of Function after Brain Injury. Pergamon Press, New York, 1963.
17. Merletti, R, et al: Clinical experience of electronic peroneal stimulators in 50 hemiparetic patients. Scand J Rehabil Med 11:111, 1979.
18. Carnstam, B, Larsson, L, and Prevec, TS: Improvement of gait following functional electrical stimulation. Scand J Rehabil Med 9:7, 1977.
19. Merletti, R, et al: A control study of muscle force recovery in hemiparetic patients during treatment with functional electrical stimulation. Scand J Rehabil Med 10:147, 1978.
20. Brudny, J, et al: EMG feedback therapy: Review of treatment of 114 patients. Arch Phys Med Rehabil 57:55, 1976.
21. Flom, RP, et al: Biofeedback training to overcome poststroke foot-drop. Geriatrics Dec:47, 1976.
22. Hansen, GO: EMG-controlled functional electrical stimulation of the paretic hand. Scand J Rehabil Med 11:189, 1979.
23. Fields, RW: Electromyographically triggered electric muscle stimulation for chronic hemiplegia. Arch Phys Med Rehabil 68:407, 1987.
24. Baker, LL: Clinical uses of neuromuscular electrical stimulation. In Nelson, RM and Currier, DP (eds): Clinical Electrotherapy. Appleton & Lange, Norwalk, CT, 1987.
25. Wolf, SL: Electromyographic biofeedback: An overview. In Nelson, RM and Currier, DP (eds): Clinical Electrotherapy. Appleton & Lange, 1987, p 272.
26. Booker, HE, Rubrow, RT, and Coleman, PJ: Simplified feedback in neuromuscular retraining: An automated approach using electromyographic signals. Arch Phys Med Rehabil 50:621, 1969.
27. Wolf, SL, Le Craw, DE, and Barton, LA: Comparison of motor copy and targeted biofeedback training techniques for restitution of upper extremity function among patients with neurologic disorders. Phys Ther 69:719, 1989.
28. Singer, RN: Motor Learning and Human Performance, ed 3. Macmillan, New York, 1980.
29. Burnside, IG, Tobias, HS, and Burnsill, D: Electromyographic feedback in the remobilization of stroke patients: A controlled trial. Arch Phys Med Rehabil 63:217, 1982.
30. Laughman, RK, et al: Strength changes in the normal quadriceps femoris muscle as a result of electrical stimulation. Phys Ther 63:494, 1983.
31. Selkowitz, D: Improvement in isometric strength of the guadriceps femoris muscle after training with electrical stimulation. Phys Ther 65:186, 1985.
32. Kots, Y: Notes on Electrical Muscle Stimulation. From lectures and laboratory periods. Canadian-Soviet Exchange Symposium on Electro-stimulation of Skeletal Muscles (translated by Bibkin, I and Tintsenko, N). Concordia University, Montreal, Quebec, December 6–15, 1977.
33. Middaugh, SJ: EMG Feedback as a muscle reeducation technique. Phys Ther 58:15, 1978.
34. Bowman, BR and Bajd, T: Influence of Electrical Stimulation on Skeletal Muscle Spasticity. Proceedings of the International Symposium on External Control of Human Extremities. Belgrade, Yugoslav, Committee for Electronics and Automation, 1981, p 561.
35. Lee, WJ, McGovern, JP, and Duvall, EN: Continuous tetanizing (low voltage) currents for relief of spasm. Arch Phys Med 31:766, 1950.
36. Alfieri, V: Electrical treatment of spasticity. Scand J Rehabil Med 14:177, 1982.
37. Kelly, JL, Baker, M, and Wolf, SL: Procedures for EMG biofeedback training in involved upper extremities of hemiplegic patients. Phys Ther 59:1500, 1977.

38. Katz, S, et al: Prognosis after strokes, Part II: Long-term course of 159 patients. Medicine 45:236, 1966.
39. Basmajian, JV: Biofeedback in rehabilitation: A review of principles and practices. Arch Phys Med Rehabil 62:469, 1981.
40. Stanic, U, et al: Multi-channel electrical stimulation for correction of hemiplegic gait. Scand J Rehabil Med 10:764, 1969.
41. Koerner, I: Observation of Human Gait. Health Sciences Audiovisual Education. University of Alberta, Edmonton, Alberta, T6G2G3.
42. Edelstein, JE: Orthotic assessment and management. In O'Sullivan, SB and Schmitz, TJ (eds): Physical Rehabilitation: Assessment and Treatment, ed 2. FA Davis, Philadelphia, 1988, p 603.
43. Kendall, FP and McCreary, EK: Fundamental principles in manual muscle testing, In Muscles: Testing and Function, ed 3. Williams & Wilkins, Baltimore, 1983.
44. Gault, WR and Gatens, PF: Use of low intensity direct current in management of ischemic skin ulcers. Phys Ther 56:265, 1976.
45. Carley, PJ and Wainapel, SF: Electrotherapy for acceleration of wound healing: Low intensity direct current. Arch Phys Med Rehabil 66:443, 1985.
46. Thurman, BF and Christian, EL: Response of a serious circulatory lesion to electrical stimulation. Phys Ther 51:1107, 1971.
47. Gould, N, et al: Transcutaneous muscle stimulation as a method to retard disuse atrophy. Clin Orthop 164:1, 1982.
48. Nash, MS: Computerized functional electrical stimulation: An emerging rehabilitation technology. Trends in Rehabil Spring: 5, 1986.
49. Ragnarsson, KT: Clinical Evaluation of Computerized Functional Electrical Stimulation in Spinal Cord Injury: A Pilot Multicenter Study (abstract). 63rd Annual Session American Congress Rehabilitation Medicine, 48th Annual Assembly, American Academy of Physical Medicine and Rehabilitation, Baltimore, October, 19–24, 1986.
50. Petrofsky, JA and Phillips, CA: Active physical therapy: A modern approach to rehabilitation therapy. J Neurol Orthop Surg 4:165, 1983.
51. Goldsmith, MF: Computerized biofeedback training aids in spinal injury rehabilitation. JAMA 253:1097, 1985.
52. Pollack, S: Endurance Training by Functional Electrical Stimulation of Muscles Paralyzed by Spinal Cord Injury (abstract). 63rd Annual Session American Congress Rehabilitation Medicine, 48th Annual Assembly, American Academy of Physical Medicine and Rehabilitation, Baltimore, October, 19–24, 1986.
53. DeVivo, MI, Fine, PR, and Stover SL: Cause of death following spinal cord injury (abstract). Arch Phys Med Rehabil 65:622, 1984.
54. Packman-Braun, R: Relationship between FES duty-cycle and fatigue in the wrist extensor muscles of patients with hemiparesis. Phys Ther 68(1):51, 1988.

APPENDIX

MOTOR POINT CHARTS

The following abbreviations are used in the motor point charts:

M = muscle
N = nerve
B = branch of nerve
C = cervical nerve roots
T = thoracic nerve roots
L = lumbar nerve roots

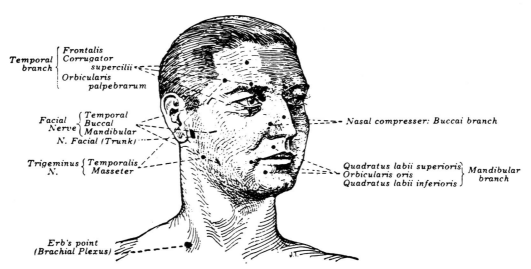

FIGURE A-1. Motor points of face. (From Siemens Burdick, Inc, Milton, WI, with permission.)

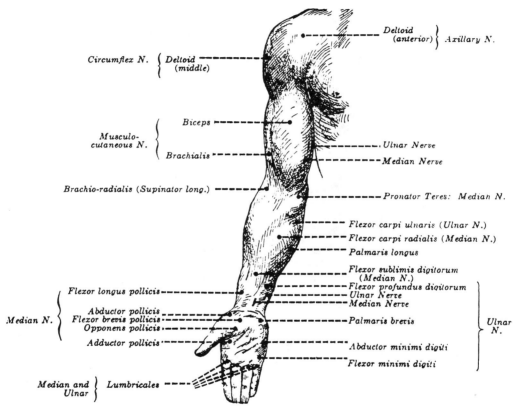

FIGURE A–2. Motor points of anterior aspect of upper limb. (From Siemens Burdick, Inc, Milton, WI, with permission.)

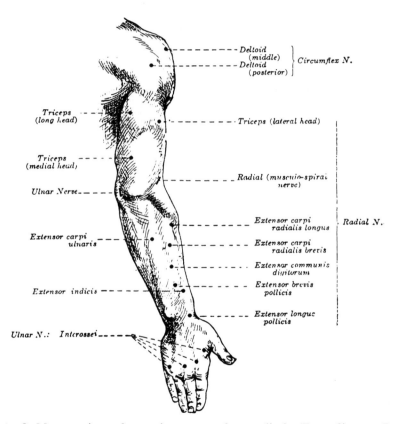

FIGURE A–3. Motor points of posterior aspect of upper limb. (From Siemens Burdick, Inc, Milton, WI, with permission.)

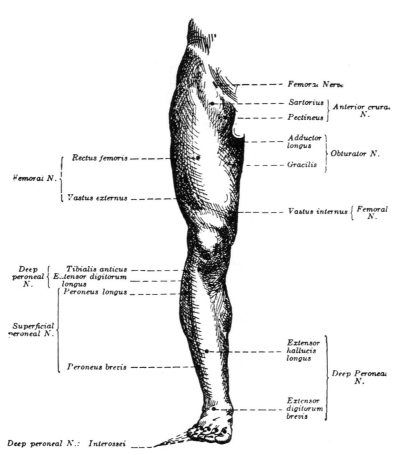

FIGURE A–4. Motor points of anterior aspect of lower limb. (From Siemens Burdick, Inc, Milton, WI, with permission.)

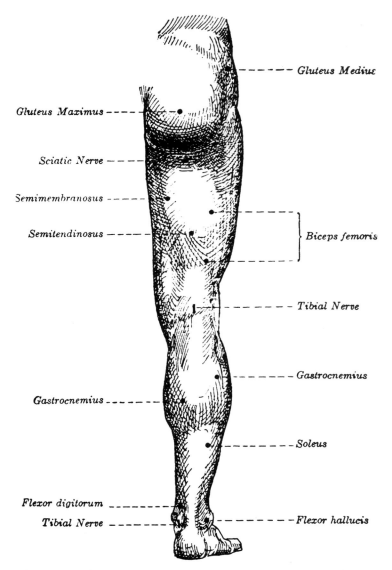

FIGURE A–5. Motor points of posterior aspect of lower limb. (From Siemens Burdick, Inc, Milton, WI, with permission.)

Index

A page number in *italics* indicates a figure; a page number followed by "t" indicates a table.